AMERICAN NURSING REVIEW

Questions & Answers
FOR NCLEX-PN

Second Edition

AMERICAN NURSING REVIEW

Questions & Answers
FOR NCLEX-PN

Second Edition

SPRINGHOUSE
Springhouse, Pennsylvania

STAFF

PUBLISHER
Judith A. Schilling McCann, RN, MSN

EDITORIAL DIRECTOR
David Moreau

CLINICAL MANAGER
Joan M. Robinson, RN, MSN, CCRN

CLINICAL PROJECT MANAGER
Beverly Ann Tscheschlog, RN

EDITORS
Cynthia Breuninger, Stacey Follin, Julie Munden, Carol Munson

COPY EDITORS
Jaime Stockslager (supervisor), Scoti Cohn, Priscilla Dewitt, Fruma Klass, Kimberly A.J. Johnson, Carolyn Petersen, Marcia Ryan, Pamela Wingrod

DESIGNERS
Arlene Putterman (associate design director), Lesley Weissman-Cook (book design), Donna S. Morris (project manager), Joseph John Clark

PROJECTS COORDINATOR
Liz Schaeffer

ELECTRONIC PRODUCTION SERVICES
Diane Paluba (manager), Joyce Rossi Biletz

MANUFACTURING
Patricia K. Dorshaw (manager), Otto Mezei (book production manager)

EDITORIAL ASSISTANTS
Beverly Lane, Beth Janae Orr, Elfriede Young

INDEXER
Manjit K. Sahai

The clinical procedures described and recommended in this publication are based on research and consultation with medical and nursing authorities. To the best of our knowledge, these procedures reflect currently accepted clinical practice; nevertheless, they can't be considered absolute and universal recommendations. For individual application, treatment recommendations must be considered in light of the patient's clinical condition and, before administration of new or infrequently used drugs, in light of the latest package-insert information. The authors and publisher disclaim responsibility for any adverse effects resulting directly or indirectly from the suggested procedures, from any undetected errors, or from the reader's misunderstanding of the text.

Printed in the United States of America.
ANRQAPN2 – D N O S A J J M A M
03 02 01   10 9 8 7 6 5 4 3 2 1

Library of Congress Cataloging-in-Publication Data
American nursing review : questions & answers for NCLEX-PN. — 2nd ed.
    p. ; cm.
  Rev. ed. of: American nursing review / Phyllis F. Healy. 1996.
  Includes bibliographical references and index.
  ISBN 1-58255-095-6 (alk. paper)
  1. Practical nursing — Examinations, questions, etc.
I. Title: Questions & answers for NCLEX-PN. II. Title: Questions and answers for NCLEX-PN. III. Healy, Phyllis F. American nursing review. IV. Springhouse Corporation.
[DNLM: 1. Nursing, Practical — Examination Questions. WY 18.2 A5125 2001]
RT62 .H43 2001
610.73′6′93076 — dc21
                      00-069234

CONTENTS

Contributors

Ann Allen, MSN, RN
Director of Performance Improvement
Lake Norman Regional Medical Center
Mooresville, N.C.

Cynthia A. Chatham, RN,C, DSN
Associate Professor
University of Southern Mississippi
Long Beach

Tobie Fleming Day, RN, MSN
Instructor of Psychosocial Nursing
Bishop State Community College
Mobile, Ala.

Carol J. Duell, MSN, CRNP
Nursing Instructor
Abington Memorial Hospital School of Nursing
Willow Grove, Pa.

Margaret M. Gingrich, RN, MSN
Associate Professor
Harrisburg (Pa.) Area Community College

Rebecca Crews Gruener, RN, MS
Associate Professor of Nursing
Louisiana State University at Alexandria

Kathleen J. Hudson, RN, MSN
Nursing Instructor
Illinois Eastern Community Colleges at Wabash Valley
Mt. Carmel

Mary Susan Hungerford, RN, MSN
Instructor of Nursing
Bridgeport (Conn.) Hospital School of Nursing

Elaine Bishop Kennedy, RN, EdD
Professor of Nursing
Wor-Wic Community College
Salisbury, Md.

Meri Beth Kennedy, RN, MS
Director of Nursing
Dakota County Technical College
Rosemount, Minn.

Patricia B. Lisk, RN, BSN
Instructor
Augusta (Ga.) Technical Institute

Gayla H. Love, RN, BSN, CCM
Case Manager
Blue Cross Blue Shield of Georgia
Atlanta

Julia A. McAvoy, RN, MSN, CCRN
Clinical Nurse Specialist, Critical Care
The Washington (Pa.) Hospital

Georgia A. O'Neal, RN, MSN
Instructor in Nursing
Jefferson State Community College
Birmingham, Ala.

Janet A. Rudolph, RN, MSN
Nursing Instructor
Brandywine School of Nursing
Coatesville, Pa.

June Schneberger, RN, MSN, CS
Process Improvement Coordinator
Baptist Health System
San Antonio, Tex.

Billie Ward, RN, MSN
Nursing Instructor
Bishop State Community College
Mobile, Ala.

We extend special thanks to the following persons, who contributed to the previous edition:

Richardean Benjamin-Coleman, RN, PhD

Carol Bininger, RN, PhD

Sandra Czerwinski, RN, MS, CCRN

Carolyn Fakouri, RN, DNS

Phyllis F. Healy, RN,C, PhD

Mary Keaveny, RN, MSN

Judy Maurer, RN, MSN

Carrie McCoy, RN, MSN, CEN

Janis Metro-Emmert, RN, MSN

Aletta Moffett, RN, MSN

Leona Mourad, RN, MSN, ONC

Larry Purnell, RN, PhD

Koreen Smiley, RN, MSN

Tamara Young, RN, BSN

Elaine Zimbler, RN, MSN

FOREWORD

The National Council Licensure Examination for Practical Nurses (NCLEX-PN) is your last step in completing the requirements to become a licensed practical nurse (LPN). To ensure a successful outcome, you must use precise preparation and planning. In preparing for the examination, you'll need to review at length the nursing content likely to be tested, understand how the NCLEX-PN is developed and administered, and learn successful strategies to answer the questions. A well-planned study program can be crucial to your success.

The second edition of *American Nursing Review: Questions & Answers for NCLEX-PN* will assist you in your study preparation. This valuable book offers:

■ practical preliminary information about the computerized adaptive test (CAT) format, providing the most up-to-date information about the test, its construction, and how it's administered

■ more than 1,000 NCLEX-style questions in all four clinical areas — including medical-surgical, maternal-neonatal, pediatric, and psychiatric nursing and covering such topics as nursing principles and procedures, disorders, nutrition, pharmacology, and diagnostic tests

■ rationales for the correct answer to each question and explanations as to why the other options are incorrect; each rationale also reveals the applicable phase of the nursing process (NP), client needs category (CN), client needs subcategory (CNS), and cognitive level (CL) of the information being tested

■ two comprehensive posttests that integrate questions of varying difficulty from all four clinical areas in a style similar to the actual examination

■ convenient two-column format with questions on the left and answers and rationales on the right that provides instant feedback.

American Nursing Review: Questions & Answers for NCLEX-PN, Second Edition, has all the elements you'll need to succeed with your study plan. To enhance effective study, each chapter contains important information to help you prepare with simple, basic topics that lead to more complex, technical concepts.

Chapter 1, Understanding the NCLEX-PN CAT, gives you helpful information about registration, test sites, and scheduling for the examination. It details the new CAT format, reviews the main components of the NCLEX-PN test plan, and offers practical test-taking strategies that will improve your success during your study and on the day of your examination.

Chapter 2, Medical-Surgical Nursing, reviews the health problems that are likely to be covered on the NCLEX-PN. You'll find various questions that explore such topics as commonly treated body system disorders, cancer, acquired immunodeficiency syndrome, and complex technical procedures.

Chapter 3, Maternal-Neonatal Nursing, focuses on maternal, fetal, and neonatal well-being, with questions of normal pregnancy and obstetric disorders, such as placenta previa, abruptio placentae, and pregnancy-induced hypertension, among other topics.

Chapter 4, Pediatric Nursing, tests your knowledge of such pediatric problems as asthma, meningitis, sickle cell anemia, and diabetes, including how to care and give instructions to a pediatric client who needs special attention for his illness.

Chapter 5, Psychiatric Nursing, covers the spectrum of mental health and illness, including electroconvulsive therapy, bipolar disorder, restraints and seclusion, obsessive-compulsive disorder, and adverse drug interactions.

Chapter 6, Posttests, exposes you to all areas of the test plan. In two 85-question posttests, you'll be challenged with questions that are arranged in the same format as the NCLEX-PN. These tests can help you identify topics that require further study. Knowing what to expect can help you assess the time it will take to complete the examination, therefore, relieving much of your anxiety.

The key to success is a carefully thought-out and executed plan. On completion of your studies, you'll confidently approach the last hurdle toward reaching your goal of becoming an LPN. I wish you well on the NCLEX-PN and welcome you into the profession of nursing.

Deborah C. Connelly, MSN, RN,C
Assistant Director of Nursing
Practical Nursing Program
Bishop State Community College
Mobile, Ala.

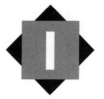

Understanding the NCLEX-PN CAT

Anyone who wants to practice as a licensed practical nurse in the United States must be licensed by the nursing licensure authority in the state or territory in which she intends to practice. To obtain this license, you must pass the National Council Licensure Examination for Practical Nurses (NCLEX-PN).

Your success on the NCLEX-PN depends on your nursing knowledge base, your study program for the test, your level of confidence, and your familiarity with computerized adaptive testing (CAT). Understandably, you may feel anxious about taking the examination on a computer, especially if you haven't had much practice with one. This chapter provides helpful information about the test, acquaints you with the new computerized format, and gives you effective strategies for passing it.

REGISTRATION, TEST SITES, AND SCHEDULES

Once you have met all eligibility requirements, you must apply to take the NCLEX-PN through your state board of nursing. Shortly after your application is approved, you'll receive an "Authorization to Test" from the Educational Testing Service (ETS) Data Center. This authorization will instruct you to make an appointment to take the examination at a Sylvan Technology Center. More than 200 of these centers are located throughout the United States, with at least one in each state or territory. Each center will have up to 10 computer terminals available for candidates. A proctor will assist you in getting started and will monitor security during the test.

The computerized NCLEX-PN, which lasts a maximum of 5 hours, is offered 15 hours every day, Monday through Saturday, throughout the year (on Sundays only when necessary to meet peak de-

mands). You'll take the test no later than 30 days from the day you call to schedule it, so make sure that you're thoroughly prepared when you call. If you're being retested after failing the examination, your test date will be within 45 days of your call. You may reschedule without charge by telephoning the test center at least 3 days before your test date.

COMPUTERIZED ADAPTIVE TESTING

In April 1994, the test format changed from a pencil-and-paper test to a computerized test in which the candidate must answer enough questions of varying levels of difficulty to demonstrate minimum competence as an entry-level nurse.

The CAT differs from the paper-and-pencil test in several ways. Of course, the most obvious difference is that, instead of sitting at a table with a test book and a pencil, you'll sit in front of a computer terminal, interacting with it as you take the NCLEX-PN.

The CAT chooses test items based on your response to the previous question; that is, the computer will "adapt" to each answer, correct or incorrect, by selecting a harder or easier item for the next question. For example, at the start of the examination, you'll be given a question of medium-level difficulty. If you answer the question correctly, the computer will then ask a more difficult question. If you answer incorrectly, the computer will ask an easier question.

The test bank contains thousands of questions, each categorized according to the NCLEX-PN test plan and assigned a level of difficulty using a complex statistical formula. Every time you answer a question, the computer searches the test bank for an appropriate next question based on the difficulty of the previous question and the accuracy of your response. This process continues until the com-

APPEARANCE OF QUESTIONS ON THE COMPUTER SCREEN

Questions on the computerized NCLEX-PN are structured in one of two ways, as shown below. Some questions are stand-alone items; others are based on brief case studies, which appear to the left of the question.

A patient has been admitted to the hospital with a diagnosis of malignant melanoma. When providing discharge instructions on ways to prevent recurrence of this type of tumor, the nurse should emphasize the importance of:	1. performing wound care. 2. wearing sunscreen and a hat. 3. performing range-of-motion exercises. 4. eating a diet high in vitamins A, B, and C.

A 40-year-old male has a large bowel obstruction. He's admitted to the hospital for treatment that involves placement of an intestinal tube connected to wall suction drainage.	Which nursing intervention would be most effective for this patient? 1. Measure abdominal girth every 12 hours. 2. Turn the patient from side to side, as prescribed. 3. Give the patient sips of water to facilitate passage of the tube through the bowel. 4. Add antacids to the intestinal tube to reduce bowel reaction.

puter can determine your competence in all areas of the test plan. Because each test is individualized, the number of questions can range from 85 to 205 (15 of these will be practice questions).

The computerized test begins with brief instructions on using the computer and then provides a short practice session. Previous computer experience isn't necessary. You'll use only two keys on the keyboard: the *space bar* and the *enter key*. All other keys will be nonfunctioning. You'll use the space bar to move the cursor among four possible options and press the enter key to record your answer. The computer will then ask you to confirm your choice by pressing the enter key a second time. This ensures that you don't select an answer unintentionally.

One question at a time will appear on the computer screen, shown in one of two formats. (See *Appearance of questions on the computer screen*.)

After carefully reading the question, press the space bar to move among the four possible options. Analyze each choice and then select the one that best answers the question. Press the enter key twice to record your choice. You must answer every question until the test ends; unlike the paper-and-pencil testing method, the computer won't allow you to skip an item or go back to a previous question.

The test center will transmit your results electronically to the ETS Data Center. Your state board will notify you of the results in 4 to 6 weeks. No test results are released over the telephone.

NCLEX-PN TEST PLAN

In April 1999, a new NCLEX-PN test plan was implemented based on a job analysis study conducted by the National Council for State Boards of Nursing. This study was conducted to ensure that the content of the examination reflected the scope of nursing practice.

The NCLEX-PN test plan incorporates new content from all phases of the nursing process (collecting data, planning care, implementing care, and evaluating care) throughout the test. Other integrated nursing concepts in the test include caring, communication, cultural awareness, documentation, self-care, and teaching and learning.

The four major client needs categories have also been reorganized so that each has two or more subcategories. These categories, as well as the percentage of test questions allocated to each subcategory, are described as follows.

1. SAFE, EFFECTIVE CARE ENVIRONMENT
■ *Coordinated care (6% to 12%):* Collaborating with other health care team members to facilitate effective patient care
■ *Safety and infection control (7% to 13%):* Protecting clients and health care personnel from environmental hazards

2. HEALTH PROMOTION AND MAINTENANCE
■ *Growth and development through the life span (4% to 10%):* Assisting the patient and significant others in the normal expected stages of growth and development from conception through advanced old age
■ *Prevention and early detection of disease (4% to 10%):* Providing client care related to prevention and early detection of health problems

3. PSYCHOSOCIAL INTEGRITY
■ *Coping and adaptation (6% to 12%):* Promoting client's ability to cope, adapt, and problem solve in situations related to illness or stressful events

- *Psychosocial adaptation (4% to 10%):* Participating in providing care for clients with acute or chronic illness

4. PHYSIOLOGICAL INTEGRITY
- *Basic care and comfort (10% to 16%):* Providing comfort and assistance in the performance of activities of daily living
- *Pharmacological therapies (5% to 11%):* Providing care related to the administration of medications and monitoring clients receiving parenteral therapies
- *Reduction of risk potential (11% to 17%):* Reducing the client's potential for developing complications or health problems related to treatments, procedures, or existing conditions
- *Physiological adaptation (13% to 19%):* Participating in providing care to clients with acute, chronic, or life-threatening physical conditions.

PREPARING FOR THE EXAMINATION

Proper preparation for the examination involves thorough study and careful planning before the test and mastery of test-taking strategies that you can use during the test. The following tips will help ensure your success on the computerized NCLEX-PN.

Study thoroughly.
- Become well versed in all of the topics that the examination is likely to cover and answer as many practice questions as you can. After answering the questions in each clinical area of this book, take the posttests in Chapter 6, which will ensure your exposure to all areas of the test plan.
- Complete the self-evaluation form after the posttests to help you determine why you may have answered a question incorrectly. This analysis will enable you to pinpoint topics that may require further study.
- Become familiar with all parts of a test question. (See *Parts of a test question.*)
- Supplement this book with other resources, such as *American Nursing Review for NCLEX-PN,* 3rd ed., a complete study guide for the test.
- Take a review course or organize a study group with others planning to take the examination.
- Ask a nursing instructor or colleague for help or clarification if you encounter material that is unfamiliar or difficult to understand.

Plan carefully.
- Schedule your examination at a test site near your residence, if possible, so that you can familiarize yourself with parking facilities and travel time before the test date.
- If you must travel a lengthy distance and stay overnight, make hotel arrangements well in advance of the test date to ensure that you have a convenient place to stay.

PARTS OF A TEST QUESTION

Multiple-choice questions on the NCLEX-PN are constructed according to strict psychometric standards. As shown below, each question has a stem and four options: a key (correct answer) and three distractors (incorrect answers). A brief case study may precede the question.

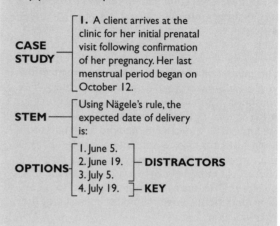

CASE STUDY — 1. A client arrives at the clinic for her initial prenatal visit following confirmation of her pregnancy. Her last menstrual period began on October 12.

STEM — Using Nägele's rule, the expected date of delivery is:

OPTIONS —
1. June 5.
2. June 19. — **DISTRACTORS**
3. July 5.
4. July 19. — **KEY**

- Schedule your examination for the time of day that coincides with your peak performance. Some people work best in the early morning; others, in late afternoon or early evening.
- Get a good night's sleep the night before the test. Staying up late to do last-minute cramming will probably hurt — rather than help — your performance.
- Eat a nutritious breakfast on the day of the test.
- Wear layered clothing so that you can easily adapt to the room temperature at the test center.
- Keep your admission ticket and identification where you can easily retrieve them when you leave for the test site. You must present your "Authorization to Test" from the ETS Data Center and two forms of identification with your signature, including one photo identification. Without them, you won't be permitted to take the test.
- Try to avoid last-minute anxiety that could sap your energy or disturb your concentration. Although mild anxiety is normal and can actually heighten your awareness, too much anxiety can impair your performance. If test anxiety has been a problem in the past, practice relaxation techniques (such as guided imagery) as you study and be ready to use them during the actual test.

Apply test-taking strategies.
- Read case studies carefully. They contain information that you'll need to answer the question correctly.
- *Pay special attention to such words as best, most, first, and not when reading the stem of the question.* These words (which may be italicized, capitalized, or otherwise highlighted in some way) usually

provide clues to the correct response. For example, consider the question, "What should the nurse do *first*?" All of the listed options may be appropriate nursing actions for the given circumstances, but only one action can take top priority.

■ Try to predict the correct answer as you read the stem of the question. If your predicted answer is among the four options, it's probably the correct response.

■ Read each question and all options carefully before making your selection.

■ Reread two options that seem equally correct; there must be some difference between them. Also reread the stem. You may notice something that you missed before that will aid in your selection. If you're still unsure, make an educated guess. The computer won't allow you to skip a question.

■ Remain calm if a question focuses on an unfamiliar topic. Try to recall clients who have had problems similar to those in the question. Determine the nursing principles involved in your former clients' care and how they may apply to the test question. This may help you eliminate some options and increase your chances of selecting the right answer.

■ Take the necessary time for each question without spending excessive time on any one item. You'll have up to 5 hours to take the test. Pace yourself accordingly.

■ Pay no attention to other candidates or the time they need to complete their tests. Because each test is individualized, some tests contain more questions than others.

■ Take advantage of breaks during the test to give your mind and body a needed rest. The first mandatory break is given after 2 hours of testing and lasts 10 minutes. Candidates may take an optional break 90 minutes after testing resumes. If you tend to get hungry, bring a small snack with you to eat during the breaks. Do some stretching exercises, too, during breaks to help you relax.

Developing and following an organized study plan will provide the best assurance that you're fully prepared to succeed on the NCLEX-PN. Approach the test with confidence. Good luck and congratulations on choosing nursing as a career.

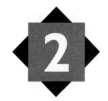

Medical-Surgical Nursing

1 A 60-year-old female client has been diagnosed with a sliding hiatal hernia. The nurse can improve the client's comfort by teaching her to:
- ☐ 1. drink carbonated cola beverages with meals.
- ☐ 2. lie down immediately after eating.
- ☐ 3. eat three large high-carbohydrate meals each day.
- ☐ 4. sleep with her head elevated 30 degrees.

CORRECT ANSWER: 4
With a hiatal hernia, sleeping with the head of the bed elevated 30 degrees (about 3″ or 4″ [7.6 or 10.2 cm]) prevents stomach acids from refluxing into the esophagus. Option 1 would create gas and possibly irritate the herniated area as the client begins to tolerate bland foods. Option 2 would facilitate the reflux of stomach acids, causing irritation and possible aspiration. Option 3 is wrong because small meals are recommended for clients with hiatal hernias.
NP: Implementing care
CN: Physiological integrity
CNS: Basic care and comfort
CL: Application

2 What is the priority nursing goal for a client who has had a barium enema?
- ☐ 1. To prevent fecal incontinence
- ☐ 2. To monitor for bleeding
- ☐ 3. To prevent constipation
- ☐ 4. To limit fluid intake

CORRECT ANSWER: 3
Barium should be promptly eliminated from the client's system after it has been introduced into the colon to prevent mass formation and possible bowel obstruction. Therefore, laxatives or enemas are commonly given after a barium enema to prevent the client from becoming constipated. Option 1: Fecal incontinence isn't an issue because the passage of stool is desired. Option 2: Bleeding isn't commonly anticipated after a barium enema. Option 4: The client should be encouraged to increase, not decrease, fluid intake.
NP: Planning care
CN: Physiological integrity
CNS: Reduction of risk potential
CL: Application

3 A client has a nasogastric tube in place after gastric surgery. The tube is connected to low intermittent suction. Which nursing action should the nurse anticipate for this client?
☐ 1. Provide mouth care every 2 hours.
☐ 2. Check the client's gag reflex each shift.
☐ 3. Reposition the tube by pulling it 1″ to 2″ (2.5 to 5 cm) each shift.
☐ 4. Give the client sips of water, as desired, for comfort.

CORRECT ANSWER: 1
Frequent mouth care helps to lessen discomfort and relieve the dry, parched mouth and lips associated with tube placement and breathing through the mouth. Option 2: Checking the gag reflex isn't indicated and would only increase the client's discomfort. Option 3: Tubes are placed by the surgeon after gastric surgery and shouldn't be adjusted by the nurse. Option 4: Giving water as desired is contraindicated because too much water could lead to fluid and electrolyte imbalance.
NP: Planning care
CN: Physiological integrity
CNS: Basic care and comfort
CL: Application

4 A client in a nursing home is receiving continuous nasogastric (NG) feedings of Vivonex. At the start of the shift, the nurse finds the client turned on her side with the bed flat. The feeding is running with a volumetric pump at 75 ml/hour, as ordered. The formula container is filled with 150 ml of fluid. Based on this information, which action should the nurse take?
☐ 1. Add 500 ml to the formula container.
☐ 2. Raise the bed to semi-Fowler's position.
☐ 3. Turn the client onto her back.
☐ 4. Clamp the NG tube.

CORRECT ANSWER: 2
Clients receiving tube feedings should be placed in semi-Fowler's position to prevent aspiration. Option 1: Formula is highly prone to bacterial contamination; therefore, only a 4- to 6-hour amount of formula should be exposed to room temperature in the container. Option 3: A side-lying position is desired to also prevent aspiration if the client experiences vomiting or reflux of the formula. Option 4: There is no reason to stop the feedings if they're ordered continuously.
NP: Implementing care
CN: Safe, effective care environment
CNS: Safety and infection control
CL: Application

5 A client with a history of duodenal ulcers tells the admitting nurse that he takes antacids once in a while to relieve the pain. Which statement by the client should be reported immediately?
☐ 1. "I've had a lot more pressure at work lately."
☐ 2. "My bowel movements have been sticky and black."
☐ 3. "I have this bad taste in my mouth after taking my antacid and feel like I have to vomit."
☐ 4. "I have this gnawing pain in my belly a few hours after I eat that causes me to feel nauseated."

CORRECT ANSWER: 2
Bleeding is a common complication of peptic ulcers. When bleeding occurs high in the GI tract, the stools appear black and sticky. Such hemorrhaging can be mild or life-threatening and must be reported promptly. Option 1: Stress is a common precipitating factor associated with peptic ulcer disease. The nurse should anticipate such a report during the initial assessment. Option 3: Nausea and vomiting are common with peptic ulcers and should be reported; however, they aren't indicative of a serious complication such as bleeding. Option 4: Abdominal pain and nausea are common symptoms of duodenal ulcers.
NP: Collecting data
CN: Physiological integrity
CNS: Physiological adaptation
CL: Application

6 A client who suffered a head injury is in a rehabilitation center. He's receiving 30 ml of aluminum hydroxide (Amphojel) through a nasogastric tube every 4 hours because of his increased risk for a stress ulcer. Which potential adverse effect should the nurse monitor for with this client?
☐ 1. Constipation
☐ 2. Urine retention
☐ 3. Nausea and vomiting
☐ 4. Diarrhea

CORRECT ANSWER: 1
Constipation is a potential adverse effect of antacids that contain aluminum. Options 2 and 3 aren't adverse effects of this drug. Option 4: Diarrhea occurs with use of magnesium-containing antacids.
NP: Collecting data
CN: Physiological integrity
CNS: Pharmacological therapies
CL: Application

7 The nurse is preparing to ambulate a 320-lb (145-kg) female client who underwent gastroplasty (gastric stapling) yesterday. The client has an I.V. line in place, a nasogastric (NG) tube connected to suction, and oxygen running at 6 L/minute by way of a nasal cannula. The physician has ordered patient-controlled analgesia (PCA) with 2 mg of morphine sulfate. What is the best way to plan for this client's walking activity?
☐ 1. Seek assistance from another person to support the client during the walk.
☐ 2. Ask the client to withhold using her PCA for 45 minutes before the walk to prevent orthostatic hypotension.
☒ 3. Obtain a portable oxygen unit to maintain the oxygen delivery during the client's ambulation.
☐ 4. Connect the NG tube to a portable suction machine while the client is walking.

CORRECT ANSWER: 3
Because the client's oxygen demands will increase with activity and oxygen delivery must be maintained, obtaining a portable oxygen unit is best. Option 1: To manage such a large client who has several tubes in place, the nurse would need adequate help. Two persons wouldn't provide enough assistance to ensure safety. Option 2: The client needs the morphine to relieve her pain so she can ambulate. Option 4: The NG tube doesn't need to be connected to suction while the client is walking; it should be "plugged" or clamped to keep the drainage from running out.
NP: Planning care
CN: Safe, effective care environment
CNS: Coordinated care
CL: Application

8 The nurse is caring for a client who has just had a liver biopsy. Which nursing intervention is most applicable after the biopsy?
☐ 1. Position the client on the left side with a pillow across the puncture site.
☐ 2. Take the client's vital signs every 2 hours.
☐ 3. Have the client cough and deep-breathe every 15 minutes for the 1st hour after the biopsy.
☐ 4. Keep the client on bed rest, lying on the right side.

CORRECT ANSWER: 4
Because the liver is a highly vascular organ, the client is at increased risk for hemorrhage. Lying on the right side exerts some pressure on the liver, which may help prevent bleeding. Option 1: The liver is located on the right, not left, side. Option 2: Vital signs need to be taken more frequently (for example, every 15 minutes for the first 2 hours). Option 3: Coughing isn't indicated.
NP: Implementing care
CN: Safe, effective care environment
CNS: Safety and infection control
CL: Application

9 A 24-year-old male client had a hemorrhoidectomy. After the packing is removed, the nurse begins preparations for a sitz bath. The client is reluctant to take the sitz bath and says to the nurse, "What good is it anyway?" Which response would be most appropriate?

☐ 1. "It will help soften your stool so that it won't be painful when you pass it."

☐ 2. "It helps prevent bleeding, which may occur after the packing is removed."

☐ 3. "The sitz bath helps reduce swelling in the rectal area, which helps relieve the discomfort."

☐ 4. "Sitting in a sitz bath is more comfortable than sitting on a chair."

CORRECT ANSWER: 3
A sitz bath increases circulation, thereby reducing congestion, swelling, and pain after a hemorrhoidectomy. Option 1: Stool softeners, not a sitz bath, are commonly given to soften the stool and relieve pain with the first bowel movement after surgery. Option 2: Clients must be checked frequently for rectal bleeding. A sitz bath doesn't prevent bleeding. Option 4: A sitz bath may not be more comfortable than sitting on a chair that has been padded with foam or a pillow.
NP: Implementing care
CN: Physiological integrity
CNS: Basic care and comfort
CL: Application

10 A client with ascites underwent a paracentesis in which 1,500 ml of fluid was removed. After the procedure, the nurse must observe the client for:

☐ 1. increasing respiratory distress.

☐ 2. increased pulse rate.

☐ 3. abdominal distention.

☐ 4. urine retention.

CORRECT ANSWER: 2
Removal of large quantities of fluid at one time can cause shifts between the vascular and extravascular compartments and result in shock. An increased pulse rate is one of the signs of shock. Option 1: The removal of the fluid should reduce the ascites and relieve respiratory distress. Option 3: The removal of the fluid should reduce the client's ascites and abdominal girth. Option 4: Urine retention isn't a problem in this situation. However, the client may be at risk for a perforated bladder if he didn't void before the procedure. The nurse should monitor for evidence of blood in the urine, a sign of perforation.
NP: Collecting data
CN: Physiological integrity
CNS: Physiological adaptation
CL: Application

11 The nurse is assisting with the placement of a nasogastric (NG) tube in a 56-year-old client with alcoholic cirrhosis. What is the best way to determine whether the NG tube is in his stomach?

☒ 1. Apply suction to the tube with an Asepto syringe and observing for the return of gastric contents.

☐ 2. Irrigate the tube with normal saline solution and observe for the return of the solution combined with gastric juices.

☐ 3. Place the "pigtail" end of the tube in water and observe for air bubbles.

☐ 4. Instill air into the tube and palpate for the tube over the epigastric area.

CORRECT ANSWER: 1
Aspirating gastric contents without inserting liquid is a safe way to determine if the tube is in the stomach. Option 2: If saline solution were inserted and the tube was in the trachea, solution would be introduced into the lungs. Option 3: A Levine tube doesn't have a "pigtail," but a Salem sump tube does. Also, if the tube were placed in water while it was in the trachea, the client could inhale water. Option 4: If air is instilled, the nurse should use a stethoscope to listen for a "whooshing" sound over the stomach (left upper quadrant) area. The tube can't be palpated over the epigastric area.
NP: Evaluating care
CN: Safe, effective care environment
CNS: Safety and infection control
CL: Application

12 A client underwent a cholecystectomy and exploration of the common bile duct this morning. She returned to the unit with an I.V. line, a Penrose drain, and a T tube in place. To evaluate the effectiveness of the T tube, the nurse should understand that the primary reason for a T tube in this situation is to:
☐ 1. promote wound drainage.
☐ 2. provide a means to irrigate the incision.
☐ 3. maintain drainage of bile from the common bile duct.
☐ 4. deliver an antibiotic irrigation to the surgical site.

CORRECT ANSWER: 3
Because the common bile duct may become edematous from the trauma of exploratory surgery, a T tube is introduced to maintain the duct's patency and to allow for the flow of bile. Without the tube, the bile may back up into the liver. Option 1: A Penrose drain would remove any drainage from the incision site. Option 2: The T tube isn't irrigated. Furthermore, the tube is inserted into the common bile duct, not the incision. Option 4: The tube is used for bile drainage, not surgical site irrigation.
NP: Evaluating care
CN: Physiological integrity
CNS: Physiological adaptation
CL: Comprehension

13 A client with advanced cancer of the mouth has a tongue that is swollen, necrotic, and seeping. Which nursing diagnostic category should be a priority in planning care?
☐ 1. *Imbalanced nutrition: Less than body requirements*
☐ 2. *Impaired oral mucous membrane*
☐ 3. *Impaired verbal communication*
☐ 4. *Ineffective airway clearance*

CORRECT ANSWER: 4
In clients with advanced mouth cancer, the priority nursing concerns are maintaining a patent airway and monitoring for signs of hemorrhage. Essential nursing measures include aspirating the client's oral secretions and maintaining a side-lying position to keep the airway open. Options 1, 2, and 3: These are areas of concern but they aren't immediately life-threatening and, therefore, aren't the priority.
NP: Planning care
CN: Safe, effective care environment
CNS: Coordinated care
CL: Application

14 A client has a colostomy in the descending colon after surgical removal of a tumor. Which of the following should the nurse anticipate when the client resumes a regular diet?
☐ 1. Formed, soft stools
☐ 2. Mushy, semiliquid stools
☐ 3. Several liquid stools a day
☐ 4. Hard stools with considerable flatus

CORRECT ANSWER: 1
By the time stool reaches the descending colon, much of the moisture has been absorbed and the stool should be formed and soft. Options 2 and 3: Liquid or semiliquid stools would be expected if the colostomy were located in the ascending or transverse colon. Option 4: Hard stools wouldn't be expected. If the stools are hard, the nurse should consult the dietitian.
NP: Collecting data
CN: Physiological integrity
CNS: Physiological adaptation
CL: Application

15 The physician inserts a Miller-Abbott tube in a client with a suspected small-bowel obstruction who has been vomiting fecal-like material. Which intervention would the nurse expect to perform after the insertion of the tube?
☒ 1. Ambulate the client and turn him from side to side every 2 hours.
☐ 2. Securely tape the tube to the client's nose.
☐ 3. Remove the mercury from the tube when drainage is observed.
☐ 4. Pin the tubing to the bedding to prevent it from becoming tangled.

CORRECT ANSWER: 1
Ambulation and turning are desired to facilitate passage of the tube through the pylorus and to increase peristalsis, which would help pass the tube along the intestinal tract. Options 2 and 4: The tube should never be taped to the client's face or bedding while it's being advanced through the intestinal tract because advancement would be prevented. Option 3: Mercury should be withdrawn only after the decompression is terminated; it facilitates the passage of the tube through the tract by gravity.
NP: Planning care
CN: Physiological integrity
CNS: Basic care and comfort
CL: Application

16 The nurse is preparing a client for a colectomy and an ileostomy to treat ulcerative colitis. Which statement by the client indicates the need for more teaching?
- ☐ 1. "I'll have little control over the drainage."
- ☐ 2. "I'll still be able to have children if I want."
- ☐ 3. "I'll have to make a few changes in my diet such as drinking more fluids."
- ☒ 4. "I'll have this ostomy temporarily while my bowel heals."

CORRECT ANSWER: 4
An ileostomy for ulcerative colitis is considered a curative measure, and the ostomy is permanent (a total colectomy involves the removal of the entire colon and rectum). Options 1, 2, and 3 indicate the client's understanding of anticipated changes.
NP: Evaluating care
CN: Health promotion and maintenance
CNS: Prevention and early detection of disease
CL: Application

17 A client with advanced colon cancer is receiving total parenteral nutrition (TPN) with 50% dextrose through a central line. What should the nurse caring for this client plan to do?
- ☐ 1. Turn off the TPN pump when the client is sitting upright in a chair.
- ☐ 2. Monitor the client's capillary blood glucose levels every 6 hours.
- ☐ 3. Change the central line dressing once weekly.
- ☐ 4. Monitor the client's urine for ketones every 12 hours.

CORRECT ANSWER: 2
The nurse must check the glucose levels periodically to determine whether the client can tolerate the 50% dextrose solution. The nurse should notify the physician if the client's glucose levels are elevated because this may indicate the need for insulin. Excessively high glucose levels may indicate hyperosmolar hyperglycemic nonketotic coma. Option 1: The delivery rate of TPN should never be disrupted. Option 3: Central line dressings should be changed every 7 days using sterile technique. Option 4: This client isn't diabetic, so ketone levels don't need to be checked.
NP: Planning care
CN: Physiological integrity
CNS: Pharmacological therapies
CL: Application

18 A female client who underwent a hemorrhoidectomy 6 hours ago still hasn't voided. What should the nurse do?
- ☐ 1. Check with the charge nurse for a catheterization order.
- ☐ 2. Force fluids because urine retention is a common problem after hemorrhoidectomy.
- ☐ 3. Remove the rectal packing, which may be causing pressure in the area and decreasing the urge to void.
- ☐ 4. Auscultate over the bladder with a stethoscope to determine if the client's bladder is full.

CORRECT ANSWER: 2
Many clients have difficulty voiding after hemorrhoid surgery. However, 6 hours with no report of client distress would indicate a need to begin forcing fluids; running water from the faucet into the sink while the client is in the bathroom may also promote the urge to void. Option 1: Catheterization shouldn't be considered until the client is encouraged to void on her own. Option 3: Removal of the rectal packing, without a physician's order and so soon after surgery, could cause hemorrhage. Option 4: Auscultation with a stethoscope over the bladder wouldn't indicate bladder fullness. Palpation over the bladder would be appropriate.
NP: Implementing care
CN: Physiological integrity
CNS: Basic care and comfort
CL: Application

19 A 20-year-old man is in the same-day-surgery recovery area after repair of an inguinal hernia. He's alert and taking fluids well. He feels the need to void and has tried using the urinal twice without success. He's anxious to be discharged soon. Which action should the nurse take?
- ☐ 1. Assist the client to stand and use the urinal or toilet.
- ☐ 2. Obtain an order to increase the client's I.V. fluids.
- ☐ 3. Check the client's chart to see whether he has had voiding difficulties in the past.
- ☐ 4. Withhold pain medication until the client voids.

CORRECT ANSWER: 1
Difficulty voiding is a common problem that is easily managed by assisting the client to stand and void. This client is alert and planning discharge, so he can be assisted to stand without endangering his condition. Option 2: The client is taking oral fluids, which can be increased, if necessary. Option 3: The client is alert and can communicate if he has had prior difficulty with voiding. Option 4: Pain medication shouldn't be withheld because the client should remain as comfortable as possible during the postoperative period.
NP: Implementing care
CN: Physiological integrity
CNS: Basic care and comfort
CL: Application

---

20 The nurse is preparing a client for discharge after a permanent colostomy. The discharge instructions indicate that the client will irrigate the colostomy at home. Which statement by the client indicates that teaching about the irrigation has been effective?
- ☐ 1. "I'll use sterile water for the irrigation."
- ☐ 2. "I'll hang the irrigation bag from the shower curtain rod, which is about 1' above my head."
- ☐ 3. "I'll put some cloth over the stoma after the irrigation."
- ☒ 4. "I'll use about a quart of warm water for irrigation."

CORRECT ANSWER: 4
About 1,000 ml of tap water that is 100° to 105° F (37.8° to 40.6° C) is recommended for a colostomy irrigation. Option 1: Sterile water is unnecessary. Option 2: The bottom of the irrigation bag should be at the client's shoulder level. If the bag is higher, the solution will enter the bowel too rapidly. Option 3: The client can expect drainage from the stoma for 1 hour after the irrigation and, therefore, will need to remain in the bathroom or cover the stoma with a pouch while all the returns are eliminated.
NP: Evaluating care
CN: Health promotion and maintenance
CNS: Growth and development through the life span
CL: Application

---

21 A 40-year-old female client with a long history of type 1 diabetes mellitus recently had an amputation and is in the rehabilitation unit. When the nurse enters the room to administer her daily NPH insulin, the client is diaphoretic, reports having a headache, and has slurred speech. What should the nurse do next?
- ☐ 1. Give the client insulin, bring her breakfast tray immediately, and help her eat.
- ☐ 2. Give the client insulin, bring her a glass of orange juice, and report her findings to the head nurse.
- ☐ 3. Withhold the client's insulin, bring her some milk and crackers, and report the findings to the head nurse.
- ☐ 4. Withhold the client's insulin, bring her a glass of orange juice, and report her findings to the head nurse.

CORRECT ANSWER: 4
The client is showing classic signs of hypoglycemia. Orange juice will help reverse the hypoglycemia. The head nurse needs to be informed for continuity of assessment and intervention. Options 1 and 2: The insulin should be withheld until further assessment and treatment of the hypoglycemia. Option 3: Milk and crackers don't work as fast as orange juice to alter the glucose levels.
NP: Implementing care
CN: Physiological integrity
CNS: Physiological adaptation
CL: Application

22 A 21-year-old female client has recently been diagnosed with type 1 diabetes. She's receiving 5 units of regular insulin and 15 units of NPH insulin every morning before breakfast at 7 a.m. Which statement regarding her insulin is correct?

☐ 1. The regular insulin will begin to act rapidly (within 30 to 60 minutes) and peak in 8 hours.

☒ 2. The NPH insulin will begin to act in 1 to $1\frac{1}{2}$ hours and will peak in 4 to 12 hours (by mid-afternoon).

☐ 3. The regular insulin will begin to act in 1 to $1\frac{1}{2}$ hours and will peak in 5 hours (at about lunch time).

☐ 4. The NPH insulin will begin to act in 4 to 8 hours and will peak in 18 hours (by early evening).

CORRECT ANSWER: 2
NPH insulin has an onset of 1 to $1\frac{1}{2}$ hours and peaks in 4 to 12 hours. Regular insulin has an onset of 30 minutes to 1 hour and peaks in $2\frac{1}{2}$ to 5 hours.
NP: Collecting data
CN: Physiological integrity
CNS: Pharmacological therapies
CL: Knowledge

23 An insulin-dependent diabetic client has a leg infection that is being treated with antibiotics, wet-to-dry dressings, and whirlpool therapy. Since the infection began, her blood glucose levels have been unstable. Which observations are likely to indicate impending severe hyperglycemia?

☐ 1. Flushed cheeks, dry mouth, and a breath odor of overripe bananas (acetone)

☐ 2. Mental changes, fever, and hand tremors

☐ 3. Headache, sweating, and nervousness

☐ 4. Periods of rapid breathing followed by absence of breathing, picking at the bed linen, and nausea

CORRECT ANSWER: 1
Diabetic ketoacidosis is characterized by flushed skin; signs of dehydration (dry mouth); and fast, deep, labored respirations with a smell of acetone on the breath. Options 2, 3, and 4 include a variety of vague symptoms and don't include the classic signs of hyperglycemia (dehydration, flushed appearance, and Kussmaul's respirations with acetone breath).
NP: Collecting data
CN: Physiological integrity
CNS: Physiological adaptation
CL: Comprehension

24 The nurse prepares to administer regular insulin to a client based on the physician's order for "Regular insulin 6 units U100." Which statement regarding the insulin is true?

☐ 1. The insulin is cloudy.

☐ 2. The insulin should be rolled and gently rotated before drawing the medication into the syringe.

☒ 3. U100 means that there are 100 units in each milliliter of the insulin, and 6 units are to be administered.

☐ 4. The insulin should be drawn up in a tuberculin syringe.

CORRECT ANSWER: 3
There are 100 units of insulin in each milliliter of U100 insulin and it should be drawn up in a U100 syringe (orange needle cap). Options 1 and 2: Regular insulin is clear. Cloudy insulin has a zinc precipitate that must be evenly distributed in the solution. Option 4: Insulin syringes are the only type of syringe used for drawing up insulin.
NP: Implementing care
CN: Safe, effective care environment
CNS: Safety and infection control
CL: Knowledge

Reg insulin onset = 30 to 60 min
peak - 5 hours
NPH insulin onset = 1 to 1½ hours
peak - 4 to 12 hours

25 A diabetic client who had a stroke has right-sided paralysis and incontinence and is in the rehabilitation center. Which action should be the nurse's priority in caring for this client?
- ☐ 1. Apply body powder every 4 hours to keep the client dry.
- ☐ 2. To conserve energy, maintain bed rest when the client isn't in therapy.
- ☐ 3. Insert an indwelling urinary catheter to keep the client continent.
- ☐ 4. Wash the client's skin with soap and water, gently patting it dry.

CORRECT ANSWER: 4
The skin of a diabetic client should be kept dry to prevent breakdown and infection. Option 1: The nurse should avoid excessive use of powders, which can cake with perspiration and cause irritation. Option 2: Clients undergoing rehabilitation should be upright in a chair, except for short rest periods during the day, to promote optimal recovery. Option 3: Diabetic clients are especially prone to infections. Urinary tract infections are commonly caused by the use of indwelling catheters. Other methods should be used to encourage continence.
NP: Planning care
CN: Physiological integrity
CNS: Basic care and comfort
CL: Application

26 A 55-year-old type 2 diabetic is obese and hasn't been successful at controlling the condition by diet alone. The physician has prescribed glipizide (Glucotrol). The nurse knows that glipizide is commonly used for type 2 diabetes because it:
- ☐ 1. is an oral form of insulin.
- ☐ 2. stimulates the pancreas to secrete more insulin.
- ☐ 3. promotes weight reduction, which lowers the blood glucose level.
- ☐ 4. is a sulfa drug that treats pancreatic infections.

CORRECT ANSWER: 2
Oral antidiabetic drugs work by stimulating the beta cells of the pancreas to secrete more insulin and decrease insulin resistance at the receptor sites. Option 1: Oral insulin would be destroyed in the GI tract. Option 3: Weight reduction would help to reduce the blood glucose level; however, glipizide is classified as an oral antidiabetic drug, not an appetite suppressant. Option 4: Oral antidiabetics are sulfa-based drugs; however, they aren't indicated in diabetes for their anti-infective actions.
NP: Evaluating care
CN: Physiological integrity
CNS: Pharmacological therapies
CL: Application

27 The nurse knows that dietary management is part of the treatment regimen for clients with diabetes. Which information should the nurse include in client-teaching sessions with diabetic clients?
- ☐ 1. Diabetes is caused by eating too much sugar.
- ☐ 2. Sugar is primarily found in desserts.
- ☐ 3. A diabetic should stop eating sugary foods.
- ☐ 4. Meals should be eaten at consistent times each day.

CORRECT ANSWER: 4
Maintaining a regular eating pattern to avoid hunger and the temptation to snack on high-calorie foods is crucial for clients with diabetes. An insulin-dependent diabetic needs to adjust insulin doses according to food intake throughout the day. A non-insulin-dependent diabetic should limit total calories but not skip meals. Option 1: Diabetes results from inadequate insulin or improper insulin utilization to control glucose. Once diabetes occurs, eating too much sugar can cause the glucose level to rise. Option 2: Various forms of sugar are available in different foods, not just desserts. Diabetic clients should be taught to scrutinize all food labels for the sugar content. Option 3: Not all sugars should be removed; for example, natural sugars in fruits should be eaten, whereas concentrated sweets should be avoided.
NP: Implementing care
CN: Health promotion and maintenance
CNS: Prevention and early detection of disease
CL: Application

28 A female client has been diagnosed with hyperthyroidism. In planning her care, the nurse should give priority to which goal?
☐ 1. Keeping the client warm
☐ 2. Reducing the client's caloric intake
☐ 3. Providing adequate rest and sleep
☐ 4. Forcing fluids and roughage

CORRECT ANSWER: 3
Clients with hyperthyroidism are typically anxious, diaphoretic, nervous, and fatigued. They need a calm, restful environment to relax and get adequate rest and sleep. Option 1: Clients with hyperthyroidism are usually warm and diaphoretic and need a cool environment. Option 2: Those with hyperthyroidism require a high-caloric diet and should eat four to six small meals per day. Option 4: Hyperthyroidism causes diarrhea from hypermotility of the GI tract. Excess fluids and foods high in roughage should be avoided.
NP: Planning care
CN: Physiological integrity
CNS: Basic care and comfort
CL: Knowledge

29 A 35-year-old male client is returned to his room after a thyroidectomy. Which nursing measure is most important on the evening after surgery?
☐ 1. Asking the client to say a few words to check his voice for tone and hoarseness
☐ 2. Removing the dressing if the client reports tightness around the surgical incision site
☐ 3. Keeping the Jackson-Pratt drain partially compressed to avoid too much pressure on the incision site
☐ 4. Monitoring for hemorrhage by examining the front of the dressing every 2 hours

CORRECT ANSWER: 1
Paralysis of the recurrent laryngeal nerve is a possible complication after thyroid surgery. Therefore, the nurse should be careful to assess the client's ability to speak. Option 2: The compression dressing shouldn't be removed. If the client reports tightness, the dressing may be loosened when the nurse checks for bleeding. Option 3: The drainage device must be fully compressed for maximum effectiveness. Option 4: Oozing of blood may occur around the back of the neck. The nurse should feel around the client's neck to check for dampness. Also, the client should be turned to monitor for bleeding.
NP: Implementing care
CN: Physiological integrity
CNS: Reduction of risk potential
CL: Application

30 An 86-year-old female client who has been on long-term steroid therapy now has drug-induced Cushing's syndrome. She's residing in an extended-care facility because of her multiple chronic health problems. Which condition is closely related to chronic use of steroids?
☐ 1. Periods of hypoglycemia
☐ 2. Muscle wasting in the abdominal area
☐ 3. Thin, easily damaged skin
☐ 4. Weight loss

CORRECT ANSWER: 3
Clients taking steroids on a long-term basis lose subcutaneous fat under the skin and are especially vulnerable to skin breakdown and easy bruising. Such clients should take great care when performing tasks that may injure the skin and should anticipate delayed healing when injuries occur. Option 1: Clients taking steroids long-term are likely to have hyperglycemia. Option 2: Typically, these clients experience weight gain in the abdomen and thinning of the extremities while on steroids. Option 4: Such clients should be monitored for weight gain and edema.
NP: Collecting data
CN: Physiological integrity
CNS: Pharmacological therapies
CL: Application

31 During a shift report, the nurse is told that a postoperative diabetic client is on a "sliding scale." What does the "sliding scale" indicate?
- [ ] 1. Administration of regular insulin is based on periodic blood glucose readings.
- [ ] 2. The laboratory will obtain a blood glucose level 2 hours after each meal, and the insulin dose will be based on these test results.
- [ ] 3. The client's diet is based on fasting blood glucose levels.
- [ ] 4. An insulin order must be obtained from the physician every day.

CORRECT ANSWER: 1
With a sliding scale, capillary blood is assessed for glucose on a regular basis and short-acting regular insulin is administered based on the glucose levels for short-term glucose management after surgery. Option 2: A blood glucose level 2 hours after a meal describes a 2-hour postprandial glucose test. Option 3: A sliding scale refers to insulin, not dietary, orders. Option 4: The physician typically leaves orders for the administration of specific units of regular insulin based on ranges of blood glucose levels that usually don't alter until the client is off the sliding scale.
NP: Implementing care
CN: Physiological integrity
CNS: Physiological adaptation
CL: Comprehension

32 A 70-year-old male client is admitted to the hospital after an episode of right-sided weakness, difficulty speaking, and blurred vision. The physician diagnoses a stroke in evolution. Why does the nurse ask the client to squeeze her hand?
- [ ] 1. To assess his ability to follow simple commands
- [ ] 2. To determine if he's right- or left-handed
- [ ] 3. To evaluate his orientation to person
- [ ] 4. To assess his response to pain

CORRECT ANSWER: 1
Asking the client to squeeze the nurse's hand assesses the client's ability to follow commands, thereby determining his level of consciousness during a stroke in evolution. This also allows the nurse to evaluate the strength of the client's grip. Option 2: The client's handedness reflects his dominant side of the brain and would be determined during the client history. Option 3: Orientation to person is determined by a client's recognition of himself and others. Option 4: Asking the client to squeeze the nurse's hand wouldn't induce pain. Furthermore, because his level of consciousness is only slightly diminished, eliciting a pain response wouldn't be necessary.
NP: Collecting data
CN: Physiological integrity
CNS: Physiological adaptation
CL: Application

33 A client has lost the ability to express words. The nurse should plan to:
- [ ] 1. use complex statements to acknowledge the client's intelligence.
- [ ] 2. communicate with the client's family, who can answer the nurse's questions.
- [ ] 3. provide opportunities for the client to repeat words and point to objects.
- [ ] 4. limit communications to speech therapy sessions so the client doesn't become tired.

CORRECT ANSWER: 3
Speech should be promoted at all times. Opportunities should be provided for verbal as well as nonverbal forms of communication, such as pointing and nodding. Options 1 and 2 would lead to frustration. The client should be treated with dignity and encouraged to speak for himself. Option 4: Although speech therapy is important, such sessions are limited and the client needs to practice beyond the set times with the speech therapist.
NP: Planning care
CN: Psychosocial integrity
CNS: Coping and adaptation
CL: Application

34 A 22-year-old male client has a history of seizures. While he's being transported to the medical imaging laboratory for a brain scan, he cries out, his muscles become rigid, and he falls to the floor. What should the nurse do first?
☐ 1. Elevate the client's head.
☐ 2. Move furniture away from the client.
☐ 3. Insert a padded tongue blade between the client's teeth.
☐ 4. Run to a phone to notify the physician.

CORRECT ANSWER: 2
The nurse should first move anything in the environment that could injure the client. Option 1: The client should be turned on his side, if possible, to prevent aspiration of saliva. The head should be turned, not elevated. Option 3: An airway may be inserted but only before the tonic (rigid) phase of a seizure. Option 4: The nurse must always stay with the client.
NP: Implementing care
CN: Safe, effective care environment
CNS: Safety and infection control
CL: Application

35 After a client experiences a generalized tonic-clonic seizure, what is the priority nursing action?
☐ 1. Turn the client on his back.
☐ 2. Ask the client when he last took his prescribed medication.
☐ 3. Place the client in a darkened room and check on him in 30 minutes.
☐ 4. Check the client's vital signs and remove restrictive clothing.

CORRECT ANSWER: 4
It's important to assess the client's blood pressure and pulse immediately after the seizure and every 30 minutes until the client is awake. Changes from the baseline should be reported. Restrictive clothing should be removed to prevent injury in the event of another seizure. Option 1: The client should be turned on the side to prevent aspiration during the postictal state. Option 2: Clients are typically confused and drowsy after a seizure. They should be reassured and made comfortable, not asked questions. Option 3: The room should be dim with minimal noise, but the client should be checked more frequently in case of recurring seizure activity.
NP: Implementing care
CN: Safe, effective care environment
CNS: Coordinated care
CL: Application

36 A 35-year-old female client with chronic epilepsy of the tonic-clonic type has taken phenytoin sodium (Dilantin) for several years. Which statement by her indicates the need for further teaching about phenytoin?
☐ 1. "I take the drug with food to keep my stomach from becoming upset."
☐ 2. "I always use a soft toothbrush and floss my teeth every day; my dentist says that my mouth is in good shape."
☐ 3. "My blood levels are tested regularly to see how the drug is affecting me."
☐ 4. "I've been taking the drug for so long now that taking half the dose from time to time won't cause any problems."

CORRECT ANSWER: 4
A client should never decrease the dosages of an anticonvulsant medication without the physician's approval because such a decrease may result in seizures. Option 1: The drug is alkaline and may cause gastric distress unless taken with large amounts of fluid or food. Option 2: Overgrowth of gum tissue can occur with phenytoin. Using a soft toothbrush, flossing, and seeing the dentist regularly for examination and treatment may prevent oral problems. Option 3: Regular blood tests are necessary to determine the drug's therapeutic level and to detect early signs of adverse effects such as liver problems.
NP: Evaluating care
CN: Health promotion and maintenance
CNS: Prevention and early detection of disease
CL: Application

37 The physician prescribes levodopa-carbidopa (Sinemet) for a client with Parkinson's disease to control symptoms. Which information should the nurse include while teaching the client about this drug?

- [ ] 1. A loading dose is given and the dosage is gradually decreased until a therapeutic level is achieved.
- [ ] 2. Antiembolism stockings are useful to prevent orthostatic hypotension, which is an adverse effect of this medication.
- [ ] 3. The desired effect of the medication is to increase mental alertness.
- [ ] 4. Urinary incontinence is a common adverse effect of this medication.

CORRECT ANSWER: 2

Antiembolism stockings can help control orthostatic hypotension, a common adverse effect of this medication. Option 1: The dosage is gradually increased until a therapeutic level is achieved. Option 3: The drug decreases tremors, rigidity, and bradykinesia, which are symptoms of Parkinson's disease. Option 4: Urine retention, not incontinence, is a potential adverse effect of this drug.

NP: Implementing care
CN: Health promotion and maintenance
CNS: Prevention and early detection of disease
CL: Analysis

38 The Glasgow Coma Scale is used to assess levels of consciousness in neurologic clients. Using this scale, which of the following assessment responses would give the lowest score and should be reported immediately to the physician?

- [ ] 1. Moves arm or leg and opens eyes to pain with no verbal response
- [ ] 2. Opens eyes to speech, is confused, and responds to localized pain
- [ ] 3. Obeys commands, opens eyes spontaneously, and is oriented
- [ ] 4. Makes incomprehensible sounds, tries to remove painful stimuli, and opens eyes to speech

CORRECT ANSWER: 1

The responses included in option 1 would yield a low score of 6 out of a possible 14 (normal response) on the Glasgow Coma Scale. Option 2 would yield a score of 11. Option 3 is a normal response, with a score of 14. Option 4 would yield a score of 9.

NP: Collecting data
CN: Physiological integrity
CNS: Physiological adaptation
CL: Application

39 On evening rounds at the nursing home, the nurse finds an unresponsive female client with deep, gurgling respirations and puffiness on her right cheek. The client has no voluntary motion or muscle tone of her right arm and leg. What should the nurse do first?

- [ ] 1. Turn the client on her left side and place the bed in semi-Fowler's position.
- [ ] 2. Summon someone to notify the nursing supervisor.
- [ ] 3. Lower the head of the bed 30 degrees and elevate the client's legs 20 degrees.
- [ ] 4. Turn the client on her right side and elevate the head of the bed 15 degrees.

CORRECT ANSWER: 4

This client is showing signs of a stroke with respiratory distress. To maintain airway patency, the nurse should turn the client on her affected side so that any secretions can run out her mouth. Also, elevating the head of the bed will promote intracranial drainage. Option 1: Turning the client on the unaffected side will hinder the drainage of oral secretions. Option 2: The supervising nurse needs to be informed after the safety of the client has been established. Option 3: Lowering the client's head may increase intracranial pressure.

NP: Implementing care
CN: Physiological integrity
CNS: Reduction of risk potential
CL: Application

40 The nurse is assisting the physician with a lumbar puncture. The client appears worried and anxious. After the procedure, which statement is most appropriate for the nurse to make?
☐ 1. "Just relax. There are no bad aftereffects and the worst is over."
☐ 2. "I'll put the head of the bed up so you can watch your favorite television programs. There is a good baseball game on now."
☐ 3. "I want you to lie flat for a while. I'll close the curtain and perhaps you can rest. I'll be quiet when I check on you in a few minutes."
☐ 4. "I'll fluff your pillows so you can sit and drink some juice. Call me if you need me."

CORRECT ANSWER: 3
Headaches are common after a lumbar puncture. Lying flat in a darkened room may help to relieve or prevent the discomfort. Checking on the client frequently will make the client feel secure. Options 1, 2, and 4 may promote a headache.
NP: Implementing care
CN: Physiological integrity
CNS: Reduction of risk potential
CL: Application

41 An 86-year-old female client with generalized arthritis arrives at the clinic for her regular check-up. She takes aspirin several times per day. Because of the client's heavy use of aspirin, the nurse should gather information about:
☐ 1. constipation and fatigue.
☐ 2. fragile skin and weight gain.
☐ 3. orange color and fruity smell of urine.
☐ 4. easy bruising and reports of unusual bleeding.

CORRECT ANSWER: 4
Because salicylates interfere with the blood's clotting mechanism, the client may show signs of bruising and bleeding. Additionally, salicylates can cause GI irritation, which may lead to GI bleeding. Options 1, 2, and 3 aren't commonly found with long-term salicylate use.
NP: Collecting data
CN: Physiological integrity
CNS: Pharmacological therapies
CL: Application

42 A female client who fell while washing her outside windows has a fractured right ankle and is being fitted with a cast. After assisting with the cast application, what instructions should the nurse give the client?
☐ 1. Go home and stay in bed for about 5 days.
☐ 2. Keep the cast covered with plastic until it feels dry.
☐ 3. Move the right toes for several minutes every hour.
☐ 4. Expect some swelling and blueness of the toes.

CORRECT ANSWER: 3
Moving the toes is encouraged to facilitate circulation and prevent swelling. By moving the toes, the client will be aware of any numbness or swelling and can take appropriate action, such as elevating the extremity and reporting the findings to her physician. Option 1: Usually, clients are instructed to remain in bed for 24 hours while the cast dries. Prolonged immobility creates problems for the client. Option 2: While the cast is still damp, the ankle should be elevated on a pillow that is protected with plastic; the cast itself should be left open to the air. Option 4: Swelling and a bluish color of the toes indicate compromised circulation and should be reported immediately.
NP: Implementing care
CN: Physiological integrity
CNS: Reduction of risk potential
CL: Application

43 A client with advanced cancer has been receiving chemotherapy and is now experiencing stomatitis. To promote comfort and nutrition while the client's mouth is sore, the nurse should plan to speak with the client's family about:
- ☐ 1. providing hot fluids, such as tea and broth, between meals.
- ☐ 2. brushing the client's teeth with a firm toothbrush.
- ☐ 3. encouraging the client to eat his favorite Mexican foods.
- ☐ 4. rinsing the client's mouth with diluted hydrogen peroxide every 2 hours.

CORRECT ANSWER: 4
Frequent rinsing of the mouth with a nonirritating solution helps maintain moisture and promotes comfort. Option 1: Hot liquids would be uncomfortable for the client. Option 2: A soft toothbrush is recommended. Option 3: Small, frequent feedings of a soft, bland diet is generally better tolerated by clients with stomatitis.
NP: Planning care
CN: Health promotion and maintenance
CNS: Prevention and early detection of disease
CL: Application

44 A female client is receiving chemotherapy through a central line catheter. The nurse who is helping with her bath notes that the infusion pump is frequently indicating a slowing of the infusion rate. Which action should the nurse take?
- ☐ 1. Turn off the pump until the bath is finished.
- ☐ 2. Check the line for kinks.
- ☐ 3. Check for blood return in the catheter.
- ☐ 4. Change the central line dressing.

CORRECT ANSWER: 2
The I.V. line may have become kinked or tangled in the bedding during the bath. Straightening the tubing may reestablish the flow rate. Option 1: The client's chemotherapy shouldn't be stopped. Option 3: Checking for blood isn't indicated. A blood return with a central catheter is obtained only by applying negative pressure. Option 4: The dressing should be changed once every 7 days. Although some tubing may have become coiled under the dressing, this is more likely to occur with the exposed I.V. line.
NP: Implementing care
CN: Physiological integrity
CNS: Basic care and comfort
CL: Application

45 A client reports urinary frequency and burning. The physician diagnoses cystitis and prescribes co-trimoxazole (Bactrim DS). What advice should the nurse give the client?
- ☐ 1. Expect the urine to be dark green.
- ☐ 2. Discontinue the medication when the symptoms are gone.
- ☐ 3. Take the medication with 6 to 8 oz (177 to 237 ml) of water.
- ☐ 4. Encourage exposure to the sun for vitamin D absorption.

CORRECT ANSWER: 3
Adequate fluid intake is required with sulfa drugs to prevent crystalluria. The minimum urine output should be 1.5 L/day while on the drug. Option 1: The urine shouldn't turn green. Option 2: The nurse should stress the importance of taking the entire prescription, warning that symptoms typically disappear before the bacteria are eliminated from the system. Option 4: The client should avoid prolonged sun exposure because the drug may cause a photosensitivity reaction.
NP: Planning care
CN: Health promotion and maintenance
CNS: Prevention and early detection of disease
CL: Application

46 A 76-year-old male client underwent a transurethral resection of the prostate (TURP) for benign prostatic hyperplasia. He has an indwelling urinary catheter in place and is on continuous irrigations. Which finding is most desirable on the first postoperative day?
- ☐ 1. Light pink urine
- ☐ 2. Passage of bright red blood around the catheter
- ☐ 3. Catheter patency established with 1,500 ml of sterile water
- ☐ 4. Moderate scrotal edema

CORRECT ANSWER: 1
The client's urine should be light pink to clear after 24 hours. Option 2: Passage of blood around the catheter would indicate bladder spasms and the need for pain or spasm relief. Option 3: Overzealous use of irrigating fluid may induce bleeding and cause bladder spasms. Also, water absorption may cause electrolyte imbalances. Option 4: Scrotal edema is abnormal with TURP and should be reported.
NP: Evaluating care
CN: Physiological integrity
CNS: Physiological adaptation
CL: Application

47 An 86-year-old female client has a fractured left hip. Her left leg is in Buck's traction while she's being prepared for a hip pinning. The nurse who is planning to insert an indwelling urinary catheter would:
- ☐ 1. choose a #12 French catheter.
- ☐ 2. instruct the client to turn on her right side with both legs flexed.
- ☐ 3. instruct the client to cough and deep-breathe during catheterization.
- ☐ 4. add tape to the catheter tray for taping the indwelling catheter to the client's abdomen.

CORRECT ANSWER: 3
Coughing and deep breathing help to relax the client, in general, and the sphincter, in particular, and prevent spasms. Option 1: A #16 or #18 French catheter is used for an adult. Option 2: The client couldn't be turned on her right side. Buck's traction is being used to keep the left extremity aligned. Option 4: The catheter should be taped to the unaffected thigh.
NP: Planning care
CN: Safe, effective care environment
CNS: Coordinated care
CL: Application

48 The nurse is preparing a client for surgery. The physician has ordered a preoperative injection of 65 mg of meperidine (Demerol). Prefilled syringes containing 100 mg in 2 ml are available. How much solution should the nurse give?
- ☐ 1. 0.7 ml
- ☐ 2. 1.3 ml
- ☐ 3. 1.5 ml
- ☐ 4. 1.7 ml

CORRECT ANSWER: 2
Because 65 mg is desired and 100 mg in 2 ml is on hand, the nurse should administer 1.3 ml (2 × 65 ÷ 100 = 1.3).
NP: Implementing care
CN: Safe, effective care environment
CNS: Safety and infection control
CL: Comprehension

49 A client returns from surgery with an I.V. solution of dextrose 5% in saline. The order is for 125 ml of I.V. solution per hour. The I.V. set delivers 15 drops/ml. How many drops per minute should the I.V. solution run?
- ☐ 1. 15 drops/minute
- ☐ 2. 21 drops/minute
- ☐ 3. 31 drops/minute
- ☐ 4. 41 drops/minute

CORRECT ANSWER: 3
The I.V. rate would be 31 drops/minute (15 × 125 = 1,875 divided by 60 minutes = 31.25). Options 1, 2, and 4: These rates are incorrect.
NP: Implementing care
CN: Safe, effective care environment
CNS: Safety and infection control
CL: Comprehension

50 A female client who is at risk for blood clots after bone surgery is to receive subcutaneous heparin. A multidose vial of heparin contains 20,000 units in 5 ml. How many milliliters should the nurse administer for an ordered dose of 5,000 units?
- ☐ 1. 0.25 ml
- ☐ 2. 1.25 ml
- ☐ 3. 4 ml
- ☐ 4. 20 ml

CORRECT ANSWER: 2
The nurse should administer 1.25 ml of heparin (5 × 5,000 [desired dose] = 25,000 divided by 20,000 units = 1.25). Options 1, 3, and 4: These options are incorrect.
NP: Implementing care
CN: Safe, effective care environment
CNS: Safety and infection control
CL: Comprehension

51 A client is in the postanesthesia care unit (PACU) after abdominal surgery. While assessing the client for discharge to the medical-surgical nursing unit, the nurse should report which finding indicative of a potential complication?
- ☐ 1. Temperature of 97.8° F (36.6° C)
- ☐ 2. Client responding to name but falling back asleep
- ☐ 3. Urine output of 20 ml/hour
- ☐ 4. Client complaints of pain

CORRECT ANSWER: 3
Adequate urine output is at least 30 ml/hour. Anything less indicates a potential problem of retention. Option 1: The temperature must be at least 96.8° F (36° C) before a client is discharged from the PACU. Option 2: The client's responding to his name indicates an appropriate level of consciousness. Falling back to sleep isn't a complication. Option 4: Postoperative clients typically experience pain.
NP: Collecting data
CN: Physiological integrity
CNS: Physiological adaptation
CL: Analysis

52 A male client has been admitted to the hospital with heart failure. On entering the room, the nurse notices that the client is having difficulty breathing. Which position would be the most appropriate to help his breathing?
- ☐ 1. Place the client flat in bed with his feet elevated.
- ☐ 2. Place the client in semi-Fowler's position.
- ☐ 3. Turn the client on his side.
- ☐ 4. Place the client in high Fowler's position.

CORRECT ANSWER: 4
High Fowler's position facilitates adequate lung expansion by aiding gravity to pull the organs away from the chest and decreases venous return to the heart. Options 1, 2, and 3: These positions promote venous return to an already overloaded heart and restrict lung expansion.
NP: Implementing care
CN: Physiological integrity
CNS: Basic care and comfort
CL: Application

53 A client is on the surgical unit after orthopedic surgery. The physician has ordered 8 mg of morphine sulfate I.M. for pain. The Tubex reads "MS gr $^1/_6$ = 1 cc." How much should the nurse inject?
- ☐ 1. 0.8 ml
- ☐ 2. 0.3 ml
- ☐ 3. 0.4 ml
- ☐ 4. 0.5 ml

CORRECT ANSWER: 1
The nurse should inject 0.8 ml of morphine. The nurse should know that MS gr $^1/_6$ = 10 mg = 1 cc (or 1 ml). Therefore, 8 mg ÷ 10 mg × 1 ml = 0.8 ml. The other answers are incorrect.
NP: Implementing care
CN: Safe, effective care environment
CNS: Safety and infection control
CL: Application

54 The nurse knows that client teaching about hypertension has been effective when the client states:
- ☐ 1. "I shouldn't adjust my medication without my physician's advice."
- ☐ 2. "I can stop taking my medication when I no longer have headaches."
- ☐ 3. "I should stop taking my medication if I have adverse effects."
- ☐ 4. "I only have to take the medication when I feel bad."

CORRECT ANSWER: 1
Medication for blood pressure control must not be adjusted or stopped without the physician's approval. Any changes in medication require close monitoring of the client. Options 2 and 4: Medication must be continued on a regular schedule, or the blood pressure will rise. Option 3: If serious adverse effects occur, the physician should be notified. Other medications can be substituted without the adverse effects.
NP: Evaluating care
CN: Health promotion and maintenance
CNS: Prevention and early detection of disease
CL: Analysis

55 A male client is receiving digoxin (Lanoxin) and furosemide (Lasix) as treatment for heart failure. He complains of feeling weak and having muscle cramps. His apical pulse is 76 beats/minute; respirations, 16 breaths/minute; and blood pressure, 148/86 mm Hg. What action should the nurse take?
- ☐ 1. Tell the client that he's probably weak from inactivity.
- ☐ 2. Look at the chart for his last potassium level and contact the physician.
- ☐ 3. Look at the chart for his last digoxin level and notify the physician.
- ☐ 4. Notify the physician that the client is experiencing heart failure.

CORRECT ANSWER: 2
Muscle weakness and cramping are signs of hypokalemia, which can be a adverse effect of furosemide. Option 1: The client's hypokalemia will worsen if the nurse doesn't follow up on his complaints. Options 3 and 4: The client isn't exhibiting symptoms indicative of digoxin toxicity or heart failure.
NP: Collecting data
CN: Physiological integrity
CNS: Pharmacological therapies
CL: Analysis

56 A male client has arteriosclerosis with intermittent claudication. The nurse has worked with him to develop a walking program. Which statement by the client indicates that he understands the program?
- ☐ 1. "I should stop walking and elevate my legs when pain occurs."
- ☐ 2. "I should stop walking and rest before pain occurs."
- ☐ 3. "I should walk further each day even if pain occurs."
- ☐ 4. "I should walk until pain occurs, then rest."

CORRECT ANSWER: 4
Pain should be the guide to the amount of activity the client performs. When pain occurs, the tissues aren't being oxygenated adequately, so the client should stop and rest to allow the tissues to become oxygenated. Option 1: The legs should remain dependent to aid gravity in delivering oxygenated blood to the tissues. Legs are typically elevated for venous problems. Option 2: The client should exercise until pain occurs to develop collateral circulation and promote circulation. Option 3: The client shouldn't walk past the point of pain because the tissues aren't being oxygenated adequately.
NP: Evaluating care
CN: Health promotion and maintenance
CNS: Prevention and early detection of disease
CL: Analysis

57 A client with pneumonia has a nursing diagnosis of *Ineffective airway clearance related to increased secretions and ineffective cough.* Which intervention would facilitate effective coughing?
- ☐ 1. Lying in semi-Fowler's position
- ☐ 2. Sipping water, hot tea, or coffee
- ☐ 3. Inhaling and exhaling through pursed lips
- ☐ 4. Using thoracic breathing

CORRECT ANSWER: 2
Sips of water, hot tea, or coffee may stimulate coughing. Option 1: The best position is sitting in a chair with the knees flexed and the feet placed firmly on the floor. Option 3: The client should inhale through the nose and exhale through pursed lips. Option 4: Diaphragmatic, not thoracic, breathing helps to facilitate coughing.
NP: Planning care
CN: Physiological integrity
CNS: Basic care and comfort
CL: Application

58 On entering the room of a client with chronic obstructive pulmonary disease (COPD), the nurse notices that the client is receiving oxygen at 4 L/minute by way of a nasal cannula. The nurse's actions should be based on which of the following statements?
- ☐ 1. The flow rate is too high.
- ☐ 2. The flow rate is too low.
- ☐ 3. The flow rate is correct.
- ☐ 4. The client shouldn't receive oxygen.

CORRECT ANSWER: 1
The administration of oxygen at 1 to 2 L/minute by way of a nasal cannula is recommended for clients with COPD; therefore, a rate of 4 L/minute is too high. The normal mechanism that stimulates breathing is a rise in blood carbon dioxide. Clients with COPD retain blood carbon dioxide, so their mechanism for stimulating breathing is a low blood oxygen level. High levels of oxygen may cause hypoventilation and apnea. Oxygen delivered at 1 to 2 L/minute should aid in oxygenation without causing hypoventilation. Option 4: Oxygen therapy is the only therapy that has been demonstrated to be life-preserving for clients with COPD.
NP: Implementing care
CN: Safe, effective care environment
CNS: Safety and infection control
CL: Application

59 A male client with tuberculosis (TB) has been admitted to the medical-surgical unit. What is the best measure for preventing transmission of TB?
- ☐ 1. Wash hands with antimicrobial soap.
- ☐ 2. Teach the client to cover his mouth and nose when coughing.
- ☐ 3. Require all people who enter the room to wear a face mask.
- ☐ 4. Require the client to wear a face mask.

CORRECT ANSWER: 2
TB is an infectious disease that is transmitted by airborne droplets from coughing, laughing, and sneezing. Option 1: Washing hands after contact with infected sputum is important, but hand washing without sputum control won't prevent transmission. Options 3 and 4: Masks are reportedly ineffective in preventing transmission of tuberculosis.
NP: Planning care
CN: Safe, effective care environment
CNS: Safety and infection control
CL: Knowledge

---

60 The nurse is monitoring a client's chest tube that is attached to suction through a Pleur-evac. Assessment data include 50 ml of additional output in the collecting chamber in the past hour, continuous bubbling in the water-seal and suction chambers, and a dry, intact dressing. Which nursing action is appropriate?
- ☐ 1. No action is necessary because all assessment data are within normal expectations.
- ☐ 2. Notify the physician of the excess drainage.
- ☐ 3. Check the system for an air leak.
- ☐ 4. Check the suction for a malfunction.

CORRECT ANSWER: 3
Continuous bubbling in the water-seal chamber indicates an air leak. Option 1: The nurse should act quickly to correct the air leak. Option 2: Fifty milliliters of drainage isn't excessive. Option 4: There is no indication of malfunctioning suction equipment.
NP: Implementing care
CN: Safe, effective care environment
CNS: Safety and infection control
CL: Application

---

61 To teach a client deep-breathing and coughing exercises, which technique is most correct?
- ☐ 1. Cough to clear the airway and take several deep breaths.
- ☐ 2. Cough, deep-breathe, cough, and deep-breathe.
- ☐ 3. Take a deep breath and cough until the lungs are empty of air.
- ☐ 4. Take a deep breath, cough once, take another breath, and cough.

CORRECT ANSWER: 3
This method of coughing moves secretions from the smaller airways to the larger airways. Options 1 and 2: Taking a deep breath before coughing helps to stimulate the cough reflex. Option 4: Taking a deep breath after coughing once might move the secretions deeper.
NP: Implementing care
CN: Safe, effective care environment
CNS: Safety and infection control
CL: Knowledge

---

62 The nurse knows that a client has mastered the technique needed to correctly use an incentive spirometer when the client:
- ☐ 1. blows quickly and hard into the mouthpiece.
- ☐ 2. inhales slowly and deeply through the nose.
- ☐ 3. inhales quickly and deeply through the mouthpiece.
- ☐ 4. inhales slowly and deeply through the mouthpiece.

CORRECT ANSWER: 4
The client should be taught to inhale through the mouth slowly and deeply to properly inflate the alveoli. Option 1: Blowing can cause the alveoli to collapse. Option 2: Inhalation is through the mouth, not the nose. Option 3: Inhalations should be slow, not quick.
NP: Collecting data
CN: Safe, effective care environment
CNS: Safety and infection control
CL: Analysis

63 A client is receiving oxygen by way of a nasal cannula at a rate of 2 L/minute. How should the oxygen flow meter be set?
- ☐ 1. The bottom of the ball should sit on top of the line marked "2."
- ☐ 2. The top of the ball should sit below the line marked "2."
- ☐ 3. The line marked "2" should cut the ball in half.
- ☐ 4. Any part of the ball should touch the line marked "2."

CORRECT ANSWER: 3
The oxygen flow rate is set by centering the indicator on the line marked "2." Options 1, 2, and 4 are incorrect.
NP: Implementing care
CN: Safe, effective care environment
CNS: Safety and infection control
CL: Knowledge

64 An elderly client with pneumonia has a nursing diagnosis of *Ineffective airway clearance*. Which interventions would be most appropriate?
- ☐ 1. Monitor the need for suctioning every hour.
- ☐ 2. Suction every hour.
- ☐ 3. Suction once per shift.
- ☐ 4. Ask the physician for an order to suction.

CORRECT ANSWER: 1
Suctioning should be performed only when necessary, based on the client's condition at the time of assessment. Therefore, options 2 and 3 are incorrect. Option 4: Suctioning is a nursing procedure and doesn't require a physician's order.
NP: Planning care
CN: Physiological integrity
CNS: Basic care and comfort
CL: Application

65 The nurse is collecting supplies needed to perform tracheostomy care. Which equipment should be gathered?
- ☐ 1. Sterile gloves, sterile saline solution, and hydrogen peroxide
- ☐ 2. Sterile gloves and sterile water
- ☐ 3. Sterile gloves and hydrogen peroxide
- ☐ 4. Clean gloves, water, and hydrogen peroxide

CORRECT ANSWER: 1
Tracheostomy care is a sterile procedure that requires the use of sterile gloves, hydrogen peroxide to loosen incrustations and secretions, and sterile saline solution to rinse off the hydrogen peroxide before replacing the inner cannula. All the other options are incorrect.
NP: Implementing care
CN: Safe, effective care environment
CNS: Safety and infection control
CL: Knowledge

66 A male client with a fractured femur is in Russell's traction. He asks the nurse to help him with back care. Which nursing action is most appropriate?
- ☐ 1. Tell the client that he can't have back care while he's in traction.
- ☐ 2. Remove the weight to give the client more slack to move.
- ☐ 3. Support the weight to give the client more slack to move.
- ☐ 4. Tell the client to use the trapeze to lift his back off the bed.

CORRECT ANSWER: 4
The traction must not be disturbed to maintain correct alignment. Therefore, the client should use the trapeze to lift his back off of the bed. Option 1: The client can have back care as long as he uses the trapeze and doesn't disturb the alignment. Option 2: The weight shouldn't be removed without a physician's order. Option 3: The weight should hang freely without touching anything.
NP: Implementing care
CN: Physiological integrity
CNS: Reduction of risk potential
CL: Application

67 A client has just returned from the postanesthesia care unit after undergoing internal fixation of a fractured left femoral neck. The nurse should place the client in which position?
☐ 1. On the left side with the right knee bent
☐ 2. On the back with two pillows between the legs
☐ 3. On the right side with the left knee bent
☐ 4. Sitting at a 90-degree angle

CORRECT ANSWER: 2
The operative leg must be kept abducted to prevent dislocation of the hip. Options 1 and 3 don't promote abduction. Option 4: Acute flexion of the operated hip may cause dislocation. The head of the bed may be raised 35 to 40 degrees.
NP: Implementing care
CN: Physiological integrity
CNS: Reduction of risk potential
CL: Application

68 When performing neurovascular checks on a client after surgical repair of a fractured leg, which assessment isn't considered a routine part of the checks?
☐ 1. Level of consciousness and pupil reaction
☐ 2. Bilateral leg comparison for pulse, color, and temperature
☐ 3. Ability to wiggle toes
☐ 4. Capillary refill in the toes

CORRECT ANSWER: 1
Neurovascular checks are performed on the area affected by the client's condition. Level of consciousness and pupil reaction would be performed on a client with a condition involving the head, not the leg. Options 2, 3, and 4 would all be performed.
NP: Collecting data
CN: Physiological integrity
CNS: Reduction of risk potential
CL: Analysis

69 A client has been fitted for crutches, and the nurse is evaluating the outcome of patient-teaching sessions for crutch walking. Which outcome is desired?
☐ 1. The client's weight is being born by the axilla.
☐ 2. The client is wearing slippers.
☐ 3. The elbows are bent at a slight angle.
☐ 4. When descending stairs, the unaffected leg moves first.

CORRECT ANSWER: 3
The elbows shouldn't be locked open but rather bent at a slight angle if the crutches are fitted correctly. Option 1: Weight shouldn't be born on the axilla; this could cause nerve damage. It should be born by the heel pad of the hand. Option 2: Crutches shouldn't be used in stocking feet, slippers, or high heels. Only sturdy, low-heeled shoes should be worn to prevent injuries. Option 4: For proper support, the client leads off with the unaffected foot when ascending stairs and with the affected foot and crutches when descending. The client should remember "Down with the bad and up with the good."
NP: Evaluating care
CN: Safe, effective care environment
CNS: Safety and infection control
CL: Analysis

70 The nurse is evaluating a client's use of a cane before discharge from the hospital. Which finding indicates proper use of a cane?
☐ 1. The cane is used on the side of the unaffected leg.
☐ 2. The cane moves with the unaffected leg.
☐ 3. The cane moves first and is followed by both legs.
☐ 4. The client is bent forward at the waist.

CORRECT ANSWER: 1
The cane is used on the unaffected side, with the cane and affected leg moving together. Therefore, options 2 and 3 are incorrect. Option 4: Good posture is encouraged with the use of assistive devices.
NP: Evaluating care
CN: Safe, effective care environment
CNS: Safety and infection control
CL: Analysis

71 When assessing the abdomen of a client with intestinal obstruction, in what order should the assessment proceed?
☐ 1. Palpation, auscultation, and inspection
☐ 2. Auscultation, inspection, and palpation
☐ 3. Auscultation, palpation, and inspection
☐ 4. Inspection, auscultation, and palpation

CORRECT ANSWER: 4
Collecting data of the abdomen always proceeds from inspection to auscultation to palpation. Any other order can change the assessment data.
NP: Collecting data
CN: Safe, effective care environment
CNS: Coordinated care
CL: Knowledge

72 A female client who has been diagnosed with colon cancer expresses concern about what this means for the future. What is the nurse's best initial response?
☐ 1. "Cancer can be treated and has a good cure rate today."
☐ 2. "You seem troubled; tell me more about how you're feeling."
☐ 3. "Your physician can answer your questions better than I can."
☐ 4. "You have a wonderful family. I'm sure they'll be supportive."

CORRECT ANSWER: 2
Open communication and trust need to be established, and the client needs to talk about what is troubling her. Option 2 lets the client know that the nurse is supportive and encourages the client to ventilate her concerns. Options 1, 3, and 4 close communication and convey nonsupport.
NP: Implementing care
CN: Psychosocial integrity
CNS: Coping and adaptation
CL: Application

73 The nurse inserting a nasogastric tube should ask the client to:
☐ 1. hold his breath.
☐ 2. swallow.
☐ 3. breathe deeply through the nose.
☐ 4. blow outward through pursed lips.

CORRECT ANSWER: 2
Swallowing helps to advance the tube into the stomach by closing the opening to the trachea. Options 1, 3, and 4 leave the trachea open and increase the chance of misplacing the tube.
NP: Implementing care
CN: Physiological integrity
CNS: Basic care and comfort
CL: Knowledge

74 The nurse has inserted a nasogastric (NG) tube and is checking for proper placement. Which of the following indicates that the tube isn't in the stomach?
☐ 1. A bubbling sound is heard with a stethoscope over the epigastric area when air is injected into the tube.
☐ 2. Stomach contents are aspirated through the tube.
☐ 3. The client speaks with a whisper.
☐ 4. The client complains about the tube being in his nose.

CORRECT ANSWER: 3
When the NG tube passes into the trachea, the client is unable to speak in a normal voice. Options 1 and 2 are acceptable methods of verifying tube placement and indicate proper placement. Option 4: The NG tube is uncomfortable, even when properly placed.
NP: Collecting data
CN: Physiological integrity
CNS: Reduction of risk potential
CL: Analysis

75 The nurse is assessing a client who is receiving a continuous nasogastric (NG) tube feeding. Which of the following data suggests the need for nursing action?
☐ 1. Respirations are quiet and nonlabored.
☐ 2. The feeding pump is operating at 60 ml/hour.
☐ 3. The feeding bag has been hanging for 8 hours.
☐ 4. The client is sleeping with the head of the bed flat.

CORRECT ANSWER: 4
When a client is receiving feeding through an NG tube, the head of the bed should be elevated at all times to prevent aspiration. Options 1, 2, and 3 indicate no need for nursing action.
NP: Collecting data
CN: Safe, effective care environment
CNS: Safety and infection control
CL: Analysis

76 When teaching the client to apply a colostomy pouch, the nurse should cut the opening in the pouch face plate so that:
☐ 1. it fits snugly around the stoma.
☐ 2. about $1/8''$ (0.3 cm) is left between the stoma and the face plate.
☐ 3. about $1/4''$ (0.6 cm) is left between the stoma and the face plate.
☐ 4. about $1/2''$ (1.3 cm) is left between the stoma and the face plate.

CORRECT ANSWER: 2
The face plate shouldn't touch the stoma to prevent irritation; however, it should cover the skin to prevent breakdown. Option 2 provides enough protection. Options 1, 3, and 4 are incorrect.
NP: Implementing care
CN: Health promotion and maintenance
CNS: Prevention and early detection of disease
CL: Comprehension

77 The nurse is teaching a client how to apply an abdominal binder. What is the proper position of the client while the binder is being applied?
☐ 1. Lying on the back
☐ 2. Sitting on the side of the bed
☐ 3. Standing
☐ 4. Bending forward

CORRECT ANSWER: 1
By lying on the back, the abdominal organs become properly positioned by gravity, thereby enabling the client to fasten the binder. Options 2, 3, and 4 cause the abdomen and its contents to protrude, making fastening difficult.
NP: Implementing care
CN: Health promotion and maintenance
CNS: Prevention and early detection of disease
CL: Knowledge

78 Which findings are indicative of increasing intracranial pressure (ICP)?
☐ 1. Decreased level of consciousness (LOC), elevated blood pressure, and elevated pulse rate
☐ 2. Decreased blood pressure, decreased pulse rate, and decreased LOC
☐ 3. Widened pulse pressure, decreased respirations, decreased pulse rate, and decreased LOC
☐ 4. Decreased respirations, increased pulse rate, and decreased LOC

CORRECT ANSWER: 3
As ICP increases, pressure is exerted on the brain stem, causing a widening pulse pressure, apneic periods, bradycardia, and a decreased LOC. Options 1, 2, and 4 are incorrect.
NP: Collecting data
CN: Physiological integrity
CNS: Physiological adaptation
CL: Comprehension

79 A client who had a cerebrovascular accident is having difficulty swallowing while taking medications with water. Which nursing action is best initially?
☐ 1. Administer the medications with pudding.
☐ 2. Administer the medications dissolved in juice.
☐ 3. Have the pharmacy provide liquid forms of the medications.
☐ 4. Administer the medication by another route.

CORRECT ANSWER: 1
Soft foods, such as pudding, are easier to swallow than liquids, such as juice (Option 2) and liquid medications (Option 3). Option 4: Administering the medication by another route is necessary only after all other options have been explored.
NP: Implementing care
CN: Physiological integrity
CNS: Basic care and comfort
CL: Application

80 The nurse enters the room of a client who is having a seizure. Which initial response by the nurse would be appropriate?
- ☐ 1. Insert a padded tongue blade into the client's mouth.
- ☐ 2. Turn the client's head to the side.
- ☐ 3. Yell for help.
- ☐ 4. Call a code.

CORRECT ANSWER: 2
During a seizure, the nurse should turn the client's head to the side to allow for drainage of secretions and an open airway. After the seizure, the client may be placed on his side. Option 1: During a seizure, the jaw is clenched. The nurse should never force the jaw open to insert objects. Option 3: The nurse's primary goals during a seizure are to protect the client and to observe the incident closely for later documentation. No other help is needed. Option 4: Codes are called for clients whose respirations and heartbeats have stopped.
NP: Implementing care
CN: Safe, effective care environment
CNS: Safety and infection control
CL: Application

81 A male client with acute glomerulonephritis tells the nurse that he has been increasing his water intake because he knows that it's important to drink a lot when he has an infection. What should be the nurse's initial reaction?
- ☐ 1. "That is good. I'm glad to know that you're interested in doing what is good for you."
- ☐ 2. "Fruit juices would be better for you. What kind of juice do you like?"
- ☐ 3. "Didn't your physician tell you that you can't drink anything?"
- ☐ 4. "With most infections, it's good to drink a lot of fluids. In this situation, however, your fluid intake must be restricted."

CORRECT ANSWER: 4
In clients with glomerulonephritis, fluid intake must be restricted to equal fluid output to ensure that fluid isn't retained while kidney function is impaired. Options 1 and 2 don't convey the importance of restricting fluids. Option 3: Total restrictions of fluids is unnecessary.
NP: Implementing care
CN: Physiological integrity
CNS: Physiological adaptation
CL: Application

82 During the first 24 hours after a transurethral prostatectomy, the nurse checks the client for symptoms of transurethral resection (TUR) syndrome. These include:
- ☐ 1. hypertension, bradycardia, confusion, and tachypnea.
- ☐ 2. urine retention, bladder distention, and pain.
- ☐ 3. excessive bleeding, hypotension, and tachycardia.
- ☐ 4. retrograde ejaculation and inability to form an erection.

CORRECT ANSWER: 1
TUR syndrome is caused by excessive absorption of irrigating solution, which causes a fluid volume excess and electrolyte imbalances. Symptoms include hypertension, bradycardia, confusion, and tachypnea. Options 2, 3, and 4 aren't symptoms of TUR syndrome.
NP: Collecting data
CN: Physiological integrity
CNS: Physiological adaptation
CL: Application

83 Which statement made by a client beginning hemodialysis shows an understanding of the treatment?
- ☐ 1. "I'll feel better immediately after dialysis."
- ☐ 2. "I can eat and drink whatever I want because I'm on dialysis."
- ☐ 3. "Dialysis is a complication-free procedure."
- ☐ 4. "The dialysis takes about 4 hours and must be done 3 days per week."

CORRECT ANSWER: 4
Hemodialysis usually takes 3 to 5 hours and is performed three times per week. Option 1: Most clients feel best the day after dialysis. Option 2: Protein, sodium, and potassium are usually restricted, and calories and carbohydrates are increased. Fluids are restricted. Option 3: Complications can occur.
NP: Evaluating care
CN: Health promotion and maintenance
CNS: Growth and development through the life span
CL: Application

84 The nurse is preparing to insert a urinary catheter into a client who has bowel incontinence. Which nursing intervention is appropriate?
- ☐ 1. Clean the urinary meatus with soap and water and insert the catheter.
- ☐ 2. Clean the urinary meatus with povidone-iodine (Betadine) and insert the catheter.
- ☐ 3. Clean the urinary meatus with soap and water and Betadine, and then insert the catheter.
- ☐ 4. Clean the client, change the soiled garment and linens, and begin inserting the catheter.

CORRECT ANSWER: 4
The nurse must take special precautions to ensure that no organisms are introduced into the client's bladder. Options 1, 2, and 3: The client must be clean before the procedure begins.
NP: Implementing care
CN: Safe, effective care environment
CNS: Safety and infection control
CL: Application

85 The nurse is preparing a teaching plan that will be used for clients with hyperthyroidism. What should be included in this plan?
- ☐ 1. Increase the room temperature if feeling cold.
- ☐ 2. Eat a high-calorie, high-protein, high-carbohydrate diet.
- ☐ 3. Add fiber to the diet.
- ☐ 4. Use over-the-counter laxatives as needed.

CORRECT ANSWER: 2
Metabolism is increased in clients with hyperthyroidism. Therefore, weight loss will occur if intake isn't greatly increased. Options 1, 3, and 4 are interventions for clients with hypothyroidism.
NP: Planning care
CN: Health promotion and maintenance
CNS: Prevention and early detection of disease
CL: Application

86 The nurse found a stage 1 pressure ulcer on a client. Which wound covering would be appropriate?
- ☐ 1. Enzymatic debriding agent
- ☐ 2. Wet-to-dry gauze
- ☐ 3. Clear plastic dressing
- ☐ 4. Absorptive gel

CORRECT ANSWER: 3
Clear plastic dressings provide a moist, protective environment that speed healing of stage 1 ulcers. Options 1, 2, and 4 are appropriate for stages 2, 3, and 4.
NP: Implementing care
CN: Safe, effective care environment
CNS: Safety and infection control
CL: Application

87 A client has been receiving chemotherapy for ovarian cancer, but the treatment has been ineffective and produced many adverse effects. She has decided to end the treatment and live the remainder of her life free from the adverse effects. After the nurse talks with the client and realizes that she's making an informed decision, what should the nurse do?
- ☐ 1. Tell the client that she's making a mistake.
- ☐ 2. Tell the client she has no choice; treatment must continue.
- ☐ 3. Tell the client that her family won't accept her decision.
- ☐ 4. Offer to help explain her decision to her family.

CORRECT ANSWER: 4
After the client has made an informed decision, the nurse should be supportive in whatever way the client wishes. Option 1: This approach makes the client feel unaccepted and closes communication with the nurse. Option 2: Treatment can't continue without the client's consent. Option 3: The nurse needs to convey acceptance and support by listening and offering to help.
NP: Implementing care
CN: Psychosocial integrity
CNS: Coping and adaptation
CL: Application

88 The nurse is evaluating the outcome of a client with a nursing diagnosis of *Dysfunctional grieving related to loss of right breast*. Which of the following indicates that the goal "The client will adjust to her altered breast appearance" has been reached?
- ☐ 1. The client talks repeatedly about her surgical experience when the nurse enters the room.
- ☐ 2. The client states the correct wound care procedure to use when she's discharged.
- ☐ 3. The client looks at her incision and demonstrates proper wound care.
- ☐ 4. The client states that she doesn't want to see her husband.

CORRECT ANSWER: 3
Being able to look at the surgical site is a sign that the client is adjusting to a change in body image. Option 1: Talking repeatedly about a topic indicates anxiety. Option 2: The client must demonstrate the procedure, not state it, for the nurse to know that it can be done. Option 4: This indicates a problem with self-concept.
NP: Evaluating care
CN: Health promotion and maintenance
CNS: Growth and development through the life span
CL: Application

89 The nurse is gathering supplies to change a central line dressing. Which supplies should be included?
- ☐ 1. Dressing kit
- ☐ 2. Dressing kit and a mask
- ☐ 3. Dressing kit and two masks
- ☐ 4. Dressing kit, two masks, and gown

CORRECT ANSWER: 2
The nurse should obtain a prepackaged dressing kit and wear a mask to cover the mouth and nose, thereby preventing organisms from causing infection. All other necessary supplies for changing the dressing are included in the dressing kit. Option 1: A mask is also needed. Option 3: The client doesn't wear a mask during the dressing change but instead turns the head to the side. Option 4: A gown isn't needed for this type of dressing change.
NP: Planning care
CN: Safe, effective care environment
CNS: Safety and infection control
CL: Application

90 A client who is being tested for tuberculosis has a positive Mantoux result, a negative chest X-ray, and no clinical symptoms. The physician recommends 300 mg of isoniazid daily for preventive therapy. The nurse should explain to the client that the isoniazid:
- ☐ 1. should be taken daily for 9 to 12 months to prevent active disease.
- ☐ 2. should be taken until the Mantoux skin test reverts to normal.
- ☐ 3. produces no serious adverse effects.
- ☐ 4. provides active immunity to the disease as long as it's taken.

CORRECT ANSWER: 1
Isoniazid is a bactericidal agent that stops the growth of the bacilli. It should be taken long-term (9 to 12 months) to prevent the disease. Option 2: Mantoux skin tests remain positive for years as long as living bacilli remain in the body. Option 3: Serious adverse effects of isoniazid include neuritis and hepatitis, which require continued evaluation. Option 4: Isoniazid doesn't provide active immunity; it's a bactericidal agent that inhibits growth of the bacilli.
NP: Implementing care
CN: Safe, effective care environment
CNS: Safety and infection control
CL: Analysis

91 Which intervention would best help to decrease intracranial pressure (ICP) in a client with a head injury?
- ☐ 1. Elevating the body temperature above 99° F (37.2° C)
- ☐ 2. Increasing cerebral venous outflow
- ☐ 3. Increasing partial pressure of arterial carbon dioxide levels in the blood
- ☐ 4. Dilating cerebral blood vessels

CORRECT ANSWER: 2
Elevating the head of the bed helps to increase cerebral venous return and decrease ICP. Option 1: Elevating the body temperature also increases the metabolic rate and thereby increases the oxygen needs of the body. However, it doesn't decrease ICP. Option 3: Increasing the carbon dioxide levels in the blood causes vasodilation and thus increases ICP. Option 4: Dilating cerebral blood vessels increases ICP.
NP: Implementing care
CN: Physiological integrity
CNS: Physiological adaptation
CL: Analysis

92 A client is being discharged from the hospital with a permanent cardiac pacemaker that is set at 72 beats/minute. The nurse should instruct the client to report which pulse rate immediately to the physician?
- ☐ 1. 88 beats/minute
- ☐ 2. 64 beats/minute
- ☐ 3. 72 beats/minute
- ☐ 4. 96 beats/minute

CORRECT ANSWER: 2
A demand pacemaker guarantees approximately 72 beats/minute. Whenever a client's rate falls below this mark, the cardiac pacemaker initiates a beat. A rate above 72 beats/minute is normal and indicates that the client's heart is initiating the beats. A rate below 72 beats/minute should be reported because it means that the pacemaker isn't functioning at the preset rate.
NP: Collecting data
CN: Health promotion and maintenance
CNS: Prevention and early detection of disease
CL: Application

93 A female client who works in a day-care center is diagnosed with meningococcal meningitis. Her supervisor asks the nurse if this poses any danger to the children. What is the nurse's best response?
- ☐ 1. "All people who had contact with her will need to take an oral antibiotic."
- ☐ 2. "Bacterial meningitis is contained within the cranium and isn't contagious."
- ☐ 3. "Children under age 5 are at risk for bacterial meningitis."
- ☐ 4. "Although oral antibiotics aren't useful in prevention, the children should see their physicians."

CORRECT ANSWER: 1
Bacterial meningitis is transmitted by droplets from the nasopharynx. All people who have had direct contact with the infected person should be treated with oral antibiotics, such as rifampin, to prevent infection. Option 2: This disease is contagious. Option 3: Anyone who has had contact with the infected person is at risk. Option 4: If given promptly, oral antibiotics reduce or prevent the spread of infection.
NP: Implementing care
CN: Safe, effective care environment
CNS: Safety and infection control
CL: Application

94 Which of the following methods correctly elicits Brudzinski's sign?
- ☐ 1. Tapping the facial nerve lightly
- ☐ 2. Dorsiflexing either foot
- ☐ 3. Extending the lower leg from a 90-degree angle to the thigh
- ☐ 4. Lifting the client's head rapidly from the bed

CORRECT ANSWER: 4
Rapid, forward head flexion produces flexion of both thighs at the hips and flexure movements of the ankles and knees, indicating a positive Brudzinski's sign and meningeal irritation. Option 1: This elicits Chvostek's sign, which indicates a low calcium level. Option 2: This elicits Homan's sign, which indicates possible thrombophlebitis. Option 3: This elicits Kernig's sign, which is also indicative of meningeal irritation.
NP: Collecting data
CN: Physiological integrity
CNS: Physiological adaptation
CL: Knowledge

95 In a client with a head injury, the nurse must keep the body temperature normal because hyperthermia causes:
- ☐ 1. carbon dioxide retention.
- ☐ 2. increased cerebral oxygen demands.
- ☐ 3. cerebral bleeding.
- ☐ 4. diaphoresis.

CORRECT ANSWER: 2
Hyperthermia increases metabolism and thereby increases the oxygen needs of the body and the brain. Options 1, 3, and 4 are incorrect.
NP: Evaluating care
CN: Physiological integrity
CNS: Physiological adaptation
CL: Comprehension

96 A male client arrives in the emergency department lethargic with paralysis of his left arm and leg. Which finding is most pertinent to this client's condition?
☐ 1. Pupil accommodation
☐ 2. Alertness
☐ 3. Motor function
☐ 4. Reflex activity

CORRECT ANSWER: 2
Level of consciousness is most indicative of cerebral oxygenation and must be determined immediately. Options 1, 3, and 4: Assessment of pupil reaction to light, motor function, and reflex activity are also important but not the priority.
NP: Collecting data
CN: Safe, effective care environment
CNS: Coordinated care
CL: Analysis

97 A client who is diagnosed with a right subarachnoid hemorrhage should be placed in which position?
☐ 1. With the head of the bed elevated
☐ 2. On the right side
☐ 3. On the left side
☐ 4. Flat in bed

CORRECT ANSWER: 1
Elevating the head of the bed enhances cerebral venous return and thereby decreases intracranial pressure (ICP). Options 2, 3, and 4: The other positions wouldn't decrease ICP.
NP: Implementing care
CN: Safe, effective care environment
CNS: Safety and infection control
CL: Application

98 During a generalized seizure, what is the nurse's first priority?
☐ 1. Observe and record the incident.
☐ 2. Support the family.
☐ 3. Elevate the head of the bed 45 degrees.
☐ 4. Insert an oropharyngeal airway.

CORRECT ANSWER: 1
Client safety and assessment are the priority concerns of the nurse during a seizure. Option 2: This isn't a priority during a seizure. Option 3: The client should be flat and positioned on the side to facilitate drainage of secretions, unless contraindicated. Option 4: During a generalized seizure, the jaws are tightly clenched; forcing an airway could injure the client.
NP: Implementing care
CN: Safe, effective care environment
CNS: Safety and infection control
CL: Application

99 Which nursing intervention should be included in preparing a client for an electroencephalogram?
☐ 1. Keep the client on nothing-by-mouth status for 6 hours before the test.
☐ 2. Force fluids the day before the test.
☐ 3. Withhold antidepressants and tranquilizers 24 to 48 hours before the test.
☐ 4. Shave the scalp in three round $2^{3}/_{8}$" (6-cm) areas.

CORRECT ANSWER: 3
These medications alter brain activity and could affect test results; therefore, they should be withheld. Option 1: Normal meals should be consumed because a lowered serum glucose level may alter the results. Option 2: This isn't necessary; however, coffee, tea, and cola should be avoided. Option 4: The hair should be clean and dry, but shaving is unnecessary.
NP: Implementing care
CN: Safe, effective care environment
CNS: Coordinated care
CL: Analysis

100 When assessing the pupil's ability to constrict, which cranial nerve is being tested?

☐ 1. II
☐ 2. III
☐ 3. IV
☐ 4. V

CORRECT ANSWER: 2

Cranial nerve III, the oculomotor nerve, controls pupil constriction. Option 1: Cranial nerve II is the optic nerve, which controls vision. Option 3: Cranial nerve IV is the trochlear nerve, which coordinates eye movement. Option 4: Cranial nerve V is the trigeminal nerve, which innervates the muscles of chewing.

NP: Collecting data
CN: Physiological integrity
CNS: Physiological adaptation
CL: Application

101 A client is prescribed 10 mg of oral prednisone. Which consideration is most important to the nurse at this point?

☐ 1. It should be taken on an empty stomach.
☐ 2. It should be taken at bedtime.
☐ 3. It commonly causes a fluid volume deficit.
☐ 4. It shouldn't be withdrawn abruptly.

CORRECT ANSWER: 4

Prednisone should be gradually withdrawn, allowing the adrenal gland to resume normal excretion of the hormone. Option 1: This drug should be taken with food to avoid GI upset. Option 2: If taken at bedtime, prednisone can cause insomnia and irritability. Option 3: Fluid volume excess can occur with long-term use.

NP: Implementing care
CN: Safe, effective care environment
CNS: Coordinated care
CL: Application

102 Which finding would the nurse expect when observing a client who has had emphysema for 5 years?

☐ 1. Decreased anteroposterior (AP) diameter of the thorax
☐ 2. Prolonged inspiration
☐ 3. Clubbing of the fingers
☐ 4. Increased excursion of the chest with respiration

CORRECT ANSWER: 3

Clubbing of the fingers is common in clients with chronic obstructive pulmonary disease and is thought to be caused by chronic hypoxia and capillary congestion in the digits. Option 1: Increased AP diameter of the thorax is evident with this disease. Option 2: Prolonged expiration is observed as the client is trying to eliminate air. Option 4: Decreased chest excursion is seen as the thorax assumes a barrel shape.

NP: Collecting data
CN: Physiological integrity
CNS: Physiological adaptation
CL: Application

103 A client with chronic obstructive pulmonary disease (COPD) is on the nursing unit. The client's arterial blood gas results are pH, 7.42; PaO_2, 68 mm Hg; $PaCO_2$, 50 mm Hg; HCO_3^-, 29 mEq/L. Which action is most appropriate?

☐ 1. The nurse should do nothing because these results are expected in clients with COPD.
☐ 2. Notify the physician at once.
☐ 3. Increase the oxygen to 3 L and notify the physician.
☐ 4. Prepare for an impending cardiac arrest.

CORRECT ANSWER: 1

These results indicate compensated respiratory acidosis (buffering of retained carbon dioxide by the kidneys), which is common in those with chronic respiratory disease; no nursing action is necessary. Option 2: Notifying the physician is unnecessary. Option 3: Increasing the oxygen might decrease the client's stimulus to breathe, which is already low given the PaO_2 level. Option 4 is unnecessary.

NP: Evaluating care
CN: Physiological integrity
CNS: Physiological adaptation
CL: Application

104 A client is scheduled for a laryngoscopy to rule out cancer of the larynx. The purpose of a laryngoscopy is to:
☐ 1. remove any polyps or tumors.
☐ 2. visualize the larynx and obtain a biopsy.
☐ 3. prevent the spread of the tumor.
☐ 4. facilitate gas exchange.

CORRECT ANSWER: 2
Laryngoscopy allows for direct visualization of the larynx and for biopsy of any masses. Option 1: Although polyps may be removed during a laryngoscopy, tumors are resected surgically. Options 3 and 4 are incorrect.
NP: Evaluating care
CN: Physiological integrity
CNS: Reduction of risk potential
CL: Knowledge

105 Which of the following should be emphasized during preoperative teaching of a client scheduled for a total laryngectomy?
☐ 1. Type of anesthesia to be used
☐ 2. Pain control methods
☐ 3. Financial concerns
☐ 4. Alternate communication methods

CORRECT ANSWER: 4
The client will be unable to speak postoperatively and must have a method to communicate needs. Option 1: A detailed discussion of anesthetic agents is unnecessary. Option 2: Although pain control is an important part of preoperative teaching, it isn't the primary focus. Option 3: Financial concerns are addressed as necessary if the client expresses a concern, but they aren't the focus of preoperative teaching.
NP: Planning care
CN: Health promotion and maintenance
CNS: Growth and development through the life span
CL: Application

106 Which nursing diagnostic category is the priority during the immediate postoperative period after a total laryngectomy?
☐ 1. *Ineffective breathing pattern*
☐ 2. *Disturbed self-esteem*
☐ 3. *Ineffective airway clearance*
☐ 4. *Acute pain*

CORRECT ANSWER: 3
A tracheostomy tube is placed to maintain an airway during a laryngectomy. Frequent assessment and suctioning are essential to maintain patency. Options 1, 2, and 4 are important and relevant, but they aren't the priority.
NP: Planning care
CN: Safe, effective care environment
CNS: Safety and infection control
CL: Analysis

107 What is the primary goal of chest physiotherapy when prescribed for a client with lobar pneumonia?
☐ 1. To clear the upper airway
☐ 2. To prevent infection
☐ 3. To retrain the client's breathing pattern
☐ 4. To mobilize secretions

CORRECT ANSWER: 4
Chest physiotherapy is a combination of percussion, coughing, and deep breathing, which is effective in mobilizing secretions. Option 1: This type of therapy helps to clear lower airway obstructions. Option 2: In pneumonia, infection is already present. Option 3: Chest physiotherapy doesn't retrain breathing but may restore an effective breathing pattern.
NP: Planning care
CN: Physiological integrity
CNS: Basic care and comfort
CL: Comprehension

108 A male client is admitted to the hospital with increased shortness of breath at rest. Which information obtained during the history is most specific in determining the client's risk factors for lung disease?
- [ ] 1. His father died of lung cancer at age 78.
- [ ] 2. He has smoked two packs of cigarettes per day for 20 years.
- [ ] 3. He's employed as an accountant.
- [ ] 4. He received a flu shot last month.

CORRECT ANSWER: 2
The client has a 40-pack-year history of smoking (years of smoking multiplied by packs per day), which is a primary risk factor in lung disease. Option 1: There is no direct link between family history of lung cancer and the development of lung disease, although the information is relevant. Option 3: Although this occupation implies limited exercise, it doesn't suggest environmental pollutants. Option 4: Annual flu shots reduce the risk of developing pneumonia and aren't considered risk factors.
NP: Collecting data
CN: Health promotion and maintenance
CNS: Prevention and early detection of disease
CL: Analysis

109 In planning care for a client with a cuffed tracheostomy tube, the priority nursing diagnosis should be:
- [ ] 1. *Ineffective breathing pattern*
- [ ] 2. *Impaired gas exchange*
- [ ] 3. *Ineffective airway clearance*
- [ ] 4. *Risk for aspiration*

CORRECT ANSWER: 3
A client with a tracheostomy tube can't perform Valsalva's maneuver and has a limited ability to cough and deep-breathe; such a client can't effectively clear the airway. Options 1 and 2 are relevant to this situation but they aren't the priority. Option 4: When inflated, a tracheostomy cuff prevents aspiration.
NP: Planning care
CN: Safe, effective care environment
CNS: Safety and infection control
CL: Comprehension

110 A female client is having a chest tube inserted and connected to a Pleur-evac closed chest drainage system. The nurse explains that the purpose of the chest tube is to:
- [ ] 1. remove drainage from the bronchial tubes.
- [ ] 2. prevent collapse of the affected lung.
- [ ] 3. reestablish negative pressure in the pleural space.
- [ ] 4. promote pulmonary alveolar drainage.

CORRECT ANSWER: 3
The chest catheter is inserted in the pleural space to remove air or drainage (or both) and to restore negative pressure. Option 1: The catheter drains the pleural space, not the bronchial tubes. Option 2: A chest tube is inserted when a portion or all of the lung has collapsed. Although a properly functioning chest tube system prevents further lung collapse, its primary function is to restore negative pressure in the pleural space. Option 4: A chest tube doesn't drain alveolar secretions.
NP: Implementing care
CN: Physiological integrity
CNS: Physiological adaptation
CL: Comprehension

111 A client who has a chest tube connected to a closed chest drainage system calls the nurse because the chest tube has become disconnected from the Pleur-evac tubing. What should be the nurse's initial action?
- [ ] 1. Reconnect the chest tube to the Pleur-evac tubing.
- [ ] 2. Clamp the chest tube near the chest wall.
- [ ] 3. Place the end of the chest tube in a glass of water.
- [ ] 4. Clamp the chest tube and call the physician.

CORRECT ANSWER: 1
Reconnecting the chest tube to the Pleur-evac reestablishes a closed drainage system. Options 2 and 4: Chest tubes are never routinely clamped unless ordered by the physician because air and pressure will build in the pleural space and collapse the lung. Option 3: Placing the catheter in a glass of water allows drainage from the pleural space and prevents air from entering; however, in this situation, this isn't the best option.
NP: Implementing care
CN: Safe, effective care environment
CNS: Safety and infection control
CL: Application

112 When assessing the closed chest drainage system (Pleur-evac) of a client who has just returned from a lobectomy, the nurse must ensure that the:
- ☐ 1. fluid in the water-seal chamber rises with inspiration and falls with expiration.
- ☐ 2. tubing remains looped below the level of the bed.
- ☐ 3. drainage chamber does not drain more than 100 ml in 8 hours.
- ☐ 4. suction-control chamber bubbles vigorously when connected to suction.

CORRECT ANSWER: 1
Rise and fall of the water-seal chamber immediately after surgery indicates patency of the chest tube drainage system. Option 2: The tubing should be coiled on the bed, without dependent loops, to promote drainage. Option 3: Up to 500 ml of drainage can occur in the first 24 hours after surgery. Option 4: Gentle bubbling is indicated for the suction-control chamber to prevent excessive evaporation.
NP: Collecting data
CN: Physiological integrity
CNS: Physiological adaptation
CL: Application

---

113 A 74-year-old male client has his blood pressure checked at a community screening program. The nurse records a measurement of 146/90 mm Hg. What should the nurse advise him?
- ☐ 1. This is normal for his age.
- ☐ 2. He should schedule a follow-up appointment immediately because this reading is high.
- ☐ 3. The reading is high and needs to be evaluated by a physician.
- ☐ 4. He needs to follow a weight-reduction diet to lower his blood pressure.

CORRECT ANSWER: 1
For people over age 65, hypertension is defined as a systolic pressure over 160 mm Hg or a diastolic pressure over 95 mm Hg. Options 2 and 3: The client's blood pressure isn't elevated, so follow-up is unnecessary. Option 4: There is no evidence that the client is overweight. Furthermore, weight reduction may not change his blood pressure, which in older adults is often related to the loss of elasticity of the blood vessels due to the aging process.
NP: Collecting data
CN: Health promotion and maintenance
CNS: Prevention and early detection of disease
CL: Analysis

---

114 Continual assessment is an important component in cardiopulmonary resuscitation (CPR). Before initiating CPR, the nurse should always assess for:
- ☐ 1. evidence of breathlessness.
- ☐ 2. an open airway.
- ☐ 3. pulselessness.
- ☐ 4. responsiveness.

CORRECT ANSWER: 4
The first assessment is determining responsiveness by shaking the client and asking, "Are you okay?" The sequence continues with opening the airway (Option 2), determining breathlessness (Option 1), performing rescue breathing, determining pulselessness (Option 3), and providing circulation with chest compressions.
NP: Collecting data
CN: Safe, effective care environment
CNS: Coordinated care
CL: Application

---

115 A client who had a myocardial infarction is being discharged with a prescribed daily dose of 0.25 mg of digoxin by mouth. What should the nurse should instruct the client to do?
- ☐ 1. Skip the daily dose if the pulse rate is below 60 beats/minute.
- ☐ 2. Report any flashes of light or color.
- ☐ 3. Avoid foods high in potassium, such as bananas and potatoes.
- ☐ 4. Take the medication on an empty stomach.

CORRECT ANSWER: 2
These are symptoms of digoxin toxicity and need to be reported immediately. Option 1: The dose is withheld until the physician is notified but never skipped unless directed by the physician. Option 3: Digoxin promotes diuresis and potassium excretion; therefore, potassium-rich foods are encouraged. Option 4: The medication doesn't need to be taken on an empty stomach.
NP: Implementing care
CN: Health promotion and maintenance
CNS: Prevention and early detection of disease
CL: Application

116 The physician has ordered digoxin for a client with pulmonary edema. The nurse knows that digoxin has a direct and beneficial effect on myocardial contraction in the failing heart. This effect:
☐ 1. decreases cardiac output.
☐ 2. decreases ventricular emptying capacity.
☐ 3. increase the circulating blood volume.
☐ 4. slows the conduction of impulses through the atrioventricular (AV) node.

CORRECT ANSWER: 4
Digoxin's physiologic effect on the heart slows impulse conduction through the AV node. Options 1 and 2: Digoxin increases cardiac output and ventricular emptying capacity. Option 3: Digoxin promotes diuresis, thereby decreasing the circulating blood volume.
NP: Evaluating care
CN: Physiological integrity
CNS: Pharmacological therapies
CL: Analysis

117 A 42-year-old man with a history of two previous myocardial infarctions is diagnosed with acute pulmonary edema. He has severe dyspnea with noisy, wet respirations. The nurse's initial action should be to:
☐ 1. place him in high Fowler's position.
☐ 2. perform nasotracheal suctioning to relieve congestion.
☐ 3. determine the cause of the attack.
☐ 4. monitor the cardiac rhythm.

CORRECT ANSWER: 1
High Fowler's position reduces venous congestion and eases dyspnea. Option 2: Suctioning isn't a priority. Option 3: After the acute phase is stabilized, further assessments can be made. Option 4: Cardiac monitoring is indicated, but it isn't the nurse's priority in this situation.
NP: Implementing care
CN: Safe, effective care environment
CNS: Coordinated care
CL: Application

118 A male client has been complaining of chest pain and shortness of breath for the past 2 hours. He has a temperature of 99° F (37.2° C), a pulse rate of 96 beats/minute, respirations that are irregular and 16 breaths/minute, and a blood pressure of 140/96 mm Hg. He's placed on continuous cardiac monitoring to:
☐ 1. prevent cardiac ischemia.
☐ 2. assess for potentially dangerous arrhythmias.
☐ 3. determine the degree of damage to the heart muscle.
☐ 4. evaluate cardiovascular function.

CORRECT ANSWER: 2
Continuous cardiac monitoring can detect life-threatening arrhythmias, including ventricular tachycardia and fibrillation. Options 1, 3, and 4: Such monitoring doesn't prevent ischemia, measure heart muscle damage, or evaluate cardiovascular function.
NP: Implementing care
CN: Physiological integrity
CNS: Physiological adaptation
CL: Application

119 A client who has just been diagnosed with myocardial infarction (MI) begins to cry and tells the nurse that his brother died of a heart attack last year. Which response by the nurse is most appropriate?
☐ 1. "Just because your brother died doesn't mean that you will."
☐ 2. "Don't worry, we're all here to help you. We won't let you die."
☐ 3. "Do you want to talk about your family?"
☐ 4. "You sound as though you think you're going to die."

CORRECT ANSWER: 4
The client's questions and concerns should be acknowledged and addressed by the nurse after an MI. Options 1 and 2 give false reassurance. Option 3 doesn't directly address the client's immediate concern.
NP: Implementing care
CN: Psychosocial integrity
CNS: Coping and adaptation
CL: Application

120 The nurse can evaluate the effectiveness of morphine sulfate when the client demonstrates a:
☐ 1. restful sleep pattern.
☐ 2. decreased pulse rate.
☐ 3. decreased respiratory rate.
☐ 4. change in cardiac rhythm.

CORRECT ANSWER: 1
Morphine is given to decrease pain. The drug is working when the client can rest or sleep comfortably. Option 2: Morphine isn't given to decrease the pulse rate. Option 3: Although morphine may decrease the respiratory rate, this isn't the desired effect. Option 4: The effectiveness of morphine isn't measured by a change in the cardiac rhythm.
NP: Evaluating care
CN: Physiological integrity
CNS: Pharmacological therapies
CL: Application

121 A client who has been experiencing severe chest pain tells the nurse that the pain has diminished and asks to go to the bathroom to have a bowel movement. What action should the nurse take?
☐ 1. Offer a bedpan.
☐ 2. Walk the client to the bathroom.
☐ 3. Ask the client to wait until the condition stabilizes.
☐ 4. Allow the use of a bedside commode.

CORRECT ANSWER: 4
A bedside commode reduces straining and vasovagal responses. Option 1: A bedpan requires more straining due to positioning in bed. Option 2: Limited energy expenditure is essential to decrease the oxygen needs of the heart; therefore, walking to the bathroom would be contraindicated. Option 3: The client shouldn't wait to have a bowel movement because pressure from stool in the colon can cause discomfort and vagal stimulation.
NP: Implementing care
CN: Physiological integrity
CNS: Basic care and comfort
CL: Application

122 The nurse is explaining the use of transdermal nitroglycerin (Transderm-Nitro), which is to be applied twice daily. The nurse confirms the client's understanding when the client states:
☐ 1. "I should apply the patch in the same spot all the time."
☐ 2. "My wife should be careful not to touch the patch with her fingers if she helps me."
☐ 3. "I will know the medication is working if I have a headache after applying it."
☐ 4. "I'm using the transdermal nitroglycerin to lower my blood pressure."

CORRECT ANSWER: 2
The client's wife should be extremely careful to avoid getting the drug on her skin, where it's easily absorbed. Option 1: The application site should be rotated for better absorption and to prevent skin irritation. Option 3: Only some clients experience a headache with application of this drug. A headache isn't expected if the dosage is effective. Option 4: The desired effect of transdermal nitroglycerin is to increase the client's blood flow and oxygenation to the heart muscle.
NP: Evaluating care
CN: Physiological integrity
CNS: Pharmacological therapies
CL: Application

123 The nurse is caring for a 23-year-old female client who is paralyzed from the waist down after an automobile accident. The client cries and says to the nurse, "Now I'll never be able to have children." What is the nurse's best response?
☐ 1. "Are children really important to you?"
☐ 2. "Adoption is always possible."
☐ 3. "You need to worry about getting better first; then we'll talk about children."
☐ 4. "A spinal cord injury doesn't affect a woman's ability to conceive."

CORRECT ANSWER: 4
Female clients retain fertility after spinal cord injury. Problems with sexual function may be related to positioning and the lack of vaginal lubrication or to preexisting infertility. Option 1: Children are obviously important to her, and the response should relate to why she thinks she can't have children. Option 2: This response is inaccurate and nontherapeutic. Option 3: This response blocks communication and is nontherapeutic.
NP: Implementing care
CN: Psychosocial integrity
CNS: Coping and adaptation
CL: Comprehension

124 A female client is being transported to the emergency department after a two-car accident. Diagnostic tests reveal a cervical fracture. Which finding is most important to determine?
☐ 1. Motor ability of the arms and hands
☐ 2. Adequate respiratory function
☐ 3. Presence of pain or altered sensation
☐ 4. Presence of any bleeding or shock

CORRECT ANSWER: 2
Any cervical injury can produce respiratory distress. In this case, the nurse should take immediate action to maintain a patent airway and adequate oxygenation. Option 1: Assessing the motor ability of the client's hands and arms is important in cervical injuries, but it isn't the priority in this case. Option 3: Assessments of pain and altered sensation are also important but aren't the priority. Option 4: Assessing for hemorrhage and shock is essential, but airway and breathing are most important.
NP: Collecting data
CN: Physiological integrity
CNS: Physiological adaptation
CL: Comprehension

125 A female client is diagnosed with a C7 fracture and placed in a halo traction device. She asks the nurse why she needs the device. The nurse correctly explains:
☐ 1. "This will allow you to turn in bed more easily."
☐ 2. "Because you're a poor surgical risk, this will support your spine until you heal."
☐ 3. "The halo jacket immobilizes the spine and allows you to move around safely."
☐ 4. "The halo device is only needed until you're able to ambulate."

CORRECT ANSWER: 3
The halo jacket allows for early mobilization and rehabilitation while maintaining cervical alignment. It's never removed unless ordered by the physician. Option 1: The primary purpose of the device is maintenance of cervical alignment and early ambulation. Option 2: Surgery isn't always indicated for stabilized or aligned fractures. Option 4: The halo device promotes mobility, thereby preventing problems associated with prolonged bed rest.
NP: Implementing care
CN: Physiological integrity
CNS: Reduction of risk potential
CL: Analysis

126 A 42-year-old construction worker was admitted to the hospital with complaints of lower back pain and numbness down his right leg. He's being evaluated for a herniated intervertebral lumbar disk. He returns from the radiology department, where he underwent a myelogram using a water-soluble dye. How should the nurse position him?
☐ 1. Flat in bed in the supine position
☐ 2. With the head of the bed elevated 15 to 30 degrees
☐ 3. In any comfortable position
☐ 4. On his left side, with a pillow between his legs

CORRECT ANSWER: 2
Placing the head of the bed at a 15- to 30-degree angle allows the dye to pool at the lower level of the lumbar spinal canal, where it can be gradually absorbed by the arachnoid villi in the brain. Adequate hydration is essential to dilute the dye to prevent chemical meningitis. Option 1: Putting the client flat in bed allows the dye to rise undiluted to the meninges. The client may be placed flat in bed 8 to 12 hours after the myelogram to prevent cerebrospinal fluid leakage. Options 3 and 4: Elevating the head of the bed is recommended.
NP: Implementing care
CN: Physiological integrity
CNS: Reduction of risk potential
CL: Analysis

127 A male client is scheduled for a lumbar fusion from L4 to S1. A bone graft will be obtained from his left anterosuperior iliac crest. Which intervention is imperative when the client is returned to his room?
☐ 1. Assess the client's ability to grip both hands on command.
☐ 2. Assess the client's ability to ambulate using a walker.
☐ 3. Encourage deep breathing and forceful coughing every 2 hours.
☐ 4. Check the surgical dressings for drainage.

CORRECT ANSWER: 4
The nurse must immediately assess both surgical sites (the lumbar and donor areas) for bleeding or leakage of cerebrospinal fluid. Option 1: Although the assessment of grips is very important in cervical fusion, lower leg mobility is more specific to lumbar fusion. Option 2: Clients with lumbar fusions are frequently on bed rest for several days, after which they are ambulated with a brace to provide stability to the lumbar fusion site. Option 3: Deep breathing is important after surgery, but forceful coughing and bearing down can put pressure on the fusion site and displace the graft.
NP: Collecting data
CN: Physiological integrity
CNS: Reduction of risk potential
CL: Comprehension

128 A 40-year-old female client who is taking nifedipine (Procardia) for hypertension tells the nurse that she has noticed a "little swelling" in her ankles. How should the nurse respond?
☐ 1. "Tell me about your salt intake."
☐ 2. "This is a common adverse effect of this medication."
☐ 3. "The physician may need to change your medication."
☐ 4. "When did you first notice this?"

CORRECT ANSWER: 2
A common adverse effect of this calcium channel blocker is peripheral edema. Other adverse effects include headache, vertigo, and fluid retention. Option 1: All clients should be advised to reduce their salt intake. However, not all hypertensive clients respond to salt restriction. Option 3: The physician probably won't change the client's medication unless she has other adverse effects or an adverse reaction to the medication. Option 4: The client will probably report that she noticed the edema after she started taking the medication.
NP: Evaluating care
CN: Physiological integrity
CNS: Pharmacological therapies
CL: Application

129 When assisting with an electrocardiogram (ECG), the nurse would expect to place the client in which position?
☐ 1. Fowler's
☐ 2. Supine
☐ 3. Lateral
☐ 4. Prone

CORRECT ANSWER: 2
The most appropriate way to position a client undergoing an ECG is lying flat, as long as the client can tolerate being in a supine position. Otherwise, the client may be positioned with the head of the bed slightly elevated.
NP: Implementing care
CN: Physiological integrity
CNS: Reduction of risk potential
CL: Application

130 When planning care for a client with lobar bacterial pneumonia, which outcome is most desired?
☐ 1. Breath sounds clear with coughing
☐ 2. Minimum sputum production
☐ 3. Pulse oximetry reading of 80%
☐ 4. Dyspnea on exertion

CORRECT ANSWER: 1
The client with pneumonia may have crackles, wheezes, or bronchial breath sounds from consolidation. The breath sounds should clear if the client has an effective cough and is able to cough up sputum. Option 2: Most clients with bacterial pneumonia have significant sputum production. Option 3: Normal pulse oximetry readings should be above 90% unless the client has underlying lung disease. In that case, the reading should return to the client's baseline level. Option 4: A client who is responding appropriately to therapy should no longer have dyspnea.
NP: Planning care
CN: Physiological integrity
CNS: Physiological adaptation
CL: Application

131 The nurse understands that the primary purpose of administering furosemide (Lasix) to a client with pulmonary edema is to:
☐ 1. decrease urine output.
☐ 2. increase cardiac output.
☐ 3. remove fluid from the lungs.
☐ 4. lower blood pressure.

CORRECT ANSWER: 3
The primary reason for administering furosemide, which is a diuretic, is to reduce the amount of fluid backing up into the lungs by removing it from the vascular space. The nurse should note decreased crackles and dyspnea with this drug. Option 1: Lasix is a diuretic and is given to increase urine output. Option 2: Lasix has no effect on cardiac contractility. Option 4: One adverse effect of this drug is that it may also lower the client's blood pressure, but that isn't the primary reason it's given to the client.
NP: Evaluating care
CN: Physiological integrity
CNS: Pharmacological therapies
CL: Knowledge

132 Which position is contraindicated when caring for a client who has had a pneumonectomy for lung cancer?
☐ 1. Semi-Fowler's
☐ 2. Lying on the nonoperative side
☐ 3. Reverse Trendelenburg's
☐ 4. Prone

CORRECT ANSWER: 2
A client who has undergone a pneumonectomy doesn't have a chest tube in place. Therefore, the accumulation of any blood or fluid around the operative site could cause pressure on the operative side and compromise ventilation. Options 1, 3, and 4 are acceptable positions for this client.
NP: Implementing care
CN: Physiological integrity
CNS: Reduction of risk potential
CL: Application

133 While assessing a client with chronic obstructive pulmonary disease (COPD), the nurse notes wheezes and a prolonged expiration with each breath. Based on these findings, the nurse would formulate which diagnosis?
☐ 1. *Impaired gas exchange*
☐ 2. *Ineffective breathing pattern*
☐ 3. *Ineffective cardiopulmonary tissue perfusion*
☐ 4. *Ineffective airway clearance*

CORRECT ANSWER: 4
The primary problem with clients with COPD is ineffective airway clearance. Such clients have prolonged forced expiratory volumes on pulmonary function tests because of increased airway resistance. Options 1 and 2: Clients may also later develop impaired gas exchange and ineffective breathing patterns as their disease progresses. Option 3: These findings aren't related to perfusion.
NP: Planning care
CN: Physiological integrity
CNS: Physiological adaptation
CL: Application

134 The nurse is assessing a client who had a purified protein derivative (PPD) as a routine screening test for tuberculosis exposure. The nurse knows that the test is positive when she observes a:
- ☐ 1. 5-mm reddened area at 48 hours.
- ☐ 2. 10-mm indurated area at 48 hours.
- ☐ 3. 5-mm indurated area at 72 hours.
- ☐ 4. 10-mm reddened area at 72 hours.

CORRECT ANSWER: 2
The nurse would assess the amount of induration when checking a client's PPD response. Induration peaks at between 24 and 48 hours. The site may also be reddened, but redness alone doesn't constitute a positive test. The area must have 10 mm of induration for it to be positive.
NP: Collecting data
CN: Health promotion and maintenance
CNS: Prevention and early detection of disease
CL: Application

135 A client with a chest tube in place after a gunshot wound to the chest accidentally dislodges the tube. What should the nurse should do immediately?
- ☐ 1. Place the client in a supine position.
- ☐ 2. Shut off the suction to the tube.
- ☐ 3. Place the end of the tube in a sterile container.
- ☐ 4. Cover the insertion site with an occlusive dressing.

CORRECT ANSWER: 4
Dislodgment of the tube from the client's chest may cause a sucking chest wound. The nurse should immediately cover the wound with an occlusive airtight dressing, such as petroleum gauze, and tape it on three sides. This allows trapped air to escape but prevents air from entering, thereby preventing a tension pneumothorax. The nurse should then notify the physician. Option 1: The nurse would place the client in semi-Fowler's position to aid respirations. Option 2: Once the tube is dislodged, turning off the suction is of no value to the client. Option 3: The end of the tube is now contaminated, so there is no point in placing it in a sterile container.
NP: Implementing care
CN: Physiological integrity
CNS: Physiological adaptation
CL: Application

136 The nurse knows that a client with osteoarthritis of the knee understands the discharge instructions when the client states:
- ☐ 1. "I'll take my ibuprofen (Motrin) on an empty stomach."
- ☐ 2. "I'll try taking a warm shower in the morning."
- ☐ 3. "I'll wear my knee splint every night."
- ☐ 4. "I'll jog at least a mile every evening."

CORRECT ANSWER: 2
A client with osteoarthritis has joint stiffness that may be partially relieved with a warm shower on arising in the morning. Option 1: Ibuprofen should be taken with food, as should all nonsteroidal anti-inflammatory medications. Option 3: Splints are usually used by clients with rheumatoid arthritis. Option 4: Because the problem is one of continued stress on the joint, the client may want to try an exercise that puts less strain on the joint such as swimming.
NP: Evaluating care
CN: Physiological integrity
CNS: Basic care and comfort
CL: Application

137 The nurse must keep which safety principle in mind when teaching a client with a lower leg cast how to walk with a crutch?
- ☐ 1. Crutches and the affected leg should move together.
- ☐ 2. Client should look at both feet when moving forward with crutches.
- ☐ 3. Elbows should be locked when moving forward on crutches.
- ☐ 4. Body's weight should rest on the underarm pads.

CORRECT ANSWER: 3
The client should straighten the arms, lock the elbows, and bear weight on the palms at the handgrip, not at the underarm pads. Option 1: The crutches and unaffected leg should move forward together. Option 2: Client should look straight ahead, not at the feet, when moving forward on crutches. Option 4: Placing weight on the underarm pads can damage the nerves in the axillary area.
NP: Implementing care
CN: Physiological integrity
CNS: Basic care and comfort
CL: Application

138 The physician has just removed the cast from a 20-year-old male client's lower leg. During the removal, a small superficial abrasion occurred over the ankle. Which statement by the client indicates the need for additional client teaching?
- ☐ 1. "I can use a moisturizing lotion on the dry areas."
- ☐ 2. "The dry, peeling skin will go away by itself."
- ☐ 3. "I can wash the abrasion on my ankle with soap and water."
- ☐ 4. "I'll wait until the abrasion is healed before I swim."

CORRECT ANSWER: 1
The dry, peeling skin will heal in a few days with normal cleansing; therefore, lotions are unnecessary. Option 2: Vigorous scrubbing isn't necessary. Options 3 and 4 are correct procedures to follow after removal of a cast.
NP: Evaluating care
CN: Physiological integrity
CNS: Reduction of risk potential
CL: Application

139 When administering a tube feeding to a comatose client with a tracheostomy, which safety precaution should the nurse follow to prevent aspiration?
- ☐ 1. Warm the tube feeding to room temperature.
- ☐ 2. Deflate the tracheostomy cuff.
- ☐ 3. Instill air into the tube.
- ☐ 4. Place the client in Fowler's position.

CORRECT ANSWER: 4
Proper positioning is essential to prevent aspiration of the tube feeding. Elevating the head of the bed to Fowler's position helps to prevent gastric reflux. Option 1: Warming the tube won't aid in preventing aspiration. Option 2: The tracheostomy cuff should be inflated during a tube feeding. Option 3: Although the tube placement should be checked, instilling air into the tube isn't a foolproof method.
NP: Implementing care
CN: Physiological integrity
CNS: Basic care and comfort
CL: Application

140 A client has just been admitted to the hospital with a small-bowel obstruction. The nurse would anticipate the client's history to include:
- ☐ 1. vomiting.
- ☐ 2. diarrhea.
- ☐ 3. right lower quadrant pain.
- ☐ 4. left lower quadrant pain.

CORRECT ANSWER: 1
The most commonly reported symptom with a small-bowel obstruction is vomiting because intestinal contents can't pass the obstructed area. Option 2: The client usually doesn't have diarrhea and typically reports no stools. Options 3 and 4: The client typically reports crampy upper abdominal pain if the obstruction is high; the pain is more generalized with a lower obstruction.
NP: Collecting data
CN: Physiological integrity
CNS: Physiological adaptation
CL: Application

141 A client with ascites is scheduled to undergo paracentesis. In preparing for the procedure, the nurse would:
- ☐ 1. ask the client to void.
- ☐ 2. administer a Fleet enema.
- ☐ 3. place the client in Sims' position.
- ☐ 4. place the client on nothing-by-mouth (NPO) status.

CORRECT ANSWER: 1
The client should void before undergoing paracentesis because this procedure involves the insertion of a stylette into the abdomen and this rigid instrument could accidentally puncture a distended bladder. Option 2: There is no reason to administer an enema because the bowel isn't entered during paracentesis. Option 3: Inserting the stylette into the abdomen would be difficult if the client is in Sims' position. Option 4: The client doesn't need to be on NPO status for this procedure.
NP: Implementing care
CN: Physiological integrity
CNS: Reduction of risk potential
CL: Application

142 A client with an intestinal obstruction is scheduled for insertion of a cantor tube. In addition to the tube, which equipment should the nurse have at the client's bedside?
☐ 1. Two hemostats
☐ 2. Mercury
☐ 3. Saline-filled 10-ml syringe
☐ 4. Rubber band

CORRECT ANSWER: 2
Mercury is used to inflate the balloon of a cantor tube. It acts as a bolus of "food" to aid peristalsis, moving the tube through the intestinal tract. Options 1, 3, and 4 are incorrect.
NP: Planning care
CN: Physiological integrity
CNS: Reduction of risk potential
CL: Application

143 Before inserting a nasogastric (NG) tube, the nurse needs to determine the correct length of tubing to insert. This is done by measuring from the:
☐ 1. lip to the angle of the jaw, then from the angle of the jaw to the xiphoid process.
☐ 2. lip to the earlobe, then from the earlobe to the xiphoid process.
☐ 3. nose to the angle of the jaw, then from the angle of the jaw to the xiphoid process.
☐ 4. nose to the earlobe, then from the earlobe to the xiphoid process.

CORRECT ANSWER: 4
The nurse measures from the nose to the earlobe, then from the earlobe to the xiphoid process. Options 1 and 2 are incorrect. Option 3: Measuring from the lip to the earlobe and then to the angle of the jaw is used when measuring for an oral airway, not an NG tube.
NP: Implementing care
CN: Physiological integrity
CNS: Reduction of risk potential
CL: Application

144 Which finding would the nurse expect in a client with a third cranial (oculomotor) nerve deficit?
☐ 1. Vision loss
☐ 2. Hearing loss
☐ 3. Facial paralysis
☐ 4. Pupil dilation

CORRECT ANSWER: 4
A client with a third cranial nerve deficit would have pupil dilation, possibly lid ptosis (drooping eyelid), or problems with eye movement. Options 1, 2, and 3 are incorrect.
NP: Collecting data
CN: Physiological integrity
CNS: Physiological adaptation
CL: Application

145 During assessment of a client with a head injury, which finding indicative of increased intracranial pressure (ICP) would the nurse probably note first?
☐ 1. Vomiting
☐ 2. Slowing respirations
☐ 3. Slowing pulse
☐ 4. Increasing blood pressure

CORRECT ANSWER: 1
Vomiting is one of the earliest signs of increased ICP because increasing pressure may irritate the center that causes vomiting. Other early findings include headache and changes in mental status, such as confusion. Options 2, 3, and 4 are considered late findings.
NP: Collecting data
CN: Physiological integrity
CNS: Physiological adaptation
CL: Application

146 A client with a seizure disorder begins to have a seizure while the nurse is making the morning rounds. During the seizure, what should the nurse do?
- ☐ 1. Observe the characteristics and duration of the seizure.
- ☐ 2. Place a bite block between the client's teeth to prevent injury.
- ☐ 3. Restrain the client to prevent injury.
- ☐ 4. Administer oxygen.

CORRECT ANSWER: 1
During a seizure, the nurse should observe the client to determine the type of seizure, the seizure's focal point (the site where it originates in the body), and how long the seizure lasts. Option 2: The client typically clamps the jaws closed quickly during a seizure. Forcing something between the client's teeth could harm the client or nurse. Option 3: The nurse should never try to restrain the client. Instead, the nurse should attempt to secure the environment by raising the bed's side rails, which should be padded, or helping the client to the floor. Option 4: During a seizure, the client usually doesn't breathe. Therefore, oxygen would be unnecessary.
NP: Implementing care
CN: Physiological integrity
CNS: Physiological adaptation
CL: Application

147 Discharge planning for the client with Parkinson's disease who is receiving levodopa should include information about the need to modify intake of:
- ☐ 1. carbohydrates.
- ☐ 2. proteins.
- ☐ 3. vitamin C.
- ☐ 4. calcium.

CORRECT ANSWER: 2
Proteins interfere with the absorption of levodopa. Clients are advised to moderately restrict their protein intake while on this drug. Options 1, 3, and 4: The client's intake of carbohydrates, vitamin C, and calcium don't need to be modified.
NP: Planning care
CN: Physiological integrity
CNS: Physiological adaptation
CL: Application

148 The nurse would expect which outcome after administering mannitol to a client with a head injury?
- ☐ 1. Decreased pulse rate
- ☐ 2. Increased blood pressure
- ☐ 3. Increased urine output
- ☐ 4. Pupil dilation

CORRECT ANSWER: 3
Because mannitol is an osmotic diuretic, the nurse would expect the client to have increased urine output. Options 1 and 2: The pulse rate should increase and the blood pressure should decrease. Option 4: Dilation of the pupils indicates that the client's condition is worsening.
NP: Evaluating care
CN: Physiological integrity
CNS: Pharmacological therapies
CL: Application

149 Which position should the nurse use to prevent injury to a comatose client?
- ☐ 1. Side-lying
- ☐ 2. Supine
- ☐ 3. Fowler's
- ☐ 4. Prone

CORRECT ANSWER: 1
The side-lying position is the safest because the airway is most protected. Options 2 and 4: The airway is in danger of being occluded in the supine or prone position. Option 3: The comatose client's head may fall forward and close the airway in Fowler's position.
NP: Implementing care
CN: Safe, effective care environment
CNS: Safety and infection control
CL: Application

150 When planning care for a client with glomer-ulonephritis, which intervention should be given top priority?
☐ 1. Monitor for fluid overload.
☐ 2. Monitor for hypokalemia.
☐ 3. Provide high-protein snacks.
☐ 4. Increase the sodium intake.

CORRECT ANSWER: 1
A client with glomerulonephritis is at risk for fluid overload because the kidneys aren't working proper-ly. Option 2: Such a client is at risk for hyperkale-mia, not hypokalemia. Option 3: Proteins should be restricted because of the nitrogen retention and ele-vated blood urea nitrogen levels associated with this condition. Option 4: Sodium is restricted because of the risk for fluid overload and hypertension.
NP: Planning care
CN: Physiological integrity
CNS: Physiological adaptation
CL: Application

151 Which instruction about fluid intake would be appropriate for a client with benign prostatic hy-perplasia?
☐ 1. "You should drink at least two 8-oz glasses of fluid with each meal."
☐ 2. "You should limit your fluids at mealtimes to one 8-oz glass."
☐ 3. "You should stop drinking fluids at least 6 hours before bedtime."
☐ 4. "You should restrict your fluid intake to about four 8-oz glasses per day."

CORRECT ANSWER: 2
Total fluid intake for a client with benign prostatic hyperplasia should be about 51 to 68 oz (1,500 to 2,000 ml) per day unless restricted for other rea-sons by the physician. Therefore, the client should restrict his fluid intake to about 8 to 12 oz (240 to 360 ml) at mealtimes and sip beverages between meals throughout the day. Nocturia can be alleviat-ed but not necessarily eliminated by avoiding fluids the last 2 to 3 hours before bedtime. Options 1, 3, and 4 are incorrect.
NP: Implementing care
CN: Physiological integrity
CNS: Physiological adaptation
CL: Application

152 Which discharge instruction is most appro-priate for a client receiving continuous ambulatory dialysis?
☐ 1. "You'll need to remain on bed rest while you're performing the dialysis."
☐ 2. "Because you'll be at home, you'll be able to use clean technique."
☐ 3. "You should report cloudy dialysate return immediately to the physician."
☐ 4. "You should store your dialysis fluid in the refrigerator."

CORRECT ANSWER: 3
Cloudy dialysate indicates that the client may be developing an infection; it should be reported im-mediately. Other signs of possible infection include abdominal pain, fever, and chills. Option 1: The client doesn't need to be on bed rest during the pro-cedure. Option 2: The client should continue to use sterile technique at home because of the risk of in-fection. Option 4: Dialysis fluid doesn't need to be refrigerated.
NP: Implementing care
CN: Physiological integrity
CNS: Physiological adaptation
CL: Application

153 The nurse should take which safety precau-tion when inserting an indwelling urinary catheter?
☐ 1. Insert the catheter to the bifurcation in a fe-male client.
☐ 2. Always clean the urinary meatus with povidone-iodine solution.
☐ 3. Wait for urine flow before inflating the bal-loon.
☐ 4. Inject lubricant into the male urethra before inserting the catheter.

CORRECT ANSWER: 3
Until a urine flow is established, there is no guaran-tee that the catheter is correctly placed. Option 1: Inserting the catheter to the bifurcation is impor-tant in males, not females. Option 2: Povidone-iodine solution isn't always used because some clients are allergic to iodine. The nurse should al-ways check for allergies first. Option 4: Injecting lu-bricant into the male urethra may facilitate passage, but it isn't a safety precaution.
NP: Implementing care
CN: Physiological integrity
CNS: Reduction of risk potential
CL: Application

154 The nurse caring for a client with a nephrostomy tube would expect to find which of the following in the postoperative period?
☐ 1. Frank bleeding at the site for the first 3 to 4 hours
☐ 2. No urine output in the nephrostomy tube for the first 24 hours
☐ 3. Urine drainage on the dressing
☐ 4. A clamped indwelling urinary catheter

CORRECT ANSWER: 3
Leakage of urine on the dressing isn't unusual after insertion of a nephrostomy tube. Option 1: Although the operative site may be somewhat blood-tinged, frank bleeding shouldn't occur. Option 2: The nephrostomy tube was inserted to ensure the flow of urine; therefore, the client should have a urine output. Option 4: The indwelling urinary catheter shouldn't be clamped.
NP: Collecting data
CN: Physiological integrity
CNS: Reduction of risk potential
CL: Application

155 The nurse knows that a 40-year-old female client who is being treated for hyperthyroidism with propylthiouracil needs further instructions if she states:
☐ 1. "I'll take the drug at least 1 hour before meals."
☐ 2. "I'll notify my physician if I get a sore throat or rash."
☐ 3. "I'll keep the medication in its light-resistant container."
☐ 4. "I'll take my medication at 7 a.m., 3 p.m., and 11 p.m."

CORRECT ANSWER: 1
This antithyroid medication should be taken with food to lessen gastric irritation. Options 2, 3, and 4 indicate that the client understands the medication instructions.
NP: Evaluating care
CN: Physiological integrity
CNS: Pharmacological therapies
CL: Application

156 While assessing a client with hypothyroidism, the nurse would expect to observe:
☐ 1. hypoactive bowel sounds.
☐ 2. hypertension.
☐ 3. photophobia.
☐ 4. flushed skin.

CORRECT ANSWER: 1
Hypothyroidism is associated with a general slowing of the body systems, as indicated by hypoactive bowel sounds. Option 2: The nurse would expect to find the client hypotensive, not hypertensive. Options 3 and 4: These symptoms are associated with hyperthyroidism.
NP: Collecting data
CN: Physiological integrity
CNS: Physiological adaptation
CL: Application

157 Which roommate is most appropriate for a client with Cushing's syndrome who has a nursing diagnosis of *Risk for infection?*
☐ 1. Postmastectomy client
☐ 2. Client with a tracheostomy
☐ 3. Client with a pressure ulcer
☐ 4. Client with diarrhea

CORRECT ANSWER: 1
The postmastectomy client has the least chance of having an infection that could be transferred to the client with Cushing's syndrome. Options 2, 3, and 4 are all at higher risk for infection.
NP: Implementing care
CN: Safe, effective care environment
CNS: Safety and infection control
CL: Application

158 When preparing a 21-year-old smoker for a glucose tolerance test, the nurse should give which instruction?
- ☐ 1. "You won't be able to eat or drink anything during the test."
- ☐ 2. "You'll be able to smoke, but you'll have to walk outside to do so."
- ☐ 3. "Your test is scheduled for 8 a.m., so don't eat or drink anything after 10 p.m. the night before."
- ☐ 4. "You'll be on a low-sugar diet for 2 days before the test."

CORRECT ANSWER: 3
Because the test is performed in the morning, the client shouldn't eat or drink for 10 hours before the test. Option 1: The client will drink the diagnostic glucose solution during the test. Option 2: The client shouldn't smoke during the test. Option 4: The client may be instructed to eat a diet consisting of at least 150 g of carbohydrates for 2 days before the test.
NP: Implementing care
CN: Physiological integrity
CNS: Reduction of risk potential
CL: Application

159 The nurse is instructing a 30-year-old client with a history of kidney stones on how to collect a 24-hour urine specimen, which will be used to measure calcium and uric acid levels. The nurse should tell the client, "When you get up in the morning, void immediately, note the time:
- ☐ 1. discard the specimen, and save every specimen after that in this jug for the next 24 hours."
- ☐ 2. save the urine specimen in this jug, and save every specimen after that for the next 24 hours."
- ☐ 3. save the urine specimen in this jug, and save every specimen except the last one in this jug for the next 24 hours."
- ☐ 4. discard the first specimen, and save every specimen except the last one in this jug for the next 24 hours."

CORRECT ANSWER: 1
For a 24-hour urine specimen, the client should void, note the time, discard the voided specimen, and then save every subsequently voided specimen for the next 24 hours in a specimen jug that is usually kept on ice. At the end of 24 hours, the client voids and also saves that specimen in the jug. Options 2, 3, and 4 are incorrect.
NP: Implementing care
CN: Physiological integrity
CNS: Reduction of risk potential
CL: Application

160 When assessing a burn client who has a 20% deep partial-thickness (second-degree) burn of the arms and trunk, the nurse understands that the client has damage to what layers of skin?
- ☐ 1. Epidermis
- ☐ 2. Epidermis and part of the dermis
- ☐ 3. Epidermis and all of the dermis
- ☐ 4. Dermis and subcutaneous tissue

CORRECT ANSWER: 2
A deep partial-thickness burn affects the epidermis and part of the dermis. Option 1: A superficial partial-thickness (first-degree) burn affects the epidermis. Options 3 and 4: A full-thickness (third-degree) burn affects the epidermis and all the dermis; it also may affect the subcutaneous tissue.
NP: Collecting data
CN: Physiological integrity
CNS: Physiological adaptation
CL: Application

161 The nurse is monitoring the fluid status of an adult client with a 25% full-thickness burn of the legs and trunk. The nurse realizes that the client's fluid volume status is adequate when his:
- ☐ 1. blood pressure is 90/60 mm Hg.
- ☐ 2. pulse rate is 100 beats/minute.
- ☐ 3. urine output is 50 ml/hour.
- ☐ 4. capillary refill time is 3 seconds.

CORRECT ANSWER: 3
Urine output is the best indicator of fluid volume status. An output of 50 ml/hour is adequate. Option 1: A blood pressure of 90/60 mm Hg is low. It should be at least 100 systolic. Option 2: The client's pulse rate should be under 100 beats/minute. Option 4: The capillary refill time should be less than 3 seconds.
NP: Evaluating care
CN: Physiological integrity
CNS: Physiological adaptation
CL: Application

162 Which instruction would be appropriate when teaching a client with human immunodeficiency virus who is at high risk for altered oral mucous membranes?
☐ 1. "Brush your teeth frequently with a firm toothbrush."
☐ 2. "Use mouthwash that contains an astringent agent."
☐ 3. "Be sure to heat all your food."
☐ 4. "Lubricate your lips."

CORRECT ANSWER: 4
Lubricating the lips will keep them moist and prevent cracking. Option 1: A firm toothbrush would damage already sensitive gums. Options 2 and 3: An astringent would be painful, as would foods that are too hot.
NP: Implementing care
CN: Physiological integrity
CNS: Reduction of risk potential
CL: Application

163 The nurse would instruct a client with human immunodeficiency virus who has frequent bouts of diarrhea to avoid eating or drinking:
☐ 1. milk.
☐ 2. red licorice.
☐ 3. chicken soup.
☐ 4. broiled meat.

CORRECT ANSWER: 1
Clients with chronic diarrhea may develop intolerance to lactose, which may worsen the diarrhea. Option 2: Although red licorice may be eaten, black licorice should be avoided. Other foods that the client should avoid include fatty foods, other lactose-containing foods, caffeine, and sugar. Options 3 and 4 may be consumed.
NP: Implementing care
CN: Physiological integrity
CNS: Reduction of risk potential
CL: Application

164 When gathering data from a client who is receiving external beam radiation for lung cancer, the nurse should focus on which finding?
☐ 1. Dysphagia
☐ 2. Fatigue
☐ 3. Diarrhea
☐ 4. Bruising

CORRECT ANSWER: 1
A client undergoing radiation therapy for lung cancer receives the radiation to the chest area. Besides observing for a cough, the nurse should assess the client for dysphagia because of the proximity of the esophagus to the lungs. Options 2, 3, and 4 wouldn't occur after radiation to the chest.
NP: Collecting data
CN: Physiological integrity
CNS: Reduction of risk potential
CL: Application

165 The nurse is planning to teach a postmastectomy client exercises to increase her shoulder mobility on the affected side. Which activity of daily living would best help to increase shoulder mobility?
☐ 1. Tying a shoe
☐ 2. Fastening a button
☐ 3. Typing
☐ 4. Brushing the hair

CORRECT ANSWER: 4
Brushing the hair would best increase the client's mobility because it takes the shoulder through the full range of motion. Options 1, 2, and 3 don't exercise the shoulder.
NP: Planning care
CN: Physiological integrity
CNS: Basic care and comfort
CL: Application

166 A 40-year-old client is at high risk for body image disturbance after a mastectomy. She asks the nurse when she can wear a prosthesis. The nurse's best response would be:
☐ 1. "You'll get a prosthesis in about 4 weeks."
☐ 2. "You may wear a prosthesis in 2 months."
☐ 3. "As soon as you leave the hospital, you can wear a temporary prosthesis."
☐ 4. "You may wear a temporary prosthesis as soon as the dressing is removed."

CORRECT ANSWER: 4
A lightweight, temporary prosthesis can be worn as soon as the dressing is removed. The client can wear gauze between the prosthesis and the suture line to cushion and protect it. A permanent prosthesis is fitted in about 2 months.
NP: Implementing care
CN: Psychosocial integrity
CNS: Coping and adaptation
CL: Application

167 An 80-year-old male client with lung cancer is scheduled for surgery. According to hospital policy, the client's dentures, hearing aid, rings, and other prostheses must be removed; however, the client insists on keeping his hearing aid. What should the nurse do?
☐ 1. Insist that the hearing aid be removed.
☐ 2. Report this to the charge nurse.
☐ 3. Leave the hearing aid in, but tell the operating room nurse that the aid is in place.
☐ 4. Remove the hearing aid after performing preoperative care.

CORRECT ANSWER: 3
The nurse should notify the operating room staff and leave the hearing aid in place until the client is in surgery. This enables the client to hear instructions given before administration of the anesthetic, thereby allowing him to maintain a sense of control. Options 1, 2, and 4: Removing the client's hearing aid or reporting the incident to the charge nurse is unnecessary.
NP: Implementing care
CN: Psychosocial integrity
CNS: Coping and adaptation
CL: Application

168 The nurse knows that patient-teaching sessions involving the use of an incentive spirometer have been effective when the client:
☐ 1. exhales as rapidly and forcefully as possible through the spirometer.
☐ 2. aims for a lower number on the spirometer with each breath.
☐ 3. inhales as deeply as possible through the spirometer while watching the indicator.
☐ 4. inhales as rapidly as possible through the spirometer and holds the breath.

CORRECT ANSWER: 3
The client should inhale as slowly and deeply as possible while watching the indicator rise. At the end of each inspiration, the client should hold the breath for a count of 5, if possible. Option 2: With each successive inspiration, the client should aim for a higher number. Options 1 and 4 are incorrect.
NP: Implementing care
CN: Physiological integrity
CNS: Reduction of risk potential
CL: Application

169 The nurse preparing a client for a thoracentesis should place the client in which position?
☐ 1. Supine
☐ 2. Sitting on the side of the bed with arms on an overbed table
☐ 3. On the side with knees drawn to the chest
☐ 4. Semi-Fowler's

CORRECT ANSWER: 2
The usual position for performing a thoracentesis is with the client sitting on the side of the bed leaning forward with the arms on a pillow or an overbed table. This affords the best view for the physician performing the procedure. Options 1, 3, and 4 are incorrect.
NP: Implementing care
CN: Physiological integrity
CNS: Reduction of risk potential
CL: Application

170 When caring for a client on a mechanical ventilator, the alarm sounds. What should the nurse do first?
☐ 1. Check the ventilator.
☐ 2. Begin to ventilate the client manually.
☐ 3. Notify the respiratory therapist.
☐ 4. Check the client.

CORRECT ANSWER: 4
The nurse should always check the client first. The problem might be as simple as a disconnected tube. A client who sets off the alarm by coughing may need to be suctioned. Option 1: The procedure is to always begin checking the client first and work toward the ventilator. Condensed water in the tubing could set off an alarm. Options 2 and 3: If the problem can't be readily determined, the client may be ventilated manually with a bag mask and the respiratory therapist notified.
NP: Collecting data
CN: Physiological integrity
CNS: Physiological adaptation
CL: Application

171 The nurse enters a male client's room to give him his 9 a.m. medications. When the nurse calls the client's name and he doesn't answer, what should the nurse immediately do?
- [ ] 1. Call for help.
- [ ] 2. Check for responsiveness.
- [ ] 3. Open the airway.
- [ ] 4. Give four breaths.

CORRECT ANSWER: 2
The nurse should first check for responsiveness because the client may be asleep. Options 1 and 3: If the client is unresponsive, the nurse should call for help, open the airway, and check for breathing. Option 4 is appropriate after calling for help and determining respiratory status.
NP: Collecting data
CN: Physiological integrity
CNS: Physiological adaptation
CL: Application

172 When administering one-person cardiopulmonary resuscitation (CPR) to an adult client, the nurse should give:
- [ ] 1. one breath for every 15 compressions.
- [ ] 2. two breaths for every 15 compressions.
- [ ] 3. one breath for every 5 compressions.
- [ ] 4. two breaths for every 5 compressions.

CORRECT ANSWER: 2
When performing one-person CPR on an adult, the correct ratio is two breaths for every 15 compressions. Options 1, 3, and 4 are incorrect.
NP: Implementing care
CN: Physiological integrity
CNS: Physiological adaptation
CL: Application

173 A client with a fractured ankle is being discharged from the hospital. The nurse can tell that the client understands the correct crutch-walking technique by noting that the client places weight on the:
- [ ] 1. palms of the hands.
- [ ] 2. palms of the hands and the axillae.
- [ ] 3. axillae.
- [ ] 4. feet, which are placed wide apart.

CORRECT ANSWER: 1
The palms should bear the weight to avoid damage to the nerves in the brachial plexus of the axillae. Options 2 and 3: Pressure on the axillae may damage the nerves in the brachial plexus. Option 4: The client should avoid bearing any weight on the fractured area during the early stages of healing.
NP: Evaluating care
CN: Physiological integrity
CNS: Basic care and comfort
CL: Application

174 Which equipment should the nurse have at the bedside of a client returning from the postanesthesia recovery area after undergoing a thyroidectomy?
- [ ] 1. Thoracotomy tray
- [ ] 2. Tracheotomy tray
- [ ] 3. Paracentesis tray
- [ ] 4. Cutdown tray

CORRECT ANSWER: 2
Clients undergoing neck surgery are at risk for laryngeal edema and spasm. An emergency tracheotomy may be necessary to maintain airway patency. Option 1: A thoracotomy tray would be used to insert a chest tube. Option 3: A paracentesis tray would be used to aspirate fluid from the abdominal cavity. Option 4: A cutdown tray would be used to surgically insert an I.V. line, which isn't necessary in this case.
NP: Planning care
CN: Physiological integrity
CNS: Reduction of risk potential
CL: Application

175 A 52-year-old male client who recently arrived from another country has been diagnosed with type 2 diabetes mellitus. What is the best action for the nurse to take?
- ☐ 1. Give him a food exchange list that is written in his native language.
- ☐ 2. Observe him selecting foods from the hospital menu.
- ☐ 3. Obtain a dietary history of his usual native food habits.
- ☐ 4. Teach him food habits to be consistent with American foods.

CORRECT ANSWER: 3
A complete dietary history of native foods and habits is essential to ensure compliance when working with clients from diverse cultures. Option 1: Providing a food exchange list in the client's native language may not be effective if he doesn't eat typical American foods. Option 3: Observing him select foods from the hospital menu doesn't mean that he will be able to select appropriate choices when following his customary native food patterns. Option 4: There is no need to encourage the client to change from nonnative food practices. A client's compliance increases when he is taught about foods that he would normally eat.
NP: Planning care
CN: Health promotion and maintenance
CNS: Prevention and early detection of disease
CL: Application

176 Which nursing action would promote comfort in a male client with hyperthyroidism?
- ☐ 1. Place him in a slightly warm room.
- ☐ 2. Place him in a slightly cool room.
- ☐ 3. Encourage him to drink only cool or cold liquids.
- ☐ 4. Encourage him to drink only warm or hot liquids.

CORRECT ANSWER: 2
Clients with hyperthyroidism have a heat intolerance and prefer a cooler than usual room temperature. Option 1: A warmer room would be too uncomfortable. Options 3 and 4: Clients with hyperthyroidism may drink warm or cool liquids; extremely hot liquids are discouraged because of the risk of spills and burns.
NP: Planning care
CN: Physiological integrity
CNS: Basic care and comfort
CL: Application

177 A male client has a triple-lumen indwelling urinary catheter in place for transurethral surgery. He asks why the catheter is attached to his leg with tape. The nurse explains that the purpose of traction is to:
- ☐ 1. help hold the catheter in place.
- ☐ 2. decrease the amount of pain after the surgery.
- ☐ 3. decrease bladder spasms.
- ☐ 4. apply pressure to help prevent bleeding.

CORRECT ANSWER: 4
Traction applied to the catheter puts pressure on the bladder neck and helps prevent bleeding. Option 1: The catheter is held in place by the balloon at the end of the catheter. Option 2: Traction may increase the pain after surgery. Option 3: Traction may increase bladder spasms, but it's necessary to help prevent bleeding.
NP: Implementing care
CN: Physiological integrity
CNS: Reduction of risk potential
CL: Application

178 A female client who has been receiving hemodialysis for 3 months is now scheduled for a blood transfusion and asks the nurse why her blood count is so low. Which response is most appropriate?
- ☐ 1. "The dialysis machine destroys red cells, which makes it necessary to replace blood."
- ☐ 2. "The kidneys fail to produce a necessary substance to produce new red blood cells."
- ☐ 3. "The medicine that you regularly take prevents the bone marrow from producing red blood cells."
- ☐ 4. "You should ask your physician why a transfusion is necessary."

CORRECT ANSWER: 2
Clients with chronic renal failure don't produce erythropoietin, which is required to produce red blood cells. Option 1: The dialysis machine doesn't destroy red blood cells. Option 3: The medications that chronic renal dialysis clients receive don't prevent the bone marrow from producing red blood cells. Option 4: This doesn't answer the client's question. Providing health facts and knowledge about treatment are in the realm of nursing practice.
NP: Implementing care
CN: Physiological integrity
CNS: Physiological adaptation
CL: Application

179 A male client with a myocardial infarction (MI) asks why he's receiving I.V. injections of morphine. The nurse correctly explains that morphine:
- [ ] 1. helps control irregular heartbeats.
- [ ] 2. increases blood supply to the heart muscle.
- [ ] 3. relieves pain and decreases anxiety.
- [ ] 4. prevents further extension of the MI.

CORRECT ANSWER: 3
Morphine sulfate is a central nervous system depressant that helps relieve pain and decrease anxiety. Option 1: Morphine doesn't directly prevent irregular heartbeats. Option 2: Morphine is not a vasodilator and, therefore, doesn't increase blood supply to the heart muscle. Option 4: Morphine won't prevent the spread of MI.
NP: Implementing care
CN: Physiological integrity
CNS: Pharmacological therapies
CL: Analysis

180 A thoracotomy tube that is connected to water-seal drainage becomes obstructed. Which nursing action is most appropriate?
- [ ] 1. Arrange for an X-ray.
- [ ] 2. Milk the chest tube.
- [ ] 3. Prepare for chest tube removal.
- [ ] 4. Double-clamp the tube.

CORRECT ANSWER: 2
Milking the chest tube may remove the obstruction and promote drainage. Option 1: An X-ray would be taken only if the obstruction can't be removed and the client has respiratory symptoms. Option 3: Chest tube removal wouldn't be done unless the tube couldn't be freed from obstruction. Option 4: The nurse would clamp the tube only if the tube became disconnected from the water-seal drainage.
NP: Implementing care
CN: Physiological integrity
CNS: Physiological adaptation
CL: Application

181 A client has started a regimen of cimetidine (Tagamet) and Maalox for a stress-related ulcer. What should the instructions for taking the medicines include?
- [ ] 1. Both medications at the same time before meals
- [ ] 2. Both medications at the same time immediately after meals
- [ ] 3. Cimetidine before meals and Maalox after meals
- [ ] 4. Maalox before meals and cimetidine after meals

CORRECT ANSWER: 3
Cimetidine should be taken 1 hour before meals, and Maalox should be taken 1 to 2 hours after meals. Options 1 and 2: Taking both medications simultaneously would interfere with the absorption of the cimetidine. Option 4: Maalox should be taken after meals.
NP: Evaluating care
CN: Physiological integrity
CNS: Pharmacological therapies
CL: Application

182 What is the best postoperative position for a client who had a ruptured appendix and who now has peritonitis?
- [ ] 1. Dorsal decubitus
- [ ] 2. Lateral decubitus
- [ ] 3. Flat
- [ ] 4. Semi-Fowler's

CORRECT ANSWER: 4
Clients with peritonitis are maintained in semi-Fowler's position to keep abdominal contents below the diaphragm and to promote lung expansion. Options 1, 2, and 3: The client's head should be elevated to maintain comfort and prevent complications. Therefore, these positions would be inappropriate.
NP: Implementing care
CN: Physiological integrity
CNS: Physiological adaptation
CL: Application

183 The nurse realizes that patient-teaching instructions are effective when a male client with diabetes mellitus states that he'll ingest which of the following when he has a hypoglycemic reaction?
☐ 1. Fruit juice
☐ 2. Crackers
☐ 3. Peanut butter
☐ 4. Milk

CORRECT ANSWER: 1
A client who is having a hypoglycemic reaction needs to ingest a food that provides a quick source of glucose, such as fruit juice or instant glucose. Options 2, 3, and 4: Crackers, peanut butter, and milk don't provide the instant energy needed by someone who is experiencing a hypoglycemic reaction.
NP: Evaluating care
CN: Health promotion and maintenance
CNS: Prevention and early detection of disease
CL: Application

184 When observing a client who has been admitted with a ruptured appendix and peritonitis, the nurse would expect to find:
☐ 1. polycythemia.
☐ 2. abdominal rigidity.
☐ 3. hyperactive bowel sounds.
☐ 4. hyperkalemia.

CORRECT ANSWER: 2
One of the hallmark findings in peritonitis is a rigid, boardlike abdomen. Option 1: Polycythemia, an increased red blood cell count, isn't a typical finding in peritonitis. Option 3: In clients with peritonitis, bowel sounds would be absent. Option 4: Hyperkalemia, an increase in serum potassium levels, doesn't occur with peritonitis.
NP: Collecting data
CN: Physiological integrity
CNS: Physiological adaptation
CL: Application

185 A male client complains to the clinic nurse about abdominal discomfort, fatigue, and yellow skin. The nurse suspects that the client has jaundice and checks for:
☐ 1. crackles.
☐ 2. pruritus.
☐ 3. heat intolerance.
☐ 4. abnormal peripheral pulses.

CORRECT ANSWER: 2
Clients with jaundice commonly have pruritus, or itchy skin, due to a buildup of bile salts. Option 1: Crackles isn't a symptom of jaundice. Option 3: Heat intolerance isn't necessarily associated with jaundice. However, increased environmental temperature will increase perspiration and cause increased itching. Option 4: The nurse may check peripheral pulses as part of the routine examination, but this isn't specific to the jaundice.
NP: Collecting data
CN: Physiological integrity
CNS: Physiological adaptation
CL: Analysis

186 A client had a gastroscopy while under local anesthesia. Before resuming the client's oral fluid intake, what should the nurse do first?
☐ 1. Listen for bowel sounds.
☐ 2. Determine whether the client can talk.
☐ 3. Check for a gag reflex.
☐ 4. Determine the client's mental status.

CORRECT ANSWER: 3
After a gastroscopy, the nurse should check for the presence of a gag reflex before giving oral fluids. This is essential to prevent aspiration. Options 1, 2, and 4: The presence of bowel sounds, the ability to speak, and a clear mental status wouldn't ensure the presence of a gag reflex.
NP: Implementing care
CN: Physiological integrity
CNS: Reduction of risk potential
CL: Application

187 The nurse is giving preoperative and postoperative instructions to a male client who will undergo a liver biopsy tomorrow morning. Patient-teaching information regarding which problem is most critical in this situation?
- ☐ 1. Paralytic ileus
- ☐ 2. Hemorrhage
- ☐ 3. Renal shutdown
- ☐ 4. Constipation

CORRECT ANSWER: 2
Because the most common adverse effect of a liver biopsy is bleeding, the nurse should provide relevant information regarding the potential for hemorrhage. Option 1: There is no reason to provide a client with information about a paralytic ileus. Option 3: Renal shutdown isn't an expected complication after a liver biopsy. Option 4: The nurse would have no reason to suspect that the client will have a problem with constipation after a liver biopsy.
NP: Planning care
CN: Physiological integrity
CNS: Reduction of risk potential
CL: Application

188 During a health history, which statement by the client indicates a risk factor for renal calculi?
- ☐ 1. "I've been drinking a lot of cola soft drinks lately."
- ☐ 2. "I've been jogging more than usual."
- ☐ 3. "I've had more stress since we adopted a child last year."
- ☐ 4. "I'm a vegetarian and eat cheese two to three times each day."

CORRECT ANSWER: 4
Renal calculi are commonly composed of calcium. Diets high in calcium may predispose a person to renal calculi. Milk and milk products are high in calcium. Option 1: Cola soft drinks don't contain ingredients that would increase the risk for renal calculi. Options 2 and 3: Jogging and increased stress aren't considered risk factors for renal calculi formation.
NP: Collecting data
CN: Health promotion and maintenance
CNS: Prevention and early detection of disease
CL: Analysis

189 A newly diagnosed diabetic female client has started taking NPH insulin each morning at 7 a.m. At 3 p.m. she becomes diaphoretic and weak. Based on these symptoms, the nurse suspects that the client is experiencing:
- ☐ 1. impending diabetic coma.
- ☐ 2. hyperglycemia.
- ☐ 3. hypoglycemia.
- ☐ 4. diabetic ketoacidosis.

CORRECT ANSWER: 3
Weakness and diaphoresis are symptoms of hypoglycemia. Option 1: Diabetic coma is caused by elevated blood glucose levels. This client's symptoms are indicative of a low blood glucose level. Option 2: Symptoms of hyperglycemia include polyuria, polydipsia, and hot, dry skin. Option 4: Symptoms of diabetic ketoacidosis include elevated blood glucose level, acetone breath, and hot, dry skin.
NP: Evaluating care
CN: Physiological integrity
CNS: Physiological adaptation
CL: Analysis

190 A 68-year-old female client is diagnosed with a myocardial infarction. Her pulse rate has decreased to 44 beats/minute. Which medication would the nurse expect to administer?
- ☐ 1. atropine
- ☐ 2. lidocaine
- ☐ 3. bretylium
- ☐ 4. calcium chloride

CORRECT ANSWER: 1
Atropine is the drug of choice to increase cardiac transmission in cases of bradycardia and heart block. Option 2: Lidocaine is typically given for premature ventricular contractions. Option 3: Bretylium doesn't affect cardiac impulse transmission in the same manner as atropine. Option 4: Calcium chloride is necessary for impulse formation and cardiac contraction, but it doesn't produce the immediate increased pulse rate needed in this instance.
NP: Implementing care
CN: Physiological integrity
CNS: Pharmacological therapies
CL: Application

191 A nurse finds her neighbor lying on the front yard after his riding lawn mower exploded. He isn't breathing and his clothes are burning from the fire. What action should the nurse take first?
☐ 1. Initiate mouth-to-mouth breathing.
☐ 2. Begin cardiac compressions.
☐ 3. Establish an airway.
☐ 4. Put out the fire.

CORRECT ANSWER: 4
The nurse should extinguish the fire first to ensure the safety of both the client and the nurse. Option 1: Mouth-to-mouth resuscitation shouldn't be started until the environment is safe and an airway has been established. Option 2: Cardiac compressions aren't performed until effective breathing has been established. Option 3: In this case, establishing an airway would be delayed until the fire has been controlled.
NP: Implementing care
CN: Safe, effective care environment
CNS: Safety and infection control
CL: Analysis

192 A client has started taking doxycycline for Lyme disease that resulted from a deer tick bite. Discharge planning for this client should include instructions on the need to:
☐ 1. take the medication 1 hour before meals.
☐ 2. take the medication 1 hour after meals.
☐ 3. protect the skin from exposure to the sun while taking the medication.
☐ 4. discontinue the medication if constipation occurs.

CORRECT ANSWER: 3
Doxycycline increases photosensitivity; therefore, the client should take precautions against exposure to sunlight and ultraviolet light. Options 1 and 2: This drug should be taken with food. Option 4: Constipation isn't an adverse effect of doxycycline; however, if it should occur, the client shouldn't discontinue the medication.
NP: Planning care
CN: Physiological integrity
CNS: Pharmacological therapies
CL: Application

193 The community health nurse found an elderly female client lying in the snow, unable to move her right leg because of a fracture. What is the nurse's first priority?
☐ 1. Realign the fracture ends.
☐ 2. Reduce the fracture.
☐ 3. Immobilize the fracture in its present position.
☐ 4. Elevate the leg on whatever is available.

CORRECT ANSWER: 3
Initial treatment of obvious and suspected fractures includes immobilizing and splinting the limb. Options 1 and 2: Any attempt to realign or reset the fracture at the site may cause further injury and complications. Option 4: The leg may be elevated only after immobilization.
NP: Implementing care
CN: Physiological integrity
CNS: Physiological adaptation
CL: Application

194 Which patient-teaching information should the nurse emphasize to a client with tuberculosis (TB) to help prevent the spread of disease?
☐ 1. Cover the nose and mouth when coughing or sneezing.
☐ 2. Sterilize all eating utensils at home.
☐ 3. Don't have intimate contact with family members for 1 month.
☐ 4. Disinfect all clothes and bed linens after use.

CORRECT ANSWER: 1
TB is spread by airborne droplets; the client needs to cover the nose and mouth when coughing and sneezing. Options 2 and 4: Sterilizing utensils and disinfecting clothes and bed linens are unnecessary because the disease is transmitted by airborne particles. Option 3: After treatment begins, the client may resume intimacy with family members.
NP: Implementing care
CN: Safe, effective care environment
CNS: Safety and infection control
CL: Application

195 Which explanation about the action of heparin should the nurse provide to a client who has just started taking the drug?
☐ 1. It slows the time it takes the blood to clot.
☐ 2. It stops the blood from clotting.
☐ 3. It thins the blood.
☐ 4. It dissolves clots in the arteries of the heart.

CORRECT ANSWER: 1
Heparin prolongs the time needed for blood to clot; it doesn't thin the blood (Option 3). Option 2: If given in large doses, heparin may stop the blood from clotting; however, this isn't why heparin is usually given. Option 4: Heparin doesn't dissolve clots.
NP: Implementing care
CN: Physiological integrity
CNS: Pharmacological therapies
CL: Application

196 A male client has been admitted to the coronary care unit to rule out myocardial infarction (MI). Which symptoms during the health interview would indicate that he may be developing an infarction?
☐ 1. Epigastric pain and heartburn
☐ 2. Fatigue and headache
☐ 3. Diaphoresis and substernal pain
☐ 4. Dizziness and nausea

CORRECT ANSWER: 3
Diaphoresis and substernal or radiating chest pain are classic signs of an MI. Option 1: These symptoms are more indicative of indigestion or esophagitis. Option 2: These symptoms aren't typically reported in those with myocardial infarction. Option 4: Although these symptoms may accompany an infarction, individuals experiencing an infarction don't typically report them.
NP: Collecting data
CN: Physiological integrity
CNS: Physiological adaptation
CL: Comprehension

197 Which physical finding would the nurse expect in a client with bilateral arterial peripheral vascular disease?
☐ 1. Intermittent claudication
☐ 2. Dependent edema
☐ 3. Decreased pulses in the lower extremities
☐ 4. Increased pain sensitivity to pain in the lower extremities

CORRECT ANSWER: 3
Arterial insufficiency is caused by a decrease in blood supply by the arterial system and therefore causes weak or absent pedal pulses. Option 1: The client may experience intermittent claudication; however, this is a subjective symptom, not a physical assessment finding. Option 2: Edema relates to impaired venous circulation, not arterial. Option 4: Clients with arterial insufficiency have decreased sensitivity to pain.
NP: Collecting data
CN: Physiological integrity
CNS: Physiological adaptation
CL: Comprehension

198 What is the most comfortable position for a client with severe arterial peripheral vascular disease?
☐ 1. Supine with legs straight
☐ 2. Prone with legs elevated on a pillow
☐ 3. With the head of the bed on 6″ (15.2-cm) shock blocks
☐ 4. With the foot of bed on 6″ shock blocks

CORRECT ANSWER: 3
Clients with arterial peripheral vascular disease are more comfortable with their feet dependent, which increases the blood supply to the feet. Option 1: A supine position, with feet straight, isn't usually comfortable for those with arterial peripheral vascular disease. Options 2 and 4: Keeping the feet elevated will decrease the blood supply and increase the pain.
NP: Implementing care
CN: Physiological integrity
CNS: Basic care and comfort
CL: Application

199 An elderly male client has venous insufficiency and edematous lower extremities. The home care nurse should suggest that the client:
☐ 1. place 6″ (15.2-cm) shock blocks at the head of his bed.
☐ 2. place 6″ shock blocks at the foot of his bed.
☐ 3. wear support hose only while in bed.
☐ 4. put on his support hose 1 hour after rising in the morning.

CORRECT ANSWER: 2
Clients with venous insufficiency are usually more comfortable with the feet elevated because this helps to decrease venous engorgement. Option 1: Placing shock blocks at the head of the bed increases dependent edema. Option 3: Support hose may be worn while in bed but should be worn especially while the client is ambulating. Option 4: Support hose should be put on before getting out of bed.
NP: Implementing care
CN: Physiological integrity
CNS: Basic care and comfort
CL: Application

200 A male client is admitted to the emergency department with a sucking chest would. The nurse should apply pressure to the wound at the:
☐ 1. end of inspiration.
☐ 2. beginning of inspiration.
☐ 3. beginning of expiration.
☐ 4. end of expiration.

CORRECT ANSWER: 4
The best time to cover a sucking chest wound is at the end of expiration to prevent further inhalation of air through the wound. Option 1: This would allow air to be sucked into the chest cavity. Option 2: Applying pressure at the beginning of inspiration isn't as effective as at the end of expiration. Option 3: Some air may be sucked into the wound with this technique.
NP: Implementing care
CN: Physiological integrity
CNS: Physiological adaptation
CL: Application

201 A client who is 70 lb (31.8 kg) overweight has started taking medication for essential hypertension. Desired goals for this client should include:
☐ 1. checking the client's blood pressure every 3 months.
☐ 2. maintaining a weight-reduction diet and losing 2 lb (0.9 kg) each week.
☐ 3. following a strict weight-reduction diet until at least 30 lb (13.6 kg) are lost.
☐ 4. maintaining a high-fiber diet.

CORRECT ANSWER: 2
The most effective weight loss campaign is one that is gradual and changes eating habits. A moderate weight-reduction diet that aims for a weight loss of 2 lb each week is best for an overweight client with essential hypertension. Option 1: The client's blood pressure should be checked more frequently than once every 3 months. Option 3: A strict weight-reduction diet isn't as effective as a slow, gradual decrease in weight. Option 4: Maintaining a high-fiber diet won't control blood pressure.
NP: Planning care
CN: Health promotion and maintenance
CNS: Prevention and early detection of disease
CL: Application

202 A 22-year-old female client is experiencing a new-onset asthmatic attack. Which position is best for this client?
☐ 1. High Fowler's
☐ 2. Left side-lying
☐ 3. Right side-lying
☐ 4. Supine with pillows under each arm

CORRECT ANSWER: 1
The best position is high Fowler's, which helps lower the diaphragm and facilitates passive breathing and thereby improves air exchange. Options 2 and 3: A side-lying position won't facilitate the client's breathing. Option 4: A supine position increases the breathing difficulty of an asthmatic client.
NP: Implementing care
CN: Physiological integrity
CNS: Physiological adaptation
CL: Application

203 The nurse is advising a home health aide who will be caring for a client with a history of chronic cirrhosis from chemical hepatitis. The nurse should instruct the aide to observe the client closely for which complication?
- ☐ 1. Incontinence
- ☐ 2. Hemorrhage
- ☐ 3. Confusion
- ☐ 4. Abdominal tenderness

CORRECT ANSWER: 2
The most serious and life-threatening complication of cirrhosis is bleeding because the clotting mechanisms controlled by the liver are affected. Options 1, 3, and 4: Incontinence, confusion, and abdominal tenderness may occur with chronic cirrhosis, but they aren't life-threatening.
NP: Planning care
CN: Physiological integrity
CNS: Physiological adaptation
CL: Application

---

204 The nurse is observing a client for signs of shock. Which vital sign changes indicate that shock is imminent?
- ☐ 1. Increasing pulse rate and increasing blood pressure
- ☐ 2. Increasing pulse rate and decreasing blood pressure
- ☐ 3. Decreasing pulse rate and decreasing blood pressure
- ☐ 4. Decreasing pulse rate and increasing blood pressure

CORRECT ANSWER: 2
Vital sign changes that are indicative of imminent hypovolemic shock include a drop in blood pressure and a compensatory increase in the pulse rate. Options 1, 3, and 4 are incorrect.
NP: Collecting data
CN: Physiological integrity
CNS: Physiological adaptation
CL: Comprehension

---

205 The nurse is caring for a client who has just started therapy for diabetes insipidus. The nurse knows that the client's hydration is adequate when the urine specific gravity:
- ☐ 1. increases.
- ☐ 2. decreases.
- ☐ 3. no longer fluctuates with intake.
- ☐ 4. consistently remains above 1.030.

CORRECT ANSWER: 1
In diabetes insipidus, the client produces a large volume of urine with low specific gravity. Therapy is effective when the specific gravity starts to increase. Option 2: A decrease in specific gravity indicates that the client's condition is worsening. Options 3 and 4: Urine specific gravity fluctuates with intake and output.
NP: Evaluating care
CN: Physiological integrity
CNS: Physiological adaptation
CL: Analysis

---

206 A client has started taking amphotericin B for histoplasmosis. The nurse should monitor for which common adverse effect of this drug?
- ☐ 1. Renal toxicity
- ☐ 2. Visual disturbances
- ☐ 3. Splenic enlargement
- ☐ 4. Liver engorgement

CORRECT ANSWER: 1
Long-term administration of amphotericin B causes renal toxicity. Options 2, 3, and 4: Visual disturbances, splenic enlargement, and liver engorgement aren't common adverse effects of this medication.
NP: Evaluating care
CN: Physiological integrity
CNS: Pharmacological therapies
CL: Application

207 A male client has returned to his room after surgical repair of an inguinal hernia. The nurse notes on the client's chart that he was given spinal anesthesia for the surgery. Which nursing intervention would best help relieve or prevent the headache that commonly follows spinal anesthesia?
☐ 1. Keep the client flat in bed for at least 6 hours.
☐ 2. Apply an abdominal binder and elevate the client's legs.
☐ 3. Remove the blood patch from the puncture site.
☐ 4. Begin ambulation as soon as possible.

CORRECT ANSWER: 1
Researchers believe that the headache that commonly follows spinal anesthesia is caused by a loss of spinal fluid from the puncture site. Keeping the client flat on the back for several hours reduces pressure on the puncture site, thereby helping to prevent leakage and allowing the site to seal. If any spinal fluid loss has occurred, increasing the client's oral intake will promote cerebrospinal fluid production and alleviate the discomfort. Option 2: An abdominal binder is used to support the incision and dressing after abdominal surgery. It isn't usually used after spinal anesthesia. Elevating the legs may increase the client's headache by increasing the intra-abdominal pressure and intracranial pressure, which may result in further leakage from the puncture site. Option 3: A patch is placed over the puncture site by the anesthesiologist to seal the area and prevent leakage. Option 4: Ambulation wouldn't begin until the client has regained full muscle strength in the legs.
NP: Implementing care
CN: Physiological integrity
CNS: Reduction of risk potential
CL: Application

208 The nurse caring for a male client who is scheduled for surgery knows that the client must be fully informed of all procedures before the consent for surgery is signed. Which condition would satisfy the doctrine of informed consent?
☐ 1. The surgeon explains the procedure and the risks of the surgery to the client.
☐ 2. The client states that he understands the technique that will be used in the surgery.
☐ 3. The nurse gives the client a description of the surgical procedure.
☐ 4. The client and his spouse both sign the consent form.

CORRECT ANSWER: 1
The consent for surgery should be signed by the client having the surgery (if an adult, the client must be conscious and mentally competent) only after the physician has provided an explanation of the surgical procedure, the risks of the procedure, and what is expected during the postoperative period. Option 2: The details of the techniques of surgery aren't necessary for informed consent, although many surgeons include visual aides in their teaching. Option 3: The nurse who gives this information would be practicing outside the scope of nursing. However, the nurse may answer the client's questions or clarify information after the surgeon has explained the procedure to the client. Option 4: Only the person having surgery needs to sign the operative consent.
NP: Evaluating care
CN: Physiological integrity
CNS: Reduction of risk potential
CL: Comprehension

209 Two days after an abdominal hysterectomy, a client complains of a slight burning sensation and a "funny feeling" in her toes and left calf. What should the nurse do?
☐ 1. Keep the client on bed rest and put pillows under her knees.
☐ 2. Rub both legs and place a warm blanket over them.
☐ 3. Encourage ambulation and leg exercises while the client is in bed.
☐ 4. Maintain bed rest and immediately notify the physician.

CORRECT ANSWER: 4
This client is displaying symptoms of venous stasis and thrombophlebitis and should be kept on bed rest. Because medical assessment and intervention are necessary, the nurse should call the physician immediately. Option 1: Bed rest is appropriate. However, placing pillows under the knees should be avoided because this causes pressure on the vessels behind the knee and further compromises circulation. Blood would pool in the client's veins, increasing pressure in her calf. Option 2: Rubbing the legs may dislodge a clot. Heat to the area caused by the blanket may dilate the vessels, causing increased blood volume and more pressure in the veins. This may cause additional pain or formation of an embolus. Option 3: Ambulation and leg exercises are measures to prevent the formation of thrombi.
NP: Implementing care
CN: Physiological integrity
CNS: Physiological adaptation
CL: Application

210 The nurse is caring for a postoperative client who is oliguric and who is receiving potassium chloride I.V. The nurse should question the physician regarding the I.V. fluid because of the potential danger to the client's:
☐ 1. cardiac function.
☐ 2. respiratory function.
☐ 3. renal function.
☐ 4. brain function.

CORRECT ANSWER: 1
If the client's kidneys weren't functioning, the level of potassium would increase in the bloodstream. This would adversely affect the heart muscle, causing flaccidity, arrhythmias, and cardiac arrest. Option 2: The electrolyte potassium affects the respiratory system by weakening the muscles of respiration. However, the first organ affected would be the heart. Option 3: As potassium builds, the kidneys would be unable to excrete it. However, potassium itself doesn't damage the tubules directly. Option 4: Potassium elevation causes a deficit in neuromuscular function. Skeletal muscles may be weak, and paresthesia of the face and tongue may occur. However, the brain wouldn't be affected unless an acidotic condition were causing the increased potassium level.
NP: Collecting data
CN: Physiological integrity
CNS: Pharmacological therapies
CL: Application

211 A client is about to have an electrocardiogram (ECG). Which nursing measure would best help the client to relax?
☐ 1. Holding the client's hand
☐ 2. Encouraging the client to talk during the ECG
☐ 3. Gently stroking the client's forehead with a cool cloth
☐ 4. Carefully explaining the procedure before the test

CORRECT ANSWER: 4
Client teaching before any test is extremely important. Such teaching enhances the client's understanding of the procedure and helps to reduce anxiety. A client having an ECG must lie still because any extra movements may interfere with the ECG tracing. Knowing what to expect before the procedure helps relax the client, ensures cooperation, and produces a higher-quality ECG tracing. Options 1 and 3: The nurse should avoid touching the client during an ECG. Option 2: The client having an ECG should lie still and not talk because any muscle activity can interfere with the tracing.
NP: Implementing care
CN: Physiological integrity
CNS: Reduction of risk potential
CL: Application

212 When a client is diagnosed with essential hypertension, the mean arterial pressure (MAP) is used to establish blood pressure goals and evaluate treatment. Which formula is best for calculating the MAP?
- [ ] 1. MAP = diastolic blood pressure + $\frac{1}{3}$ pulse pressure
- [ ] 2. MAP = systolic blood pressure − diastolic pressure
- [ ] 3. MAP = diastolic blood pressure + $\frac{1}{4}$ apical pulse
- [ ] 4. MAP = systolic blood pressure + diastolic blood pressure

CORRECT ANSWER: 1
The ideal MAP is equal to or less than 100 mm Hg. The correct formula for calculating MAP is: MAP = diastolic blood pressure + $\frac{1}{3}$ pulse pressure. Option 2: The systolic blood pressure minus the diastolic blood pressure equals the pulse pressure. Options 3 and 4: These formulas are incorrect for calculating MAP.
NP: Collecting data
CN: Physiological integrity
CNS: Physiological adaptation
CL: Application

213 A male client has been admitted to the hospital to rule out an acute myocardial infarction (MI). The cardiac enzyme tests reveal a normal lactate dehydrogenase level and an elevated CK-MB level. The nurse enters the client's room and finds him pacing the floor. Which statement by the nurse would be most appropriate in this situation?
- [ ] 1. "You've had a heart attack. Get back in bed."
- [ ] 2. "You seem upset. Why don't you get into bed and, if you wish, we can talk for a while."
- [ ] 3. "You sure have a lot of energy; do you want to play cards?"
- [ ] 4. "Your physician doesn't want you up. Would you please get back into your bed?"

CORRECT ANSWER: 2
Given the laboratory data, especially the elevated CK-MB level, the nurse should realize that the client probably had an MI and that he needs to lie down and rest his heart. However, the nurse also should realize the need to respond to the client's emotional distress by acknowledging his feelings and offering to discuss his situation. Option 1: Telling the client that he had a heart attack would be giving a medical diagnosis that hasn't yet been made and would also be practicing outside the scope of nursing. Option 3: This statement acknowledges the client's pacing but not his underlying concerns. Option 4: This statement attempts to impose authority to control the client's behavior. It doesn't acknowledge the client's distress.
NP: Implementing care
CN: Psychosocial integrity
CNS: Coping and adaptation
CL: Application

214 Which classification of drugs increases cardiac output?
- [ ] 1. Diuretics
- [ ] 2. Antibiotics
- [ ] 3. Beta-adrenergic blockers
- [ ] 4. Inotropic agents

CORRECT ANSWER: 4
Inotropic agents, such as digitalis glycosides, slow the heart rate and increase the force of each heartbeat. As the myocardial function becomes more efficient, the amount of blood pumped with each heartbeat increases. Option 1: Diuretics are used to treat heart failure. They promote removal of excess water by the kidneys and therefore reduce edema and make breathing easier. Option 2: Antibiotics are used to fight infection and don't have an effect on cardiac output. Option 3: Beta-adrenergic blockers, agents such as propranolol (Inderal), have a negative inotropic action. One of the adverse effects of this action is heart failure.
NP: Collecting data
CN: Physiological integrity
CNS: Pharmacological therapies
CL: Comprehension

215 The nurse finds a client with no spontaneous respirations and no palpable carotid pulse. After calling a code, the nurse begins cardiopulmonary resuscitation (CPR) by positioning the client's head and neck, pinching the nostrils, and giving two quick breaths. The nurse observes no rise and fall of the chest. Which action should the nurse take next?

☐ 1. Insert an endotracheal tube.
☐ 2. Reposition the head and neck and check for airway obstruction.
☐ 3. Begin chest compressions.
☐ 4. Turn the client on the side and deliver quick blows between the scapulae.

CORRECT ANSWER: 2

Failure of air to reach the lungs may result from incorrect positioning of the head and neck or from an airway obstruction such as vomitus. Option 1: When a code is called, additional hospital personnel arrive. The respiratory therapist or the anesthetist would insert an endotracheal tube, if indicated. Option 3: CPR should follow the ABCs: Establish an airway, check the breathing, then check the circulation. Compressions aren't begun until an airway is established. Option 4: If a foreign body were lodged in an adult's trachea, an abdominal thrust would be used. If the airway were obstructed by vomitus, the client would be turned to the side, and a finger-sweep of the mouth would be performed.

NP: Implementing care
CN: Physiological integrity
CNS: Physiological adaptation
CL: Application

---

216 Which nursing activity requires greater caution when performed on a client with chronic obstructive pulmonary disease (COPD)?

☐ 1. Administering narcotics for pain relief
☐ 2. Increasing the client's fluid intake
☐ 3. Monitoring the client's cardiac rhythm
☐ 4. Assisting the client with coughing and deep breathing

CORRECT ANSWER: 1

Narcotics suppress the respiratory center in the medulla. Both COPD and pneumonia cause alterations in gas exchange; any further problems with oxygenation could result in respiratory failure and cardiac arrest. Option 2: Increasing the fluid intake would help to thin the client's secretions. Although the nurse would need to monitor the intake and output and watch for signs of heart failure, this isn't as critical as administering narcotics. Option 3: The cardiac rhythm provides an indication of the client's myocardial oxygenation; it should be a part of the nurse's regular assessment. Option 4: Helping with coughing and deep breathing should be included in the plan of care. The only caution would be to assess for possible rupture of emphysematous alveolar sacs and pneumothorax.

NP: Implementing care
CN: Physiological integrity
CNS: Physiological adaptation
CL: Application

---

217 A client with emphysema has dyspnea at rest, a barrel chest, grunting on expiration, peripheral cyanosis, and digital clubbing. Which arterial blood gas results would the nurse expect to find?

☐ 1. Low pH, high carbon dioxide (CO_2), and high bicarbonate (HCO_3^-)
☐ 2. Low pH, low CO_2, and low HCO_3^-
☐ 3. High pH, high CO_2, and high HCO_3^-
☐ 4. High pH, low CO_2, and low HCO_3^-

CORRECT ANSWER: 1

These parameters would indicate respiratory acidosis with compensation by the kidneys. Emphysema causes a retention of CO_2, which combines with water to form carbonic acid. This acidity drops the pH. To buffer this acidity, the kidneys form HCO_3^-. Option 2: The carbon dioxide level wouldn't be low in someone with emphysema. Option 3: A high pH would indicate alkalosis. This condition isn't usually seen in clients with chronic obstructive pulmonary disease (COPD) unless medical intervention had overcompensated the acidosis. Option 4: This situation wouldn't occur in a client with COPD.

NP: Collecting data
CN: Physiological integrity
CNS: Physiological adaptation
CL: Application

218 Which action should the nurse take when transporting a client with an anterior chest tube that is attached to an underwater seal drainage?
☐ 1. Clamp the chest tube close to the chest before moving the client.
☐ 2. Place the water-seal bottle on the stretcher between the client's legs.
☐ 3. Disconnect the chest tube and place a sterile dressing on the end.
☐ 4. Place the water-seal bottle lower than the lungs.

CORRECT ANSWER: 4
Placing the bottle lower than the lungs prevents drainage from entering the pleural space, which would cause increased pressure and a collapsed lung. Option 1: Chest tubes aren't clamped unless checking for sources of leaks. If a water-seal bottle breaks, the chest tube may be clamped close to the chest wall for a short time (1 to 2 minutes) while a new setup is prepared. Option 2: Keeping the bottle higher than the chest would allow fluid to enter the pleural space. Option 3: This would allow air in the pleural space, causing a pneumothorax.
NP: Implementing care
CN: Physiological integrity
CNS: Physiological adaptation
CL: Application

219 Which goals take priority when planning the care of a 42-year-old female client with lobar pneumonia?
☐ 1. Conserve energy and assist the body's defenses.
☐ 2. Maintain cardiac and renal function.
☐ 3. Improve nutritional status and maintain skin integrity.
☐ 4. Prevent infection and promote bowel elimination.

CORRECT ANSWER: 1
To make use of nutrients for energy, the body requires a sufficient supply of oxygen. In a client with lobar pneumonia, oxygen exchange is affected, resulting in less partial pressure of oxygen in arterial blood. Thus, the client is weak and tired. Conservation of available energy is an important nursing goal. The body's defenses are assisted by use of antibiotics or other pharmacologic agents. Option 2: Lobar pneumonia is treated with antibiotics and usually results in a cure before damage to the heart or kidneys occurs. Option 3: The nurse would provide good nutrition and maintain skin integrity, especially if the client is on bed rest. However, these aren't the priority. Option 4: The client already has an infection; preventing additional infections would be more important. Bowel function isn't usually affected in a client with pneumonia unless the medications produce adverse effects that affect the bowel.
NP: Planning care
CN: Physiological integrity
CNS: Basic care and comfort
CL: Application

220 Which patient-teaching instruction would be most appropriate for a client with a chest tube?
☐ 1. Remain as active as possible.
☐ 2. Avoid coughing.
☐ 3. Maintain bed rest.
☐ 4. Avoid the side-lying position.

CORRECT ANSWER: 1
Keeping the client active is important to prevent the hazards of immobility, which include problems with skin integrity, bowel function, and respiratory function. More important, though, the client should remain active to facilitate removal of air and secretions from the pleural space. Option 2: Coughing and deep breathing should be encouraged. If this causes pain, the nurse should teach splinting techniques. Option 3: Bed rest isn't indicated unless the client has an addition medical condition that prohibits ambulation. Option 4: The client may use a side-lying position as long as it's on the unaffected side.
NP: Implementing care
CN: Physiological integrity
CNS: Physiological adaptation
CL: Application

221 A client with pulmonary tuberculosis (TB) has been taking isoniazid and rifampin for 9 months. The nurse should instruct the client to report which symptoms of toxicity immediately to the physician?
☐ 1. Deafness or dizziness
☐ 2. Severe headache or ringing in the ears
☐ 3. Numbness, tingling, and weakness of the extremities
☐ 4. Fever and decreased visual acuity

CORRECT ANSWER: 3
Numbness, tingling, and weakness of the extremities indicate isoniazid toxicity. The client should report these findings immediately because the drug may need to be discontinued. Options 1 and 2: These are symptoms associated with streptomycin toxicity. Option 4: Fever may occur from the TB itself or from another infection. Neither medication causes loss of visual acuity.
NP: Implementing care
CN: Physiological integrity
CNS: Pharmacological therapies
CL: Application

222 Which preventative measure should the nurse teach clients with tuberculosis (TB) to help slow the transmission of disease?
☐ 1. Practicing safer sexual behavior
☐ 2. Emphasizing the need to take the entire course of drug therapy
☐ 3. Emphasizing the importance of taking the Bacille Calmette-Guérin vaccine
☐ 4. Maintaining universal precautions when handling blood

CORRECT ANSWER: 2
Failure to complete the entire course of drug therapy allows the bacillus to mutate and become resistant to the medication. Taking medication for the entire time prescribed ensures that the maximum therapeutic effect is achieved. Option 1: The tubercle bacillus is transmitted in airborne droplets by sneezing or coughing. Fluid exchanges during sexual encounters don't harbor the causative organism. Option 3: This vaccine produces variable protection and isn't widely used in the United States. It can be given to those with a negative TB test, infants born to mothers with active TB, or health care personnel at risk for exposure to undiagnosed clients. Option 4: Respiratory isolation, not universal precautions, would be indicated because pulmonary TB isn't spread through the bloodstream.
NP: Implementing care
CN: Safe, effective care environment
CNS: Safety and infection control
CL: Application

223 While monitoring a client receiving oxygen by way of a nasal cannula, the nurse notes that the flow rate is set at 3 L. The physician's orders call for 40% oxygen. What action should the nurse take?
☐ 1. None because this is the correct flow rate.
☐ 2. Reduce the flow rate to 2 L/minute.
☐ 3. Increase the flow rate to 4 L/minute.
☐ 4. Increase the flow rate to 6 L/minute.

CORRECT ANSWER: 4
A flow rate of 6 L/minute delivers 40% oxygen. Option 1: The flow rate is incorrect, and action is warranted. Option 2: A flow rate of 2 L delivers 28% oxygen. Option 3: A flow rate of 4 L delivers 35% oxygen.
NP: Implementing care
CN: Physiological integrity
CNS: Pharmacological therapies
CL: Application

224 While checking a postoperative client, the nurse notices that the Salem sump tube is connected to low suction. What should the nurse do?
- ☐ 1. Switch to high suction unless otherwise contraindicated.
- ☐ 2. Test the placement of the Salem sump tube.
- ☐ 3. Irrigate the sump tube.
- ☐ 4. Do nothing because the suction is set at the appropriate setting.

CORRECT ANSWER: 4
If suction is available from a central source such as wall suction, both intermittent and continuous suction should be set on 30 to 40 mm Hg. If the equipment is portable, continuous suction should be set on 30 mm Hg, and intermittent suction should be set on 80 to 120 Hg because suction is reduced with a cyclic setting to about 25 mm Hg by the time it reaches the gastric mucosa. Option 1: Switching the suction to a high setting may damage the gastric mucosa. Options 2 and 3: In this case, there is no need to test the placement of the tube or irrigate the tube.
NP: Implementing care
CN: Physiological integrity
CNS: Reduction of risk potential
CL: Application

225 The nurse is studying for an NCLEX examination and reviewing facts about the human body's basic needs. Which factor is most essential for survival?
- ☐ 1. Oxygen
- ☐ 2. Water
- ☐ 3. Food
- ☐ 4. Sleep

CORRECT ANSWER: 1
Cells need oxygen to live; without circulating oxygen, a person quickly dies. Option 2: Although water is necessary, a person can survive without water for some time. Option 3: Food is necessary for survival because it provides nutrients, but it isn't the most crucial need. Option 4: Sleep is needed to maintain good health, but it isn't the most important requirement.
NP: Implementing care
CN: Physiological integrity
CNS: Physiological adaptation
CL: Knowledge

226 A 51-year-old male client undergoing treatment for hyperlipidemia is receiving instructions about a low-fat diet. Which is the best food choice for this client?
- ☐ 1. Low-sodium ham, potato salad, and pudding
- ☐ 2. Skim milk, baked fish, and green beans
- ☐ 3. Fried chicken, pasta, and gelatin dessert
- ☐ 4. Grilled salmon, mashed potatoes, and cheesecake

CORRECT ANSWER: 2
Skim milk is low in fat, baked fish provides the protein that the client requires, and green beans are a good vegetable choice. Option 1: Low-sodium ham is high in saturated fat, as are pudding and potato salad, all of which can elevate the client's total cholesterol level. Option 3: The fried chicken isn't a good choice because it's cooked in oil or fat; the pasta (provided it isn't prepared with oil or butter) and the gelatin dessert are low in fat. Option 4: Grilled salmon is a fair choice but can elevate the client's total cholesterol level, mashed potatoes are low-fat as long as they aren't made with butter or whole milk, and cheesecake is high in fat so it isn't a good choice.
NP: Planning care
CN: Physiological integrity
CNS: Basic care and comfort
CL: Application

227 The nurse is instructing a 71-year-old woman with osteoporosis and a history of hyperlipidemia. The client asks the nurse which item on the sample menu would be a good choice. Which is the best choice for this client?
- ☐ 1. Rye bread
- ☐ 2. Wax beans
- ☐ 3. Carrots
- ☐ 4. Skim milk

CORRECT ANSWER: 4
Osteoporosis causes a loss of calcium from the bones, so this client needs calcium. Skim milk is the best choice for this client because it has the same amount of calcium as whole milk but has a lower fat content. Option 1: Rye bread isn't a good source of calcium. Option 3: Carrots are a good source of vitamin A but not calcium. Option 4: Wax beans aren't a good source of calcium; a green leafy vegetable would be a better choice.
NP: Planning care
CN: Physiological integrity
CNS: Basic care and comfort
CL: Application

228 A 36-year-old client who underwent an appendectomy 2 days ago presses her call button and requests something for pain. The nurse needs to administer 50 mg of meperidine (Demerol). Which site isn't appropriate for this injection?
- ☐ 1. Deltoid
- ☐ 2. Gluteus maximus
- ☐ 3. Vastus lateralis
- ☐ 4. Subcutaneously in the abdomen

CORRECT ANSWER: 4
Demerol is given intramuscularly, not subcutaneously. Options 1, 2, and 3: The deltoid, gluteus maximus, and vastus lateralis are all appropriate choices to give the injection.
NP: Implementing care
CN: Physiological integrity
CNS: Pharmacological therapies
CL: Application

229 A 55-year-old male client has been hospitalized for 1 week due to injuries sustained in a motor vehicle accident. He's weak and continues to require some assistance with activities of daily living. The nurse helps the client to maintain muscle tone by:
- ☐ 1. getting the client out of bed even if he's on bed rest.
- ☐ 2. providing range-of-motion (ROM) exercises if the client is on bed rest.
- ☐ 3. limiting the client's activity.
- ☐ 4. encouraging the client to turn himself in bed.

CORRECT ANSWER: 2
ROM exercises are used to move an extremity through its range without putting stress on the joints. Option 1: If the client is on bed rest, never get him out of bed without an order; this could cause undue harm to the client. Option 3: Limiting the client's activity isn't a good choice unless there are specific orders to do so from the physician. Option 4: Encouraging the client to turn himself may prevent skin breakdown but doesn't help to maintain muscle tone. Always check the physician's order before you initiate any care.
NP: Planning care
CN: Physiological integrity
CNS: Reduction of risk potential
CL: Application

230 A 59-year-old client underwent mastectomy of the left breast yesterday and has an I.V. catheter in her lower right arm. To check the client's blood pressure, what should the nurse do?
- ☐ 1. Use the right arm above the I.V. site.
- ☐ 2. Use the left arm and pump the cuff only as necessary.
- ☐ 3. Use the leg.
- ☐ 4. Stop the I.V. infusion and then take the blood pressure in the right arm.

CORRECT ANSWER: 1
To obtain a blood pressure reading, the nurse should always use the arm opposite the side of the mastectomy. Option 2: Never take a blood pressure reading in the arm on the affected side. Option 3: Blood pressure readings may be taken in the leg in some cases, but this isn't necessary in this case. Option 4: It isn't necessary to stop the I.V. fluid to take a blood pressure reading.
NP: Implementing care
CN: Health promotion and maintenance
CNS: Prevention and early detection of disease
CL: Knowledge

231 A client who may have pneumonia is admitted to the medical unit. He has an occasional non-productive cough. The nurse initiates standard precautions, which are used:
□ 1. only for a client with known infection.
□ 2. only for a client when ordered by the physician.
□ 3. only if the client has a known communicable disease.
□ 4. on any client if the nurse may come in contact with blood or body fluids.

CORRECT ANSWER: 4
The Centers for Disease Control and Prevention recommend using standard precautions whenever the caregiver may come in contact with blood or body fluids. Option 1: The nurse can't distinguish if there is an infectious process or not, so it's imperative that standard precautions be used. Option 2: Using standard precautions is a nursing function and doesn't require a physician's order. Option 3: Standard precautions should be used when caring for any client and not be reserved for those with known communicable diseases.
NP: Implementing care
CN: Safe, effective care environment
CNS: Safety and infection control
CL: Application

232 The nurse is caring for a 75-year-old male client with dysphagia secondary to a cerebrovascular accident. Before feeding the client, it would be most appropriate for the nurse to assess:
□ 1. the client's gag reflex.
□ 2. the client's ability to hold the fork.
□ 3. the temperature of the food.
□ 4. whether the food is in the client's field of vision.

CORRECT ANSWER: 1
The nurse needs to be sure there is a positive gag reflex; this ensures that the client is able to eat safely. Options 2, 3, and 4: Assessing the client's ability to use a fork, the temperature of the food, and whether the food is in the client's visual field isn't as critical in this case.
NP: Planning care
CN: Physiological integrity
CNS: Reduction of risk potential
CL: Knowledge

233 When planning long-term care for a client who is a paraplegic, the nurse should be aware that:
□ 1. rehabilitation should be left up to the client.
□ 2. it isn't necessary to begin rehabilitation until the client is transferred to a rehabilitation facility.
□ 3. rehabilitation should begin as soon as the client is stabilized.
□ 4. rehabilitation should begin as soon as the client is admitted to the hospital.

CORRECT ANSWER: 3
After a spinal cord injury, rehabilitation should begin as soon as the client is stabilized. Option 1: Rehabilitation can't be left up to the client, particularly because he may be depressed and uninterested in rehabilitation early in the recovery process. Option 2: Valuable time may be lost if rehabilitation isn't started until a client reaches a rehabilitation facility. Option 4: If rehabilitation is started during the acute phase of injury, activities may seriously harm the client whose injury is unstable.
NP: Planning care
CN: Physiological integrity
CNS: Physiological adaptation
CL: Application

234 A client diagnosed with diabetes several years ago is in the clinic to have his hemoglobin (Hb) A_1C level checked. He tells the nurse that he doesn't need to have his blood glucose level checked because he checked it this morning. The nurse's best response is to explain that the Hb A_1C test is used to determine the:
□ 1. need for a glucose tolerance test.
□ 2. presence of ketones in the urine.
□ 3. degree of blood glucose control over the preceding 6 to 8 weeks.
□ 4. degree of blood glucose control over the preceding 12 to 18 weeks.

CORRECT ANSWER: 3
The Hb A_1C test is a blood test used to determine how well a client followed his diabetic regimen over the last couple of months. Option 1: A glucose tolerance test is a blood test used to diagnose diabetes. Option 2: A ketostick is used to check for ketones (acetone bodies) in the urine. Option 4: The Hb A_1C test doesn't provide information about blood glucose control that occurred more than 3 months before the venipuncture.
NP: Collecting data
CN: Physiological integrity
CNS: Physiological adaptation
CL: Knowledge

235 A client comes to the clinic exhibiting the following symptoms: polyphagia, polydipsia, polyuria, nausea, and slightly irregular breathing. As the nurse is checking his blood pressure, the client begins to vomit and the nurse notes a sweet smell on the client's breath. These are symptoms of:
- ☐ 1. hypoglycemia.
- ☐ 2. catabolism.
- ☐ 3. ketoacidosis.
- ☐ 4. respiratory acidosis.

CORRECT ANSWER: 3
The signs and symptoms of ketoacidosis — acidosis caused by excessive ketone bodies in the urine — are polyphagia, polydipsia, polyuria, nausea, vomiting, abdominal pain, and hyperventilation. As ketone levels rise, the client's breath develops an acetone or fruity odor. Option 1: Hypoglycemia is a deficiency of blood glucose characterized by fatigue, restlessness, malaise, and weakness. Option 2: Catabolism is the breakdown of larger substances to smaller ones. Option 4: Respiratory acidosis is always due to inadequate excretion of carbon dioxide. It doesn't result from polyphagia, polydipsia, and polyuria, which are classic signs of diabetes mellitus.
NP: Collecting data
CN: Health promotion and maintenance
CNS: Prevention and early detection of disease
CL: Knowledge

236 A 48-year-old male client on the medical-surgical unit is complaining of polydipsia, polyphagia, and polyuria. The nurse suspects these could be signs of what condition?
- ☐ 1. Hyperglycemia
- ☐ 2. Hypoglycemia
- ☐ 3. Hyperkalemia
- ☐ 4. Hypernatremia

CORRECT ANSWER: 1
Polyphagia, polyuria, and polydipsia are classic signs of hyperglycemia (excessive glucose in the blood) and diabetes mellitus. Option 2: Hypoglycemia is a deficiency of glucose in the blood; it's characterized by fatigue, restlessness, malaise, and weakness. Option 3: Hyperkalemia is caused by excessive potassium levels; it's characterized by ventricular arrhythmias, muscle weakness, and diarrhea. Option 4: Hypernatremia is an elevated sodium level; it's characterized by thirst, a dry and swollen tongue, sticky mucous membranes, flushed skin, increased muscle tone and deep tendon reflexes, and increased body temperature.
NP: Collecting data
CN: Health promotion and maintenance
CNS: Prevention and early detection of disease
CL: Knowledge

237 A 2nd-year computer science student is diagnosed with type 1 diabetes mellitus. The nurse explains that the goal of treating type 1 diabetes mellitus is to:
- ☐ 1. phase out the amount of insulin the client requires.
- ☐ 2. maintain blood glucose and lipid levels within normal limits.
- ☐ 3. maintain the blood glucose level within normal limits through dietary regulation.
- ☐ 4. prevent the client from developing diabetes insipidus.

CORRECT ANSWER: 2
By maintaining normal blood glucose and lipid levels, the client can limit and prevent complications. Option 1: The client receives a prescription for the amount of insulin needed to control the diabetes; the insulin is never phased out. Option 3: Type 1 diabetes mellitus can't be controlled by diet. Option 4: Diabetes insipidus isn't a complication of type 1 diabetes mellitus.
NP: Planning care
CN: Physiological integrity
CNS: Reduction of risk potential
CL: Knowledge

238 A 19-year-old was recently diagnosed with type 1 diabetes mellitus. She tells the nurse that her mother has type 2 diabetes mellitus, and she'll follow the same regimen that her mother follows. Which response by the nurse is best?
- ☐ 1. "Because most people react similarly to the treatments used, your mother's regimen should work."
- ☐ 2. "Type 1 and type 2 diabetes are regulated with the same diet and medications."
- ☐ 3. "Your mother should go with you to instructional classes for diabetes."
- ☐ 4. "If your mother can assist you, you may not have to attend the instructional classes."

CORRECT ANSWER: 3
The mother should also attend the classes because treatment of diabetes is individualized according to the client's age, height, weight, lifestyle, and general health. Option 1: The treatment of diabetes is different for each client. Option 2: Type 1 and type 2 diabetes mellitus are treated differently. Option 4: The client should attend instructional classes regardless of the mother's level of knowledge.
NP: Implementing care
CN: Physiological integrity
CNS: Reduction of risk potential
CL: Knowledge

239 The nurse is providing educational material about an exercise program for a diabetic client who is 5′ 2″, 203 lb (92 kg) and is receiving oral antidiabetic drugs. An exercise program for this client should:
- ☐ 1. be designed for the individual client.
- ☐ 2. be started after the client is the appropriate weight for her height.
- ☐ 3. start out with a short jog and increase in intensity.
- ☐ 4. be started to get the client's blood glucose level under control.

CORRECT ANSWER: 1
An exercise program for a diabetic client should be individualized to meet specific needs. Option 2: Each client is different and the exercise program should be modified to match the individual's physical abilities. Option 3: An exercise program should never start with a jog. The client should start with walking and increase the intensity of the exercise as tolerated. Option 4: The client's blood glucose level needs to be under control before starting an exercise program.
NP: Implementing care
CN: Health promotion and maintenance
CNS: Prevention and early detection of disease
CL: Comprehension

240 The nurse is caring for a 26-year-old woman diagnosed with diabetes. The physician orders 6 units of regular insulin administered subcutaneously at 7 a.m. The client asks the nurse how long the medicine takes to begin working. The nurse responds that regular insulin begins to act in approximately:
- ☐ 1. ¹/₂ to 1 hour.
- ☐ 2. 1 to 2 hours.
- ☐ 3. 4 to 8 hours.
- ☐ 4. 10 to 12 hours.

CORRECT ANSWER: 1
Regular insulin usually begins acting in ¹/₂ to 1 hour. Option 2: Intermediate-acting insulins have onsets of 1 to 2 hours. Option 3: Long-acting insulins have onsets of 4 to 8 hours. Option 4: None of the insulins have an onset of 10 to 12 hours, but Humulin 70/30 and Humulin 50/50 peak in 2 to 12 hours.
NP: Evaluating care
CN: Physiological integrity
CNS: Pharmacological therapies
CL: Application

241 The nurse is caring for a 38-year-old client diagnosed with diabetes. The physician writes an order for 2 units of NPH insulin to be given at 8 a.m. How does the nurse prepare to administer the insulin?
- ☐ 1. Subcutaneously
- ☐ 2. Intramuscularly
- ☐ 3. Orally
- ☐ 4. Topically

CORRECT ANSWER: 1
All insulins are given subcutaneously, rotating sites to prevent long-term complications. Option 2, 3, and 4: Insulin is never given intramuscularly, orally, or topically.
NP: Implementing care
CN: Physiological integrity
CNS: Pharmacological therapies
CL: Application

242 A driving instructor undergoing care in a family clinic has just received her first allergy injection. She thanks the nurse, says good-bye, and starts to exit the clinic. What should the nurse's response be?
- ☐ 1. Tell the client good-bye and that she'll see her next week.
- ☐ 2. Advise the client that she needs to wait 2 hours and then be checked by the nurse before leaving.
- ☐ 3. Advise the client that she needs to wait 20 minutes and then have the arm checked by the nurse before leaving.
- ☐ 4. Advise the client that she needs to wait 30 minutes and then may leave.

CORRECT ANSWER: 3
Most clinics recommend waiting 20 minutes after the injection. The nurse should then assess the site and the client before the client leaves the clinic. Option 1: Don't allow the client to leave immediately after an allergy injection in case of an allergic reaction. Option 2: The client doesn't need to wait 2 hours; 20 minutes is enough time. Option 4: Don't allow the client to leave the clinic without assessing the injection site and documenting the reaction.
NP: Implementing care
CN: Physiological integrity
CNS: Reduction of risk potential
CL: Knowledge

243 A group of nurses are discussing disease precautions after attending a seminar with fellow health care workers. Which disease is a health care worker most at risk to contract?
- ☐ 1. Human immunodeficiency virus (HIV)
- ☐ 2. Hepatitis B
- ☐ 3. Herpes simplex
- ☐ 4. Tuberculosis (TB)

CORRECT ANSWER: 2
Health care workers are most at risk to acquire hepatitis B because it's transmitted mainly by parenteral routes and is present in all body fluids and stool of carriers. Option 1: HIV is more often spread between persons with intimate contact than between client and health care worker. Option 3: Herpes simplex is spread through sexual contact. Option 4: TB is transmitted through droplets in the air but isn't the disease with which most health care workers come in contact.
NP: Collecting data
CN: Health promotion and maintenance
CNS: Prevention and early detection of disease
CL: Comprehension

244 The physician has ordered ciprofloxin (Cipro) otic drops for a 5-year-old client in the pediatric unit. The nurse needs to administer the eardrops by pulling the pinna of the ear:
- ☐ 1. down and back.
- ☐ 2. up and back.
- ☐ 3. straight up.
- ☐ 4. straight down.

CORRECT ANSWER: 1
Pulling the pinna of the ear down and back straightens the auditory canal and allows the nurse to place the eardrops on the side of the ear canal. Option 2: Pulling the pinna of the ear up and back is correct for positioning an adult's ear, not a child's. Options 3 and 4: Pulling the pinna straight up or straight down doesn't position the ear for administration of the medication.
NP: Implementing care
CN: Physiological integrity
CNS: Pharmacological therapies
CL: Application

245 A 51-year-old male client is admitted to a city hospital with possible tuberculosis (TB). The physician has ordered a purified protein derivative (PPD) test for TB. The order reads PPD 0.1cc intradermally. Which syringe and needle should the nurse choose?
- ☐ 1. 25 to 26G, $^3/_8$" needle
- ☐ 2. 19G, 1" needle
- ☐ 3. 18G, 1" to $1^1/_2$" needle
- ☐ 4. 60-ml syringe with catheter tip

CORRECT ANSWER: 1
An intradermal injection is inserted just slightly under the skin, necessitating the use of the 25G or 26G syringe with a $^3/_8$" needle, which is very small. Options 2 and 3: 18G and 19G needles are very large and aren't used for intradermal injections. Option 4: A 60-ml syringe is generally used for irrigation.
NP: Implementing care
CN: Physiological integrity
CNS: Pharmacological therapies
CL: Knowledge

246 A 49-year-old client is admitted with renal failure. The physician has ordered epoetin (Epogen). The nurse prepares to administer this medication:
- ☐ 1. intradermally, at a 15-degree angle.
- ☐ 2. intramuscularly, at a 90-degree angle.
- ☐ 3. subcutaneously, at a 45-degree angle.
- ☐ 4. orally, after meals.

CORRECT ANSWER: 3
Epoetin is administered subcutaneously at a 45-degree angle to ensure that the medication is injected in the adipose tissue. Option 1: An injection given at 15 degrees is an intradermal injection. Option 3: An intramuscular injection is given at a 90-degree angle. Option 4: Epoetin isn't given orally.
NP: Planning care
CN: Physiological integrity
CNS: Pharmacological therapies
CL: Knowledge

247 The nurse on duty in a clinic that administers chelation therapy to treat lead poisoning is preparing to administer an injection. When selecting the proper needle, the nurse knows that the:
- ☐ 1. higher the number, the smaller the bore.
- ☐ 2. lower the number, the smaller the bore.
- ☐ 3. number has no relationship to the bore of the needle.
- ☐ 4. number is always the same on every needle.

CORRECT ANSWER: 1
The higher the number is on the needle, the smaller the bore, or opening. Options 2, 3, and 4 are all incorrect choices.
NP: Planning care
CN: Physiological integrity
CNS: Pharmacological therapies
CL: Knowledge

248 The nurse is caring for a client with type 1 diabetes mellitus. What type of breathing should the nurse expect to observe if this client develops ketoacidosis?
- ☐ 1. Cheyne-Stokes respirations
- ☐ 2. Tachypnea
- ☐ 3. Kussmaul's respirations
- ☐ 4. Stridor

CORRECT ANSWER: 3
Kussmaul's respirations is a classic symptom for clients with diabetic ketoacidosis. It's characterized by difficulty breathing, with respirations occurring at irregular intervals. Option 1: Cheyne-Stokes respirations are a waxing and waning of respirations with periods of apnea. This is commonly seen with clients in comas. Option 2: Tachypnea is abnormal, rapid respiration. Option 4: Narrowing of the airway is manifested by stridor.
NP: Collecting data
CN: Physiological integrity
CNS: Physiological adaptation
CL: Knowledge

249 The nurse is studying for an NCLEX examination and reviewing proper procedures for administering medications. What are the 5 "rights" of medication administration?
- ☐ 1. Right client, right medication, right dose, right time, and right route
- ☐ 2. Right client, right medication, right dose, right time, and right reason
- ☐ 3. Right client, right medication, right dose, right time, and right physician
- ☐ 4. Right client, right medication, right dose, right time, and right quantity

CORRECT ANSWER: 1
Before administering any medication, the nurse should make sure she has the right client by checking the identification band, check the physician's order for dosage and frequency, check that the medication is ordered for the right route, and make sure she administers the medication at the right time. Options 2, 3, and 4: The right reason, right physician, and right quantity are all incorrect answers.
NP: Implementing care
CN: Physiological integrity
CNS: Pharmacological therapies
CL: Application

250 A client develops a superficial ocular infection, and the physician orders gentamicin (Garamycin) ophthalmic ointment for the client's left eye. The nurse should apply a thin line of the ointment without touching the opposite lid with the catheter tip to the inside of the:
- ☐ 1. lower lid, in a thin line from the inner to outer canthus.
- ☐ 2. lower lid, in a thin line from the outer to inner canthus.
- ☐ 3. upper lid, in a thin line from the inner to outer canthus.
- ☐ 4. upper lid, in a thin line from the outer to inner canthus.

CORRECT ANSWER: 1
Always apply eye ointments to the lower lid, from the inner to outer canthus, without touching the eyelid or eyeball. This prevents the spread of the infection. Option 2: Never apply an eye ointment from the outer to inner canthus because this could spread other bacteria into the eye. Options 3 and 4: It would be difficult to apply eye ointment to the upper lid because the nurse wouldn't be able to stabilize the lid before administering the ointment.
NP: Implementing care
CN: Physiological integrity
CNS: Pharmacological therapies
CL: Application

251 A client underwent a colostomy for inflammatory bowel disease yesterday. Her surgical wound has eviscerated. What should the nurse do first?
- ☐ 1. Call the physician.
- ☐ 2. Take the client's blood pressure and pulse.
- ☐ 3. Call for the nurse manager on the unit.
- ☐ 4. Apply a sterile gauze moistened with sterile normal saline solution.

CORRECT ANSWER: 4
Any time a wound opens up, there is a chance for infection. Applying a sterile, wet gauze maintains some sterility to the wound and keeps it moist. Option 1: Before calling the physician, the nurse needs to use sterile technique and take care of the wound. Option 2: The client's vital signs should be taken, but this isn't the nurse's first priority. Option 3: The nurse may need some assistance, but it doesn't have to be the nurse manager.
NP: Implementing care
CN: Physiological integrity
CNS: Physiological adaptation
CL: Application

252 A 36-year-old man who transcribes insurance claims at home underwent a carpal tunnel repair on his left hand 3 days ago. The nurse suspects that the surgical site is infected. Which observations might lead the nurse to this conclusion?
- ☐ 1. Swelling and a healed suture line
- ☐ 2. Tenderness and afebrile body temperature
- ☐ 3. Redness and febrile body temperature
- ☐ 4. Bruising of the arm

CORRECT ANSWER: 3
Redness, swelling, tenderness, drainage, and fever are all classic symptoms of a wound infection. Options 1 and 2: Normally, an infected wound doesn't have a completely healed suture line and the client commonly has at least a low-grade fever. Option 4: Bruising is normal after surgery and isn't a sign of infection.
NP: Evaluating care
CN: Physiological integrity
CNS: Physiological adaptation
CL: Knowledge

253 A 76-year-old minister underwent transurethral resection of the prostate yesterday. Which observation is the nurse's greatest concern?
- ☐ 1. Increased urine output
- ☐ 2. Infection
- ☐ 3. Bleeding
- ☐ 4. Fluid and electrolyte imbalance

CORRECT ANSWER: 3
The prostate area is a very vascular area, so blood loss is a major concern. Option 1: Urine output is important, but the amount of blood loss takes precedence. Option 2: Most clients are given a prophylactic I.V. dose of antibiotic before surgery, so infection shouldn't be an issue. Option 4: Although intake of fluids and laboratory values are key indicators of potential problems, this isn't the most important option in this case.
NP: Implementing care
CN: Physiological integrity
CNS: Physiological adaptation
CL: Application

254 The nurse has just emptied the Hemovac of a client who underwent a mastectomy. What action should the nurse take when caring for a closed wound drainage system?
- ☐ 1. Clean the tip of the Hemovac with sterile water after emptying.
- ☐ 2. Wear sterile gloves to empty the container.
- ☐ 3. Empty the container every 24 hours.
- ☐ 4. Squeeze the container to create suction after emptying.

CORRECT ANSWER: 4
Suction needs to be created by squeezing the container after emptying. Option 1: The tip of the Hemovac doesn't need to be cleaned. Option 2: It isn't necessary to wear sterile gloves for this procedure; clean gloves are sufficient. Option 3: The container should be emptied every 8 hours.
NP: Implementing care
CN: Safe, effective care environment
CNS: Safety and infection control
CL: Application

255 A client who received a thyroidectomy 4 days ago is progressing well. The surgical wound edges are approximated. What type of wound drainage should the nurse expect?
- ☐ 1. Serosanguineous
- ☐ 2. Purulent
- ☐ 3. Serous
- ☐ 4. Sanguineous

CORRECT ANSWER: 3
Serous drainage is a clear yellow fluid that generally decreases as the days go by. Option 1: Serosanguineous drainage is noted for a few hours after surgery. Option 2: Purulent drainage is a sign of infection. Option 4: Sanguineous drainage is bright red and occurs immediately after surgery.
NP: Collecting data
CN: Physiological integrity
CNS: Physiological adaptation
CL: Knowledge

256 The physician has ordered a nutritional supplement to be given by gastrostomy tube to a client who has difficulty consuming enough calories orally. The nurse is teaching the client's caregiver how to administer the feeding. How does the nurse instruct the caregiver to hold the enteral feeding bag?
- ☐ 1. 2″ (5.1 cm) below the stomach
- ☐ 2. 4″ to 6″ (10 to 15 cm) below the stomach
- ☐ 3. 12″ to 18″ (30 to 46 cm) above the stomach
- ☐ 4. 30″ (76.2 cm) above the stomach

CORRECT ANSWER: 3
Holding the feeding bag 12″ to 18″ above the stomach allows gravity to infuse the feeding comfortably into the stomach. Options 1 and 2: Holding the enteral feeding bag 2″ or 4″ to 6″ below the stomach would enable the feeding to flow back into the bag. Option 4: Holding the feeding bag 30″ above the stomach could be too high and cause cramping from infusing too rapidly.
NP: Implementing care
CN: Physiological integrity
CNS: Physiological adaptation
CL: Knowledge

257 The nurse is interviewing a 17-year-old female client who is complaining of lower abdominal pain. Which question is most significant for the nurse to ask this client?
- ☐ 1. "When did the pain start?"
- ☐ 2. "When was your last menstrual period?"
- ☐ 3. "Is the pain consistent or intermittent?"
- ☐ 4. "Do you have vaginal discharge?"

CORRECT ANSWER: 2
"When was your last menstrual period?" is the most significant question because the client is in her childbearing years; treatment may have to be changed if she's pregnant. Options 1, 3, and 4: Although it's important to know when the pain started, how often it occurs, and if there is vaginal discharge, the nurse first needs to investigate the possibility of pregnancy.
NP: Collecting data
CN: Health promotion and maintenance
CNS: Growth and development through the life span
CL: Application

258 The nurse is providing client teaching to a 57-year-old male client who underwent a hemorrhoidectomy yesterday. The nurse is most likely to give instructions about:
☐ 1. sitz baths.
☐ 2. cleansing enemas.
☐ 3. catheter care.
☐ 4. bowel retraining.

CORRECT ANSWER: 1
A sitz bath allows the client to submerge the buttock area in a tub of tepid water to soothe, comfort, and clean the surgical area. Option 2: Cleansing enemas are generally given before the procedure, not after. Option 3: Catheter care is done on someone with an indwelling catheter. Option 4: Bowel retraining programs are implemented when the client is unable to have a bowel movement or has incontinent stools.
NP: Planning care
CN: Physiological integrity
CNS: Basic care and comfort
CL: Application

259 A client who underwent a hemorrhoidectomy yesterday is discharged to go home and the nurse is giving the client her discharge instructions. Which statement indicates that the client has a clear understanding of her instructions?
☐ 1. "I'll eat a low-fiber diet."
☐ 2. "I'll restrict fluids to 1,200 ml per day."
☐ 3. "I'll apply hot compresses to the rectum to soothe the pain."
☐ 4. "I'll take the stool softener daily and a sitz bath after every bowel movement."

CORRECT ANSWER: 4
Taking a stool softener daily eliminates constipation and thus prevents straining at the suture site. Taking a sitz bath keeps the rectal area clean and promotes healing. Option 1: A high-fiber diet is recommended to prevent constipation and straining at the suture site. Option 2: Restricting fluids isn't recommended because it can lead to constipation. Option 3: Applying hot compresses to the rectum isn't as effective as a sitz bath for relieving pain.
NP: Planning care
CN: Physiological integrity
CNS: Basic care and comfort
CL: Comprehension

260 A client is diagnosed with type 1 diabetes mellitus and the nurse is teaching him how to monitor his blood glucose level. The client tells the nurse that he doesn't see why he has to check his blood glucose at home because it's checked when he comes to the clinic. The best response the nurse can make is:
☐ 1. "Monitoring your blood glucose level enables you to monitor your hemoglobin (Hb) A_1C."
☐ 2. "Monitoring your blood glucose level enables you to check for ketones."
☐ 3. "Monitoring your blood glucose level enables you to take steps to control your diabetes."
☐ 4. "Monitoring your blood glucose level is necessary so that you can go to the emergency care facility if it's elevated."

CORRECT ANSWER: 3
Monitoring his blood glucose level at home enables the client to keep it within a normal range, thus decreasing some long-term complications. Option 1: The client wouldn't check his Hb A_1C because this is a blood test done by venipuncture that shows how well a diabetic client managed his blood glucose level over the previous 2 to 3 months. Option 2: The client would check for ketones in his urine, not his blood. Option 4: The client needs to be taught that it's important for him to monitor his blood glucose level at home and be told what complications could develop if he doesn't; monitoring isn't done just to detect when he should go to the emergency care facility.
NP: Planning care
CN: Physiological integrity
CNS: Reduction of risk potential
CL: Application

261 A 59-year-old male is admitted with a history of hypertension. His medications include hydrochlorothiazide (HydroDIURIL) and atenolol (Tenormin). Which statement indicates that the client needs more teaching about his medications?
- ☐ 1. "I usually call my physician if I need to take an over-the-counter (OTC) medication."
- ☐ 2. "I check my blood pressure twice per day and write it in my log."
- ☐ 3. "If it seems as if I've gained a few extra pounds during the week, I just take an extra water pill."
- ☐ 4. "I sit up slowly before I get up out of bed in the morning."

CORRECT ANSWER: 3
The client should be instructed to weigh himself once per week and report any weight gain to the physician; he should never alter his medication regimen unless instructed by the physician. Option 1: OTC medications should always be checked for compatibility with prescription drugs. Option 2: Checking his own blood pressure regularly gives a good clinical picture of how the client is responding to the medication regimen. Option 4: Atenolol can reduce blood pressure so the client should be told to sit up slowly when getting out of bed in the morning; hydrochlorothiazide can deplete the client's sodium and potassium levels, increasing the risk of arrhythmias.
NP: Implementing care
CN: Physiological integrity
CNS: Reduction of risk potential
CL: Application

262 A 65-year-old client is admitted for heart failure. The physician orders administration of furosemide (Lasix) daily. Which intervention should the nurse perform before administering the medication?
- ☐ 1. Check the client's weight.
- ☐ 2. Take the client's apical heart rate.
- ☐ 3. Ask the client whether he has any numbness.
- ☐ 4. Provide the client with extra fluids.

CORRECT ANSWER: 1
Heart failure develops because the heart is unable to move blood as quickly as it should. This causes decreased urine output and weight gain. Therefore, the client should be weighed daily. Option 2: Taking the client's apical heart rate isn't indicated before administering furosemide. Option 3: Clients may have numbness in the extremities due to increased peripheral edema, but this doesn't inhibit the administration of the medication. Option 4: The nurse doesn't provide the client with extra fluids because clients with heart failure are commonly on fluid restrictions.
NP: Planning care
CN: Health promotion and maintenance
CNS: Prevention and early detection of disease
CL: Application

263 A client is admitted with atrial fibrillation and the physician orders administration of digoxin (Lanoxin). What should the nurse do before administering the medication?
- ☐ 1. Check the client's apical pulse.
- ☐ 2. Check the client's blood pressure.
- ☐ 3. Check the client's capillary refill time.
- ☐ 4. Obtain an electrocardiogram (ECG).

CORRECT ANSWER: 1
The client's apical pulse should be checked before administering digoxin to make sure it's within normal parameters. If the apical pulse is less than 50 beats/minute, the digoxin should be withheld. Option 2: The client's blood pressure is a vital sign that should be checked, but the apical pulse is more significant when this drug is administered. Option 3: Capillary refill time is used to determine the perfusion of blood to the extremities such as the fingertips. Option 4: An ECG gives a picture of the electrical impulses of the heart but wouldn't be done every time the client receives a dose of digoxin.
NP: Planning care
CN: Health promotion and maintenance
CNS: Prevention and early detection of disease
CL: Application

264 The nurse is reviewing the histories of clients in her care. Which client is most at risk for complications during surgery or in the postoperative period?
☐ 1. 25-year-old female with rheumatoid arthritis
☐ 2. 45-year-old male with a history of intermittent alcohol abuse
☐ 3. 16-year-old male who has smoked two to three cigarettes per day for about 1 month
☐ 4. 75-year-old female diagnosed with diabetes at age 18

CORRECT ANSWER: 4
Diabetic clients are at greater risk for healing problems due to elevated levels of glucose over the years. Also, anesthesia sometimes takes longer to clear the system in an elderly client. Option 1: The 25-year-old female may be somewhat debilitated from rheumatoid arthritis, but she isn't at increased risk for complications while recovering from surgery. Option 2: The 45-year-old male could have some clotting problems during or after surgery secondary to long-term liver complications from the use of alcohol, but he isn't the most at risk. Option 3: Because of his young age and the fact that the 16-year-old male hasn't been smoking very long, he isn't the most at risk.
NP: Collecting data
CN: Physiological integrity
CNS: Reduction of risk potential
CL: Knowledge

265 A 40-year-old female underwent abdominal hysterectomy 6 hours ago. The client is somewhat sleepy but is requesting medication for pain relief. The physician has ordered morphine sulfate (Duramorph) for pain. What observation should the nurse be alert for?
☐ 1. Nausea before administering the medication
☐ 2. Nausea after administering the medication
☐ 3. Respiratory rate after administering the medication
☐ 4. Respiratory rate before administering the medication

CORRECT ANSWER: 4
A known adverse effect of the opiate morphine is respiratory depression. It's imperative that the nurse observe the client's respiratory status before administering the medication. Option 1: The nurse doesn't need to check for nausea before administering the medication because it isn't given orally and nausea isn't a contraindication for administration. Option 2: Morphine can cause nausea, which can be managed with an antiemetic, but checking for nausea is secondary to respiratory assessment. Option 3: The nurse shouldn't wait until after administering the medication to observe the client's respiratory status.
NP: Implementing care
CN: Physiological integrity
CNS: Pharmacological therapies
CL: Application

266 A client admitted for radiation therapy for bladder cancer is creating tension with the staff over having his therapy treatments done. What intervention should the nurse take in dealing with the manipulative client?
☐ 1. Don't give him any type of control.
☐ 2. Set limits and calmly respond to his undesirable behavior.
☐ 3. Let him have his way in all aspects of treatment.
☐ 4. Ask the physician to talk with him about his behavior.

CORRECT ANSWER: 2
The best approach is to give the client boundaries and allow him to vent his feelings. He can't be allowed, however, to manipulate the situation. Option 1: The client needs to feel he has some control; the nurse's goal is to meet his need for control by providing some alternative ways of coping. Option 3: The nurse can't allow the client to have complete control; she must be consistent and firm. Option 4: Asking the physician to talk to the client about his behavior won't help with the client's manipulation of the staff; the staff must deal with the client themselves.
NP: Implementing care
CN: Psychosocial integrity
CNS: Coping and adaptation
CL: Application

267 The nurse is caring for a 56-year-old man who underwent coronary artery bypass grafting yesterday. What are the two most dangerous potential postoperative complications in this case?
- [ ] 1. Shock and pulmonary embolus
- [ ] 2. Infection and fluid imbalance
- [ ] 3. Thrombophlebitis and pneumonia
- [ ] 4. Ileus and urine retention

CORRECT ANSWER: 1
Shock and pulmonary embolus are the most common complications following cardiovascular surgery. Option 2: Infections are more often seen in individuals who are obese, diabetic, or immunosuppressed. Fluid imbalance can occur from a massive loss of blood. Option 3: Thrombophlebitis and pneumonia can be seen in clients after bypass surgery, but this isn't the best answer. Option 4: An ileus is more common following GI surgery, and urine retention is more common following genitourinary surgery.
NP: Implementing care
CN: Physiological integrity
CNS: Reduction of risk potential
CL: Knowledge

268 A 45-year-old man is hospitalized with an inguinal hernia and the nurse is preparing to instruct the client about breathing exercises. Such breathing exercises are most effective if they're taught:
- [ ] 1. preoperatively.
- [ ] 2. 12 to 24 hours after surgery.
- [ ] 3. 2 to 3 days after surgery.
- [ ] 4. in the recovery area.

CORRECT ANSWER: 1
The client can learn best and practice if he's without postoperative pain or discomfort. Therefore, teaching breathing exercises preoperatively typically proves most beneficial. Options 2, 3, and 4: The client should do deep-breathing exercises after surgery to increase lung expansion, but it's better if these exercises are taught before surgery.
NP: Planning care
CN: Health promotion and maintenance
CNS: Prevention and early detection of disease
CL: Knowledge

269 The nurse is reviewing patient-care procedures. What is the simplest and most important infection-control technique to use before any procedure?
- [ ] 1. Use sterile water.
- [ ] 2. Use good hand washing.
- [ ] 3. Use sterile normal saline solution.
- [ ] 4. Change gloves.

CORRECT ANSWER: 2
Hand washing is the most important and simple infection-control technique the nurse can use before any procedure. Options 1 and 3: Using sterile water or normal saline solution isn't an infection-control technique. Option 4: Changing gloves may be needed but not before washing hands.
NP: Planning care
CN: Health promotion and maintenance
CNS: Prevention and early detection of disease
CL: Comprehension

270 The physician has ordered an X-ray to examine the spinal cord and vertebral canal after a client receives an injection of a contrast medium. The nurse teaches the client that this diagnostic procedure is called:
- [ ] 1. an arthrogram.
- [ ] 2. a computed tomography (CT) scan.
- [ ] 3. a spinal series.
- [ ] 4. a myelogram.

CORRECT ANSWER: 4
A myelogram is an X-ray of the spinal cord and vertebral column using a contrast medium. Option 1: An arthrogram is an X-ray of a joint. Option 2: A CT scan can be conducted with or without a contrast medium. Option 3: A spinal series is a noninvasive X-ray series of the spinal column that doesn't use a contrast medium.
NP: Planning care
CN: Health promotion and maintenance
CNS: Prevention and early detection of disease
CL: Knowledge

271 A 51-year-old client has undergone a total hip replacement on her right side. After surgery, the nurse should turn the client every:
☐ 1. 1 to 2 hours, from the unaffected side to the back.
☐ 2. 1 to 2 hours, from the affected side to the back.
☐ 3. 4 to 6 hours, from the unaffected side to the back.
☐ 4. 4 to 6 hours, from the affected side to the back.

CORRECT ANSWER: 1
The client should be turned at least every 2 hours and always from the unaffected side to the back. Option 2: The client should never be placed on the affected side. Options 3 and 4: Turning the client every 4 to 6 hours places her at greater risk for skin breakdown.
NP: Implementing care
CN: Physiological integrity
CNS: Reduction of risk potential
CL: Application

272 A 60-year-old male is admitted with possible chronic renal failure and the nurse observes the client having a seizure. What should the nurse do during the seizure?
☐ 1. Restrain the client.
☐ 2. Protect and observe the client.
☐ 3. Move the client to a safe environment.
☐ 4. Prevent the client from biting his tongue.

CORRECT ANSWER: 2
The nurse shouldn't interfere if the seizure is already in progress. Option 1: Don't restrain the client because this could cause more harm. Option 3: Don't move the client unless it's a life-or-death situation. Wait for the seizure to stop. Option 4: Don't place anything in the client's mouth to prevent him from biting his tongue because doing so could cause an airway obstruction.
NP: Implementing care
CN: Physiological integrity
CNS: Reduction of risk potential
CL: Application

273 A 22-year-old client has a spinal cord transection at the T4 level. The nurse can expect the client to:
☐ 1. be a paraplegic.
☐ 2. be a quadriplegic.
☐ 3. have autonomic dysreflexia.
☐ 4. have no deficits.

CORRECT ANSWER: 2
Spinal cord injuries at the T4 level affect all motor and sensory nerves below the level of injury and result in dysfunction of both arms, legs, bowel, and bladder. Option 1: Paraplegic injuries result from a lesion involving the thoracic, lumbar, or sacral region of the spinal cord. Option 3: Autonomic dysreflexia occurs because of a massive sympathetic discharge of stimuli from the autonomic nervous system. Option 4: An injury at the T4 level does cause deficits.
NP: Collecting data
CN: Physiological integrity
CNS: Physiological adaptation
CL: Application

274 A 42-year-old woman is diagnosed with multiple sclerosis (MS). Which drug does the nurse expect the physician to prescribe to treat the MS?
☐ 1. lorazepam (Ativan)
☐ 2. cyclosporine (Sandimmune)
☐ 3. atropine
☐ 4. interferon beta-1a (Avonex)

CORRECT ANSWER: 4
Interferon beta-1a is given for the treatment of MS. Option 1: Lorazepam is used in the treatment of anxiety disorders. Option 2: Cyclosporine is an immunosuppressant. Option 3: Atropine is an antispasmodic.
NP: Collecting data
CN: Physiological integrity
CNS: Pharmacological therapies
CL: Knowledge

275 A 58-year-old client with coronary artery disease is scheduled for coronary artery bypass graft surgery. What will the physician most likely order to help ensure adequate return of circulation to the client's heart and help prevent blood clots?
☐ 1. Antiembolism stockings
☐ 2. Ace bandages
☐ 3. Binders
☐ 4. Montgomery straps

CORRECT ANSWER: 1
Antiembolism stockings assist venous return and thus prevent blood clots. Option 2: Ace bandages can be used but may not provide firm and even pressure. Option 3: Binders are used to support a body part. Option 4: Montgomery straps are tape straps used for frequent dressing changes.
NP: Implementing care
CN: Health promotion and maintenance
CNS: Prevention and early detection of disease
CL: Knowledge

276 A 20-year-old woman underwent surgery to reverse an ileostomy. Which assessment is most important for the nurse in the postanesthetized client?
☐ 1. The client's dressing
☐ 2. The client's identification band
☐ 3. The client's blood pressure
☐ 4. The client's airway

CORRECT ANSWER: 4
Always remember to assess the client's ABCs (airway, breathing, and circulation). The greatest priority is to make sure the client has a patent airway and is breathing. Option 1: The client's dressing should be checked frequently but isn't the highest priority in this case. Option 2: The client's identification band should have been checked when the client was returned to the room. Option 3: Blood pressure readings are taken every 5 minutes in the recovery room, then less frequently as the client becomes stable.
NP: Collecting data
CN: Physiological integrity
CNS: Physiological adaptation
CL: Application

277 An 8-year-old child is brought to the hospital because she experienced a seizure. What test is performed to identify abnormal brain wave patterns?
☐ 1. Electrocardiogram (ECG)
☐ 2. Electromyogram (EMG)
☐ 3. Electroencephalogram (EEG)
☐ 4. Computed tomography (CT) scanning

CORRECT ANSWER: 3
An EEG records the electrical activity of the brain. Option 1: An ECG records the electrical activity of the heart. Option 2: An EMG records the contraction of the muscle as a result of electrical stimulation. Option 4: CT scanning provides a three-dimensional cross section of tissues.
NP: Planning care
CN: Health promotion and maintenance
CNS: Prevention and early detection of disease
CL: Comprehension

278 A 23-year-old female client has a brain injury due to a fall from a horse. The nurse observes a neurologic response known as decorticate posturing. What does this indicate?
☐ 1. There is damage to the cortex of the brain.
☐ 2. There is damage to the pituitary gland.
☐ 3. The client is alert and oriented.
☐ 4. The injury to the brain is resolving.

CORRECT ANSWER: 1
Decorticate posturing occurs because of an injury to the cortex of the brain; in this posture, the arms are adducted and flexed and the wrists and fingers are flexed and positioned on the chest. Option 2: Damage to the pituitary gland doesn't result in posturing. Option 3: If the client is alert and oriented, she doesn't exhibit posturing. Option 4: If the injury to the brain is resolving, the client doesn't exhibit posturing.
NP: Collecting data
CN: Physiological integrity
CNS: Physiological adaptation
CL: Comprehension

279 A 60-year-old male client has aphasia secondary to a cerebrovascular accident. In an effort to communicate with the client, the nurse may initiate all of the following except:
☐ 1. speaking loudly and quickly when facing him.
☐ 2. giving him time to respond to the questions.
☐ 3. asking the client one question at a time.
☐ 4. providing an orderly and relaxed environment for communication.

CORRECT ANSWER: 1
It isn't necessary to speak loudly. The nurse should speak with a moderate tone and at a normal pace. Options 2, 3, and 4: All of these techniques may be used to communicate with the client.
NP: Planning care
CN: Physiological integrity
CNS: Physiological adaptation
CL: Application

---

280 A 7-year-old girl is admitted to the hospital with a concussion after riding her bike into a ditch. Which of the following possible observations are the earliest signs of increased intracranial pressure (ICP)?
☐ 1. Headache and crying
☐ 2. Lethargy and decreased consciousness
☐ 3. Elevated blood pressure and bounding pulse
☐ 4. Loss of consciousness and pupil changes

CORRECT ANSWER: 2
The early signs of increased ICP are lethargy, decreased consciousness, and slow speech. Option 1: Headache isn't usually a sign of an increased ICP. Options 3 and 4: Elevated blood pressure, bounding pulse, loss of consciousness, and pupil changes are all late signs of increased ICP.
NP: Evaluating care
CN: Physiological integrity
CNS: Physiological adaptation
CL: Application

---

281 A 19-year-old male client is admitted for meningococcal meningitis. He tells the nurse that he doesn't know how he got meningitis. The best response the nurse can make is that meningococcal meningitis is transmitted:
☐ 1. by sexual contact.
☐ 2. through contact with blood.
☐ 3. through contact with urine.
☐ 4. through infected droplets.

CORRECT ANSWER: 4
Meningitis is transmitted by direct contact with infected droplets as well as with discharge from the nose and throat of carriers. Options 1, 2, and 3: Meningitis isn't transmitted by sexual contact or through contact with blood or urine.
NP: Implementing care
CN: Health promotion and maintenance
CNS: Prevention and early detection of disease
CL: Comprehension

---

282 A 55-year-old woman is admitted with a right-sided cerebrovascular accident. The nurse knows the client will require physical therapy and speech therapy in a rehabilitation facility. When should preparation for rehabilitation be initiated?
☐ 1. The day of discharge
☐ 2. The day the client has accepted her disabilities
☐ 3. The day after discharge from the acute care setting
☐ 4. The day of admission

CORRECT ANSWER: 4
Discharge planning begins the day of admission. The physician must write the order before the client can be sent to a rehabilitation facility. but the nurse needs to plan and be proactive. Option 1: On the day of discharge, the client should be transferred to the rehabilitation facility. Option 2: The nurse can't wait until the client has accepted her disabilities because there is no way to anticipate when that may be. Option 3: On the day after discharge, the client should already be in the rehabilitation facility.
NP: Planning care
CN: Safe, effective care environment
CNS: Coordinated care
CL: Application

283 A 78-year-old woman is undergoing treatment for emphysema. Which intervention can the nurse do to increase independence in the elderly client?
- ☐ 1. Give sleeping medications nightly to ensure a good night's rest.
- ☐ 2. Alter settings and routines as often as possible to provide a variety of changes.
- ☐ 3. Allow ample time to complete a task.
- ☐ 4. Provide all activities of daily living for the client.

CORRECT ANSWER: 3
The elderly client may move more slowly than other clients, so allow ample time to complete a task. Option 1: Give sleeping medications only as ordered. Giving sleeping medications nightly doesn't allow the client to develop her own routine (such as drinking warm milk and reading a book) for attaining optimal sleep at night. Option 2: Avoid changing settings and routines so the client can get used to her surroundings. Option 4: Allow the client to perform as much of her own care as possible because this fosters independence.
NP: Implementing care
CN: Health promotion and maintenance
CNS: Growth and development through the life span
CL: Application

284 An 87-year-old widow comes to the clinic for a physical examination. The nurse explains that normal aging in the musculoskeletal system of the elderly client might result in:
- ☐ 1. stronger bones.
- ☐ 2. easily movable joints.
- ☐ 3. atrophy of muscles.
- ☐ 4. erect posture.

CORRECT ANSWER: 3
A person's muscles atrophy as they age, decreasing strength, endurance, and agility. Option 1: An elderly person's bones become more brittle. Options 2 and 4: An elderly person's joints may become stiff and posture may begin to slump.
NP: Implementing care
CN: Health promotion and maintenance
CNS: Growth and development through the life span
CL: Application

285 A 43-year-old woman is undergoing treatment for colon cancer. The physician documents thrombocytopenia on the client's diagnosis list. What observations can the nurse expect?
- ☐ 1. Diarrhea
- ☐ 2. Thin, brittle hair
- ☐ 3. Bruises on the skin
- ☐ 4. Urinary urgency

CORRECT ANSWER: 3
With thrombocytopenia, there is an abnormal decrease in the number of blood platelets, which can result in bruises and bleeding. Option 1: The client may have constipation but usually not diarrhea. Option 2: Thin, brittle hair isn't a sign of thrombocytopenia but could be a sign of hypothyroidism. Option 4: Urinary urgency could be a sign of urinary tract infection but not thrombocytopenia.
NP: Collecting data
CN: Physiological integrity
CNS: Reduction of risk potential
CL: Application

286 A client receiving chemotherapy notices that her hair has begun to fall out. What is the nurse's best response regarding the client's hair loss?
- ☐ 1. "Don't worry about losing your hair. You can buy really nice wigs."
- ☐ 2. "We can use a scalp tourniquet before your treatment."
- ☐ 3. "Your hair will begin to grow again once therapy is completed."
- ☐ 4. "Your hair will never grow back."

CORRECT ANSWER: 3
The nurse should support and encourage the client during her therapy. Explain that hair growth will resume after she finishes therapy. Option 1: Don't minimize the client's feelings about losing her hair. Option 2: Tourniquets may be used, but depend on the agent used; this option may give the client false hope. Option 4: The client's hair will grow back but in a different texture.
NP: Implementing care
CN: Physiological integrity
CNS: Physiological adaptation
CL: Application

287 A physician orders radiation therapy to treat a 41-year-old cancer client. The client asks the nurse to explain the use of radiation. The nurse's teaching includes which explanation about radiation?
- ☐ 1. Radiation treatment involves using different drugs on tumor cells in different stages of cell growth.
- ☐ 2. Radiation treatment affects only the cancer cells.
- ☐ 3. Radiation treatment uses ionizing radiation to kill or limit the growth of cancer cells.
- ☐ 4. Radiation therapy injures the cell membrane but doesn't affect deoxyribonucleic acid (DNA).

CORRECT ANSWER: 3
Radiation therapy uses ionizing radiation to kill cancer cells and may be internal or external. Option 1: Chemotherapy, not radiation treatment, involves using different drugs on tumor cells in different stages of cell growth. Option 2: Radiation therapy affects normal cells as well as cancer cells. Option 4: Radiation injures both the cell membrane and DNA.
NP: Planning care
CN: Physiological integrity
CNS: Pharmacological therapies
CL: Knowledge

288 A 69-year-old client has developed skin problems secondary to radiation therapy. Which self-care measure is the nurse most likely to suggest?
- ☐ 1. Using over-the-counter antibiotic ointments on the area
- ☐ 2. Using extra soap when washing the affected area
- ☐ 3. Washing the area without soap and patting it dry
- ☐ 4. Spending extra time in the sun or heat to heal affected areas

CORRECT ANSWER: 3
Soap is irritating to the skin, so the area should be washed without soap and then patted dry. Option 1: Medicated solutions will cause irritation. Option 2: Using extra soap could cause additional drying of the skin and itching. Option 4: The client should avoid exposure to the sun and prolonged heat exposure.
NP: Planning care
CN: Safe, effective care environment
CNS: Safety and infection control
CL: Application

289 You're taking a health history from a 61-year-old woman during a routine examination. Which finding is a normal process of the genitourinary system in an aging client?
- ☐ 1. Increased bladder capacity
- ☐ 2. Increased gastric motility
- ☐ 3. Atrophy and drying of the vaginal canal
- ☐ 4. Spotty pigmentation on the abdomen

CORRECT ANSWER: 3
The vaginal canal undergoes changes, such as atrophy and drying, due to decreased production of estrogen and progesterone. Option 1: Bladder capacity decreases with aging. Option 2: Gastric motility decreases in the elderly client. Option 4: Spotty pigmentation is common but only on areas exposed to the sun, such as the hands and arms, not the abdomen.
NP: Collecting data
CN: Physiological integrity
CNS: Physiological adaptation
CL: Knowledge

290 The nurse is caring for a 29-year-old client who will undergo surgery to treat appendicitis. During preoperative teaching, the nurse explains that the purpose of general anesthesia is to:
- ☐ 1. depress the central nervous system, decrease muscle reflex activity, and cause loss of consciousness.
- ☐ 2. produce a loss of painful sensation in one area of the body.
- ☐ 3. reduce motor activity and decrease anxiety.
- ☐ 4. produce a state of analgesia, amnesia, and lack of awareness.

CORRECT ANSWER: 1
General anesthesia depresses the central nervous system, decreases muscle reflex activity, and causes a loss of consciousness. Option 2: Neuromuscular blocking agents produce a loss of sensation in a particular area of the body. Option 3: Neuroleptics reduce motor activity and decrease anxiety. Option 4: Regional anesthesia produces a state of analgesia and amnesia but not a loss of consciousness.
NP: Implementing care
CN: Physiological integrity
CNS: Physiological adaptation
CL: Knowledge

291 After exploratory laparotomy, a 51-year-old male client has just entered the postanesthesia care unit. How often should the nurse assess his vital signs?
☐ 1. Every hour
☐ 2. As needed
☐ 3. Every 30 minutes
☐ 4. Every 15 minutes

CORRECT ANSWER: 4
The nurse should check the postoperative client's vital signs every 15 minutes until they're stable. Options 1 and 2: Checking the client's vital signs hourly or as needed doesn't allow the nurse to assess for any sudden changes. Option 3: After vital signs are stable, the nurse should check them every 30 minutes.
NP: Implementing care
CN: Physiological integrity
CNS: Physiological adaptation
CL: Application

292 A 61-year-old female client has just undergone an exploratory laparotomy. The nurse realizes that the return of kidney function has occurred when the:
☐ 1. client's bladder becomes distended.
☐ 2. client's indwelling urinary catheter is removed.
☐ 3. client voids within 8 hours postoperatively.
☐ 4. client voids after 24 hours.

CORRECT ANSWER: 3
The client's kidney function should be normal within 8 hours after surgery. Option 1: A distended bladder only indicates that the bladder is full, not that kidney function has returned to normal. Option 2: Removing the client's indwelling urinary catheter doesn't confirm the return of urinary functioning. Option 4: If the client hasn't voided in 24 hours, a problem with kidney functioning may be present.
NP: Evaluating care
CN: Physiological integrity
CNS: Basic care and comfort
CL: Application

293 A 13-year-old male client has just undergone lumbar puncture to confirm a diagnosis of meningitis. Which intervention is part of the nursing care required for this client?
☐ 1. Limit the client's fluid intake.
☐ 2. Assist with range-of-motion exercises.
☐ 3. Keep the client flat for 12 to 24 hours.
☐ 4. Assess the client's vital signs only once and hold all analgesics.

CORRECT ANSWER: 3
Keeping the client flat allows the puncture area to seal. Option 1: The nurse needs to force, not limit, fluid intake. Option 2: Exercise should be avoided, but assessing sensation and movement is important. Option 4: Vital signs should be checked as per the protocol for the facility. Pain medications should be administered as needed.
NP: Implementing care
CN: Physiological integrity
CNS: Basic care and comfort
CL: Application

294 A 71-year-old male cancer client is scheduled to have a computed tomography (CT) scan. While teaching about the procedure, the nurse explains that a:
☐ 1. CT scan involves the use of one complete X-ray layer.
☐ 2. contrast medium is always used.
☐ 3. CT scan is done by a general X-ray apparatus.
☐ 4. CT scan is used to detect intracranial and spinal cord lesions.

CORRECT ANSWER: 4
A CT scan can be used to detect intracranial and spinal cord lesions. Option 1: A CT scan is done in successive layers by a narrow beam X-ray. Option 2: Contrast medium may or may not be used. Option 3: A CT scan computer collects information that is used to construct a picture of the brain or spinal column.
NP: Collecting data
CN: Safe, effective care environment
CNS: Coordinated care
CL: Knowledge

295 A 68-year-old man is hospitalized with suspected intracranial bleeding. The physician orders a test that uses a radiopaque substance to visualize cerebral vessels and detect an aneurysm or occlusion. What is this test called?
- ☐ 1. A brain scan
- ☐ 2. Ventriculography
- ☐ 3. Echoencephalography
- ☐ 4. Cerebral angiography

CORRECT ANSWER: 4
Cerebral angiography is done by X-ray after injecting a radiopaque substance into the cerebral circulation through an artery. Option 1: A brain scan is done using a radioactive isotope. Option 2: Ventriculography is done by injecting air into the ventricles. Option 3: Echoencephalography involves using ultrasound to detect a midline shift.
NP: Planning care
CN: Safe, effective care environment
CNS: Coordinated care
CL: Knowledge

296 A 24-year-old female is admitted to the intensive care unit and is unconscious due to a drug overdose. The nurse caring for her recognizes that the most important intervention is to:
- ☐ 1. keep the side rails of the bed up during morning care.
- ☐ 2. maintain a clear and patent airway.
- ☐ 3. provide nutritional support as needed.
- ☐ 4. use restraints at all times.

CORRECT ANSWER: 2
The nurse's most important intervention is to maintain a clear and patent airway because the client is unconscious. Option 1: The bed's side rails should be kept up at all times. Option 3: Nutritional support is important, but the airway must be protected first. Option 4: Restraints require an order from a physician and are used as a last resort.
NP: Implementing care
CN: Physiological integrity
CNS: Physiological adaptation
CL: Application

297 The nurse is caring for a 37-year-old male client who is unconscious following a boating accident. What intervention should the nurse include in the plan of care to prevent complications of immobility?
- ☐ 1. Apply lotions constantly to keep the skin moist.
- ☐ 2. Turn and reposition the client every 4 hours.
- ☐ 3. Perform passive range-of-motion (ROM) exercises every 4 hours.
- ☐ 4. Avoid the use of footboards and splints.

CORRECT ANSWER: 3
Passive ROM exercises need to be done for the client to prevent stiffness and contractures of the joints. Option 1: The client's skin should be kept moisturized, but not moist. Option 2: Turning and repositioning should be done every 2 hours. Option 4: Footboards and splints should be used to prevent footdrop and wristdrop.
NP: Planning care
CN: Physiological integrity
CNS: Reduction of risk potential
CL: Application

298 A 35-year-old male is admitted with a large intracranial abscess. What will the nurse expect to observe?
- ☐ 1. Decreased level of consciousness
- ☐ 2. Decreased pulse pressure
- ☐ 3. Regular respirations
- ☐ 4. Pupils that are equal, round, and reactive to light and accommodation

CORRECT ANSWER: 1
Decreased level of consciousness, confusion, and disorientation are all present with the increased intracranial pressure (ICP) that occurs in an intracranial abscess. Option 2: The client's pulse pressure would widen with increased ICP. Option 3: This client's respiratory status would be abnormal, possibly with Cheyne-Stokes respirations. Option 4: The client's pupils would be sluggish and ipsilateral with increased ICP.
NP: Implementing care
CN: Physiological integrity
CNS: Physiological adaptation
CL: Comprehension

299 A 16-year-old female client received a bone marrow transplant 5 days ago and has developed severe mucositis. The nurse explains to the client's parents that this is due to:
☐ 1. immunosuppression of the bone marrow.
☐ 2. infection.
☐ 3. poor mouth care.
☐ 4. overuse of antibiotics.

CORRECT ANSWER: 1
Mucositis is an inflammation of the mucous membranes due to immunosuppression of the white blood cells. It causes ulcerations in the mouth. Options 2, 3, and 4: Mucositis isn't an infection and isn't caused by poor mouth care or an overuse of antibiotics.
NP: Evaluating care
CN: Physiological integrity
CNS: Physiological adaptation
CL: Knowledge

---

300 The nurse is teaching a 35-year-old client how to perform proper mouth care after bone marrow transplantation. The client has developed mild stomatitis. What instruction does the nurse give the client?
☐ 1. Avoid antibiotic rinses.
☐ 2. Avoid the use of lemon and glycerin swabs.
☐ 3. Avoid the use of viscous lidocaine.
☐ 4. Perform mouth care every 8 hours.

CORRECT ANSWER: 2
Lemon and glycerin swabs can cause stinging and irritation to the oral mucosa. Options 1 and 3: Antibiotic rinses and viscous lidocaine are used to treat infections in the mouth and minimize pain. Option 4: Mouth care should be done every 2 hours.
NP: Planning care
CN: Physiological integrity
CNS: Basic care and comfort
CL: Application

---

301 A 25-year-old male sustained third-degree burns to the right upper extremity while trying to light a barbecue grill. The nurse explains that a third-degree degree burn involves the:
☐ 1. epidermis only.
☐ 2. epidermis and dermis.
☐ 3. skin layers and nerve endings.
☐ 4. skin layers, nerve endings, muscles, tendons, and bone.

CORRECT ANSWER: 3
A third-degree burn involves all of the skin layers and the nerve endings. Option 1: First-degree burns involve only the epidermis. Option 2: Second-degree burns affect the epidermis and dermis. Option 4: Fourth-degree burns involve all skin layers, nerve endings, muscles, tendons, and bone.
NP: Evaluating care
CN: Physiological integrity
CNS: Physiological adaptation
CL: Knowledge

---

302 A 45-year-old male client is brought to the hospital with smoke inhalation due to a house fire. The nurse's major intervention for this client is to:
☐ 1. check the oral mucus membranes.
☐ 2. check for any burned areas.
☐ 3. obtain a medical history.
☐ 4. ensure a patent airway.

CORRECT ANSWER: 4
The nurse's top priority is to make sure the airway is open and the client is breathing. Options 1 and 2: Checking the mucous membranes and burned areas is important but not as vital as maintaining a patent airway. Option 3: Obtaining a medical history can be pursued after ensuring a patent airway.
NP: Evaluating care
CN: Physiological integrity
CNS: Physiological adaptation
CL: Application

303 A 23-year-old male client comes to the clinic with foot pain. The nurse observes that he walks with an outward rotation. The nurse recognizes this as:
☐ 1. equines.
☐ 2. varus.
☐ 3. calcaneus.
☐ 4. valgus.

CORRECT ANSWER: 4
Valgus means that the client walks with the inner ankles in an outward rotation. Option 1: Equinus means that the client walks with the ankles in a downward rotation such as walking on the toes. Option 2: Varus means that the client walks with the ankles facing inward and the bottoms of the feet facing each other. Option 3: Calcaneus means that the client walks on the heels.
NP: Evaluating care
CN: Physiological integrity
CNS: Physiological adaptation
CL: Comprehension

304 The nurse is taking an apical pulse during the routine examination of a pediatric client. The apical pulse is obtained by:
☐ 1. listening over the apex of the heart.
☐ 2. using only auscultation.
☐ 3. using only the bell of the stethoscope.
☐ 4. listening for 30 seconds.

CORRECT ANSWER: 1
The apical pulse is assessed over the apex of the heart at the 4th and 5th left intercostal space at the midclavicular line. Options 2, 3, and 4: The apical pulse is determined by auscultation and palpation, using the bell and diaphragm of the stethoscope, and listening for at least 60 seconds.
NP: Implementing care
CN: Physiological integrity
CNS: Physiological adaptation
CL: Application

305 A 43-year-old female is admitted to the hospital with an aneurysm. She is currently taking oral propranolol (Inderal). The nurse knows that this drug is given to:
☐ 1. control pain.
☐ 2. decrease the pressure of the blood coming from the heart.
☐ 3. decrease the contractions of the heart.
☐ 4. prevent possible infection.

CORRECT ANSWER: 2
Propranolol decreases the pressure of the blood coming from the heart to the affected vessel. Options 1, 3, and 4: Propranolol hydrochloride doesn't control pain, decrease heart contractions, or prevent infection.
NP: Implementing care
CN: Physiological integrity
CNS: Pharmacological therapies
CL: Knowledge

306 A 58-year-old male is admitted to the hospital with a hypertensive crisis. The nurse on duty recognizes that this:
☐ 1. is a medical emergency.
☐ 2. will resolve on its own in a day or so.
☐ 3. won't affect any of the internal organs.
☐ 4. is a very common condition.

CORRECT ANSWER: 1
A hypertensive crisis is a medical emergency that requires immediate intervention. Options 2 and 3: A hypertensive crisis causes damage to internal organs if not treated quickly. Option 4: A hypertensive crisis is an uncommon condition.
NP: Evaluating care
CN: Physiological integrity
CNS: Physiological adaptation
CL: Knowledge

307 A 45-year-old man is diagnosed with hypertension and the physician prescribes hydrochlorothiazide. The nurse explains that this medication:
☐ 1. blocks angiotensin-converting enzymes (ACE) in the lungs.
☐ 2. inhibits the movement of calcium ions across the heart muscle.
☐ 3. blocks epinephrine and norepinephrine.
☐ 4. increases renal excretion of sodium and water.

CORRECT ANSWER: 4
Hydrochlorothiazide works by increasing renal excretion, thus decreasing the client's total fluid volume. Option 1: ACE inhibitors block angiotensin. Option 2: Calcium channel blockers inhibit the movement of calcium ions across cardiac muscle. Option 3: Beta-adrenergic blockers block epinephrine and norepinephrine, causing vasoconstriction.
NP: Implementing care
CN: Physiological integrity
CNS: Pharmacological therapies
CL: Knowledge

308 A nurse is monitoring a 17-year-old male client who is receiving a blood transfusion for volume replacement. The client complains of itching about 20 minutes after the infusion begins. The nurse should:
☐ 1. stop the infusion immediately.
☐ 2. call the physician immediately.
☐ 3. give the client diphenhydramine (Benadryl) and continue the infusion.
☐ 4. do nothing because the time has passed when a reaction could have occurred.

CORRECT ANSWER: 1
Itching is a sign of an adverse reaction, so the nurse should stop the infusion immediately. Option 2: The physician should be called, but only after the infusion has been stopped and the client is assessed. Option 3: Don't give any medications without a physician's order. Option 4: Reactions can occur up to several hours after the infusion.
NP: Implementing care
CNS: Physiological integrity
CNS: Reduction of risk potential
CL: Application

309 A 73-year-old female client is about to receive a blood transfusion in the treatment of severe anemia. She asks the nurse how long the procedure will take. The nurse explains that the treatment takes:
☐ 1. 8 hours.
☐ 2. at least 12 hours.
☐ 3. at least 24 hours.
☐ 4. 4 hours.

CORRECT ANSWER: 4
The American Association of Blood Banks recommends that blood or blood components should be transfused within 4 hours. If they aren't, they should be divided and stored appropriately in the blood bank. Options 1, 2, and 3: Any length of time over 4 hours would compromise the integrity of the transfusion components.
NP: Implementing care
CN: Safe, effective care environment
CNS: Safety and infection control
CL: Application

310 A 61-year-old male client is receiving a blood transfusion to treat volume depletion that occurred during recent surgery. What solution can safely be given during a blood transfusion?
☐ 1. Normal saline solution
☐ 2. Any I.V. antibiotic
☐ 3. Total parenteral nutrition
☐ 4. Half-normal saline solution

CORRECT ANSWER: 1
The only solution that can safely be given during a blood transfusion is normal saline solution. Options 2, 3, and 4: If given to a client during a blood transfusion, these solutions could cause incompatibility reactions.
NP: Implementing care
CN: Safe, effective care environment
CNS: Safety and infection control
CL: Application

311 A 31-year-old male is undergoing a routine examination at a community clinic. The nurse notes that the client is employed as a roofer and has a moderate sunburn in various stages of healing. While teaching the client about skin cancer, the nurse informs the client that:
☐ 1. sunlight is most intense around midday.
☐ 2. sunscreen is needed only if it's bright and sunny.
☐ 3. the best time to bask in the sun is between 11 a.m. and 3 p.m.
☐ 4. sunscreen should be used 30 minutes before sun exposure only.

CORRECT ANSWER: 1
The most intense rays of the sun are found around midday, making the client most susceptible to skin damage. Option 2: Sunscreen should be used to protect the skin even on cloudy and overcast days. Option 3: Ultraviolet rays from the sun are most powerful between 11 a.m. and 3 p.m. Option 4: Sunscreen should be applied 30 minutes before sun exposure and every 60 to 80 minutes thereafter.
NP: Planning care
CN: Physiological integrity
CNS: Reduction of risk potential
CL: Application

312 A 19-year-old woman comes to the clinic with dark red lesions on her hands, wrist, and waistline. She has scratched several of the lesions until they're open and bleeding. The nurse instructs the client to try pressing on the itchy lesions. What is the rationale for this intervention?
☐ 1. Pressing the skin spreads beneficial microorganisms.
☐ 2. Pressing is suggested before scratching.
☐ 3. Pressing the skin promotes breaks in the skin.
☐ 4. Pressing the skin stimulates nerve endings.

CORRECT ANSWER: 4
Pressing the skin stimulates nerve endings and can reduce the sensation of itching. Option 1: Scratching (not pressing) the skin spreads microorganisms and opens portals of entry for bacteria. Option 2: Scratching isn't recommended at all. Option 3: Pressing the skin doesn't promote breaks in the skin.
NP: Evaluating care
CN: Physiological integrity
CNS: Physiological adaptation
CL: Application

313 A client is admitted to the hospital with a pressure ulcer. She asks the nurse if it will heal within 3 days because she has a wedding to attend. The nurse should respond based on the fact that pressure ulcers:
☐ 1. heal quickly once treatment is started.
☐ 2. heal very slowly.
☐ 3. heal quickly and don't require surgical intervention.
☐ 4. appear like normal skin so they shouldn't interfere with her plans.

CORRECT ANSWER: 2
Pressure ulcers are caused by increased venous congestion and poor circulation; they heal very slowly. Options 1 and 3: Pressure ulcers don't heal quickly and sometimes require surgical intervention. Option 4: The skin becomes very dry and rough, losing its resiliency.
NP: Implementing care
CN: Physiological integrity
CNS: Physiological adaptation
CL: Knowledge

314 A 54-year-old male is having an anaphylactic reaction to a bee sting. Which medication does the nurse expect to administer first during the anaphylactic reaction?
☐ 1. Corticosteroids
☐ 2. epinephrine
☐ 3. Vasopressors
☐ 4. albuterol

CORRECT ANSWER: 2
Epinephrine dilates the bronchioles, increases heart contractions, and constricts blood vessels. It's the first line of defense during an anaphylactic reaction. Option 1: Corticosteroids are given to bring about an anti-inflammatory effect. Option 3: Vasopressors increase a client's blood pressure. Option 4: Albuterol is given for bronchoconstriction.
NP: Implementing care
CN: Physiological integrity
CNS: Pharmacological therapies
CL: Application

315 The nurse is caring for a 42-year-old male client with tuberculosis (TB). At what time should the nurse wear a particulate respirator mask?
- [ ] 1. During the client's coughing episode
- [ ] 2. When in the same room with the client
- [ ] 3. For 24 hours after medications are started
- [ ] 4. Until the Mantoux test is negative

CORRECT ANSWER: 2
A particulate respirator must be worn before entering the room and should be worn at all times while the nurse is with the client. Option 1: The nurse should wear the mask at all times, not just during a coughing episode. Option 3: Waiting 24 hours after the medications are started places the nurse at risk for exposure. Option 4: The Mantoux test shows exposure to TB; therefore, it's never negative after exposure, even after the client is well.
NP: Implementing care
CN: Physiological integrity
CNS: Reduction of risk potential
CL: Application

316 A 24-year-old woman is diagnosed with cytomegalovirus (CMV) and the nurse is teaching the client about the disease. What information will the nurse provide about CMV?
- [ ] 1. CMV affects only the skin.
- [ ] 2. CMV is transmitted by sexual intercourse or kissing.
- [ ] 3. CMV affects healthy individuals more frequently.
- [ ] 4. CMV is manifested by weight gain and constipation.

CORRECT ANSWER: 2
CMV is part of the herpesvirus family and invades the salivary glands. It's transmitted by sexual intercourse or kissing. Option 1: CMV can affect the brain, lung, retina, liver, and GI tract. Option 3: CMV affects individuals who are immunocompromised. Option 4: CMV is manifested by weight loss, fever, diarrhea, and malaise.
NP: Planning care
CN: Health promotion and maintenance
CNS: Prevention and early detection of disease
CL: Application

317 The physician has prescribed ganciclovir sodium (Cytovene) for a client diagnosed with cytomegalovirus (CMV). After teaching, what statement indicates that the client understands the use of ganciclovir?
- [ ] 1. "I know the physician gave me this medicine because I have a cold."
- [ ] 2. "I thought this medicine is only given to pregnant women."
- [ ] 3. "Maintenance therapy with ganciclovir is required to prevent a relapse."
- [ ] 4. "Ganciclovir is the only drug to treat CMV."

CORRECT ANSWER: 3
Ganciclovir is given to prevent a relapse of CMV. Option 1: A virus from the herpes family causes CMV; symptoms may mimic those of the common cold. Option 2: Ganciclovir isn't only given to pregnant women; in fact, it's in pregnancy risk category C (animal studies have shown an adverse effect on fetuses yet the benefits of therapy may outweigh the risks). Option 4: Foscarnet sodium (Foscavir) is also used in the treatment of CMV.
NP: Planning care
CN: Physiological integrity
CNS: Pharmacological therapies
CL: Application

318 A 41-year-old male is admitted to the hospital with acquired immunodeficiency syndrome. His appetite is poor and he's dehydrated. What nursing intervention should be provided?
- [ ] 1. Leave ice cubes at the bedside.
- [ ] 2. Decrease fluid intake to increase food intake.
- [ ] 3. Discourage the use of hard candy and chewing gum.
- [ ] 4. Encourage the client to drink fluids of his choice between meals.

CORRECT ANSWER: 4
The client should be encouraged to drink fluids between meals to increase his fluid intake and reduce dehydration. Option 1: Leaving ice cubes at the bedside doesn't provide for adequate hydration. Option 2: Fluids shouldn't be decreased to increase food intake. Likewise, extra fluids shouldn't be given with meals as this may curb the appetite. Option 3: Encourage the client to use hard candy and gum to stimulate saliva production and moisten the mouth.
NP: Implementing care
CN: Physiological integrity
CNS: Basic care and comfort
CL: Application

319 A 4-year-old female is diagnosed with a lateral curving deviation of the spine. The nurse explains to the client's parents that this condition is known as:
☐ 1. kyphosis.
☐ 2. scoliosis.
☐ 3. lordosis.
☐ 4. crepitus.

CORRECT ANSWER: 2
Scoliosis is a lateral curvature of the spine. Option 1: Kyphosis is a roundness of the thoracic spinal curvature. Option 3: Lordosis is an exaggeration of the lumbar spine. Option 4: Crepitus is a grating sensation or sound.
NP: Evaluating care
CN: Health promotion and maintenance
CNS: Growth and development through the life span
CL: Application

320 A 5-year-old male is diagnosed with a deformity known as subluxation. The nurse explains to the client's parents that this condition is:
☐ 1. an injury to the ligaments surrounding a joint.
☐ 2. an abnormal shortening of muscles.
☐ 3. a partial separation of an articular surface.
☐ 4. the contraction of a hinge joint.

CORRECT ANSWER: 3
A subluxation is a partial separation of an articular surface. Option 1: An injury to the ligaments is called a sprain. Option 2: An abnormal shortening of muscles is a contracture. Option 4: The contraction of a hinge joint is a dislocation.
NP: Implementing care
CN: Health promotion and maintenance
CNS: Prevention and early detection of disease
CL: Knowledge

321 A 12-year-old male client dislocated his shoulder while riding his skateboard. The physician plans to perform a manual manipulation of the joint. The nurse knows that this procedure is known as:
☐ 1. an open reduction.
☐ 2. diarthrosis.
☐ 3. a locomotion disorder.
☐ 4. a closed reduction.

CORRECT ANSWER: 4
A closed reduction is done by manipulating a dislocated bone back into the joint without surgical intervention. Option 1: Open reduction requires surgery. Option 2: Diarthrosis is a term that indicates joints are freely movable. Option 3: A locomotion disorder means that the client's ability to move is affected.
NP: Implementing care
CN: Physiological integrity
CNS: Physiological adaptation
CL: Application

322 The nurse is caring for a client who sustained multiple fractures in an automobile accident. A fracture that has splintering on one side and bending on the other is known as:
☐ 1. an impacted fracture.
☐ 2. a greenstick fracture.
☐ 3. a spiral fracture.
☐ 4. a comminuted fracture.

CORRECT ANSWER: 2
A greenstick fracture causes splintering of the bone on one side and bending of the other side. Option 1: An impacted fracture occurs when one portion of bone is forced into another. Option 3: A spiral fracture twists around the shaft of the bone. Option 4: A comminuted fracture has splintered bone in many fragments.
NP: Implementing care
CN: Health promotion and maintenance
CNS: Prevention and early detection of disease
CL: Knowledge

323 A 61-year-old male client has had gout for a long time and has developed nodules. While teaching the client, the nurse explains that these nodules are called:
☐ 1. cysts.
☐ 2. stones.
☐ 3. tophi.
☐ 4. calculi.

CORRECT ANSWER: 3
Tophi are nodular deposits of sodium urate crystals. They can occur as a result of chronic gout. Option 1: A cyst is a closed sac or pouch with a definite wall that contains fluid, semi-fluid, or solid material. Option 2: Stones are abnormal concretions usually composed of mineral salts. Option 4: Calculi is another name for stones formed by mineral salts.
NP: Evaluating care
CN: Physiological integrity
CNS: Reduction of risk potential
CL: Comprehension

324 The nurse is teaching a 51-year-old female client who was diagnosed with gout. Which diet is recommended for a client with gout?
☐ 1. Regular diet
☐ 2. Low-salt diet
☐ 3. Low-cholesterol diet
☐ 4. Low-purine diet

CORRECT ANSWER: 4
A low-purine diet is recommended so the client avoids such items as liver, sardines, sweetbreads, and meat gravy, which may precipitate the production of urate crystals. Options 1, 2, and 3: Regular, low-salt, and low-cholesterol diets aren't recommended for clients with gout because they may not eliminate those specific foods that precipitate the production of urate crystals.
NP: Implementing care
CN: Physiological integrity
CNS: Basic care and comfort
CL: Knowledge

325 The nurse is collecting a health history from a 63-year-old man who may have gout. What joint is most often affected in the client with gout?
☐ 1. Great toe
☐ 2. Wrist
☐ 3. Ankle
☐ 4. Knee

CORRECT ANSWER: 1
The great toe is most commonly affected in clients with gout. Options 2, 3, and 4: Gout can affect other joints but most commonly affects the great toe.
NP: Implementing care
CN: Physiological integrity
CNS: Reduction of risk potential
CL: Knowledge

326 A 58-year-old male client is diagnosed with gout. In teaching about the disorder, the nurse tells the client that gout is caused by:
☐ 1. low uric acid levels.
☐ 2. ineffective purine metabolism.
☐ 3. painful joints.
☐ 4. decreased fluid intake.

CORRECT ANSWER: 2
Gout is a metabolic disease caused by ineffective purine metabolism; the etiology of gout is unknown. Option 1: Gout is characterized by hyperuricemia, not low uric acid levels. Option 3: Joint pain doesn't cause gout, although the disorder is marked by joint inflammation. Option 4: Decreased fluid intake doesn't cause gout but may reduce urate stone formation.
NP: Implementing care
CN: Health promotion and maintenance
CNS: Prevention and early detection of disease
CL: Comprehension

327 A nurse practitioner in a community clinic is examining a client who may have Lyme disease. Which of the following organisms is the carrier of Lyme disease?
☐ 1. Black flies
☐ 2. Deer ticks
☐ 3. White mice
☐ 4. Mosquitoes

CORRECT ANSWER: 2
Lyme disease is caused by infection with spirochetes carried by deer ticks. Options 1, 3, and 4: Black flies, white mice, and mosquitoes aren't carriers of Lyme disease.
NP: Implementing care
CN: Health promotion and maintenance
CNS: Prevention and early detection of disease
CL: Knowledge

328 The school nurse is preparing to remove a deer tick from a third-grade student following a field trip to a grassy local park. The proper way to remove a tick from a client is:
☐ 1. with tweezers.
☐ 2. with cotton applicators.
☐ 3. by applying turpentine to the tick's mouthparts.
☐ 4. by applying ice to the entire area.

CORRECT ANSWER: 1
Tweezers enable the nurse to grasp the tick firmly without squeezing its body. Option 2: Cotton applicators don't allow the nurse to properly grasp the tick. Option 3: The nurse can't apply turpentine to the tick's head because the mouthparts are embedded in the client's skin. Option 4: Applying ice wouldn't remove the tick.
NP: Implementing care
CN: Health promotion and maintenance
CNS: Prevention and early detection of disease
CL: Application

329 A 19-year-old male client recently underwent an above-the-knee amputation of his left leg. The client is complaining of pain in his left lower extremity. The nurse administers the ordered analgesic but recognizes that the client's pain:
☐ 1. is normal postoperative pain.
☐ 2. is phantom limb pain.
☐ 3. is due to an infection.
☐ 4. may be relieved by another analgesic.

CORRECT ANSWER: 2
Phantom limb pain is a sensation that there is pain, soreness, and stiffness in an amputated limb; it may also feel like the missing limb is twisted or crushed. The pathophysiology is unknown and can occur immediately or 2 to 3 months after amputation. It's more common in above-the-knee amputations than in all other amputations. Options 1, 3, and 4: The client's pain isn't normal postoperative pain, pain due to an infection, or pain that is resolved by administering more of the ordered analgesic or another analgesic.
NP: Implementing care
CN: Physiological integrity
CNS: Physiological adaptation
CL: Comprehension

330 The nurse is reviewing the health history of a client diagnosed with osteomyelitis. Of the following statements, which characterizes this disease?
☐ 1. It's a viral infection.
☐ 2. It occurs in the muscles and ligaments.
☐ 3. It's an inflammation of the bone and bone marrow.
☐ 4. It's a mild, nondebilitating problem.

CORRECT ANSWER: 3
Osteomyelitis is an inflammation of the bone and bone marrow. Option 1: Osteomyelitis isn't a viral infection; rather it's caused by the bacteria *Staphylococcus aureus*, *Pseudomonas*, or *Escherichia coli*. Option 2: Osteomyelitis occurs in the bone and bone marrow, not the muscles or ligaments. Option 4: Osteomyelitis is a chronic, disabling disease.
NP: Implementing care
CN: Health promotion and maintenance
CNS: Prevention and early detection of disease
CL: Comprehension

331 The nurse is caring for a 60-year-old female client diagnosed with osteomyelitis. Which treatment is most effective for clients with osteomyelitis?
☐ 1. Surgery
☐ 2. Analgesics and rest
☐ 3. Using sterile techniques
☐ 4. Drugs specific to the organism

CORRECT ANSWER: 4
A client with osteomyelitis is treated with drugs that are effective against the particular causative organism. Option 1: Surgery isn't used to treat osteomyelitis. Option 2: Analgesics and rest help with pain but aren't effective against the infection. Option 3: Aseptic technique should be used for dressing changes.
NP: Implementing care
CN: Health promotion and maintenance
CNS: Prevention and early detection of disease
CL: Comprehension

332 A 63-year-old male is being examined in a family health center. The nurse observes that her client can't hear the ticking of his watch. This may indicate a problem with which cranial nerve?
- [ ] 1. I
- [ ] 2. VI
- [ ] 3. VIII
- [ ] 4. XI

CORRECT ANSWER: 3
Cranial nerve VIII (acoustic) affects hearing. Option 1: Cranial nerve I (olfactory) affects smell. Option 2: Cranial nerve VI (abducens) affects outward eye movement. Option 4: Cranial nerve XI (spinal accessory) affects the ability to move the shoulders.
NP: Evaluating care
CN: Health promotion and maintenance
CNS: Prevention and early detection of disease
CL: Application

---

333 The nurse is reviewing the functions of the body's nervous system and is aware that the parasympathetic system:
- [ ] 1. conducts impulses.
- [ ] 2. connects the central nervous system to the skin.
- [ ] 3. maintains vital body functions.
- [ ] 4. releases chemical regulators.

CORRECT ANSWER: 3
The parasympathetic system conserves, restores, and maintains vital body functions. Options 1 and 4: Neurotransmitters conduct impulses and release chemical regulators. Option 2: The somatic nervous system connects the central nervous system to the skin and skeletal muscles.
NP: Evaluating care
CN: Health promotion and maintenance
CNS: Prevention and early detection of disease
CL: Comprehension

---

334 The nurse is performing neurologic checks. Which test is used to observe the client's level of responsiveness and consciousness?
- [ ] 1. Ranchos Los Amigos scale
- [ ] 2. Aldrete score
- [ ] 3. Functional Independence Measure (FIM) scores
- [ ] 4. Glasgow Coma Scale

CORRECT ANSWER: 4
The Glasgow Coma Scale is used to determine the client's level of consciousness. Option 1: The Ranchos Los Amigos scale is used to assess cognitive levels. Option 2: The Aldrete score is a postanesthetic recovery score. Option 3: FIM scores describe functional mobility levels.
NP: Evaluating care
CN: Health promotion and maintenance
CNS: Prevention and early detection of disease
CL: Knowledge

---

335 A 38-year-old male client is admitted following a possible cerebrovascular accident (CVA). Which sign or symptom is exhibited by a client with a right-sided CVA?
- [ ] 1. Paralysis on the right side
- [ ] 2. Paralysis on the left side
- [ ] 3. Paralysis of both lower extremities
- [ ] 4. Communication deficits

CORRECT ANSWER: 2
A right-sided CVA affects the left side of the body. Options 1 and 3: A right-sided CVA doesn't cause paralysis on the right side or paralysis of both lower extremities. Option 4: Clients who have left-sided CVAs generally have communication problems.
NP: Evaluating care
CN: Physiological integrity
CNS: Physiological adaptation
CL: Comprehension

---

336 The nurse is caring for a client diagnosed with Huntington's disease. Which information is included when teaching members of the client's family?
- [ ] 1. There is no genetic influence.
- [ ] 2. Huntington's disease can be cured if treated early.
- [ ] 3. Huntington's disease commonly causes a facial tic.
- [ ] 4. The client won't have difficulty with his speech, swallowing, or chewing.

CORRECT ANSWER: 3
Huntington's disease is characterized by involuntary, purposeless movement of all muscles. Option 1: Huntington's disease is characterized by a genetic marker. Option 2: There is no cure for Huntington's disease. Option 4: Clients with Huntington's disease have difficulty with speech, swallowing, and chewing.
NP: Implementing care
CN: Health promotion and maintenance
CNS: Prevention and early detection of disease
CL: Comprehension

337 A 25-year-old male client is being discharged following treatment for hepatitis A. During discharge teaching, the nurse reminds the client that the transmission of hepatitis A is aided by:
☐ 1. coughing without covering the mouth.
☐ 2. exposure to bird droppings.
☐ 3. mosquitoes.
☐ 4. poor hand-washing habits.

CORRECT ANSWER: 4
Hepatitis A is transmitted through contaminated food and water. Proper hand washing decreases the spread of this infection. Options 1, 2, and 3: Hepatitis A isn't transmitted by coughing or by exposure to bird droppings or mosquitoes.
NP: Implementing care
CN: Health promotion and maintenance
CNS: Prevention and early detection of disease
CL: Application

338 A 28-year-old male enters a community health clinic exhibiting signs of possible hepatitis. What types of hepatitis have vaccines available?
☐ 1. Hepatitis A and B
☐ 2. Hepatitis C and D
☐ 3. Hepatitis D and E
☐ 4. Hepatitis C and E

CORRECT ANSWER: 1
Hepatitis A and B have vaccines and immune globulin available for treatment. Options 2, 3, and 4: Vaccines for prevention or cure aren't available for hepatitis C, D, or E.
NP: Implementing care
CN: Health promotion and maintenance
CNS: Prevention and early detection of disease
CL: Comprehension

339 A client in a community health clinic is undergoing treatment for hepatitis C. While teaching the client, the nurse explains that hepatitis C:
☐ 1. is fatal within 6 weeks.
☐ 2. is linked to cirrhosis of the liver.
☐ 3. has an incubation period of up to 1 year.
☐ 4. accounts for 10% of all hepatitis cases.

CORRECT ANSWER: 2
Hepatitis C may progress to cirrhosis and liver cancer. Option 1: Hepatitis C isn't fatal but becomes chronic in 50% of cases. Option 3: The incubation period can range from 15 to 160 days. Option 4: Hepatitis C accounts for about 20% of all cases of hepatitis.
NP: Implementing care
CN: Health promotion and maintenance
CNS: Prevention and early detection of disease
CL: Comprehension

340 A 31-year-old female client is undergoing treatment for hepatitis in a family health facility. During teaching, the nurse explains that treatment for hepatitis focuses on:
☐ 1. increasing the client's activity.
☐ 2. increasing the client's fiber intake.
☐ 3. rest and early detection of complications.
☐ 4. increasing the client's intake of iron.

CORRECT ANSWER: 3
Detecting complications is the focus for a client with hepatitis. Option 1: Rest is important for this client. Option 2: Diet modification is used to decrease the amount of bile released for digestion, but increasing the client's fiber intake doesn't decrease the release of bile. Option 4: The client's iron intake should be reduced.
NP: Implementing care
CN: Health promotion and maintenance
CNS: Prevention and early detection of disease
CL: Application

341 A 27-year-old male client is admitted to the hospital with possible hepatitis. Which test is used to check for hepatitis E?
☐ 1. None available
☐ 2. Anti-HAV
☐ 3. Anti-HCV
☐ 4. HBsAg or HBeAg

CORRECT ANSWER: 1
There is no test to check for hepatitis E. Option 2: The anti-HAV test is used to detect hepatitis A. Option 3: The anti-HCV test is used to detect hepatitis C. Option 4: The HBsAg or HBeAg test is used to detect hepatitis B.
NP: Implementing care
CN: Health promotion and maintenance
CNS: Prevention and early detection of disease
CL: Knowledge

342 A 43-year-old female client is admitted to the hospital with cholelithiasis. The nurse caring for clients with gallstones recognizes that:
- ☐ 1. all gallstones cause increasing and persistent pain.
- ☐ 2. some gallstones can pass out of the gallbladder into the duodenum.
- ☐ 3. gallstones remain in the gallbladder.
- ☐ 4. poor diet is the cause of stone formation.

CORRECT ANSWER: 2
Gallstones can pass out of the gallbladder and into the duodenum without the client knowing it. Option 1: Not all gallstones cause pain; some pain is intermittent. Option 3: Gallstones can migrate to the cystic or common bile ducts. Option 4: The cause of stone formation is unknown.
NP: Implementing care
CN: Health promotion and maintenance
CNS: Prevention and early detection of disease
CL: Application

343 A nurse practitioner in a small city is teaching a group of Girl Scouts about eating disorders. Which condition may be a complication of anorexia nervosa or bulimia?
- ☐ 1. Acne
- ☐ 2. Arrhythmias
- ☐ 3. Obesity
- ☐ 4. Chlamydia

CORRECT ANSWER: 2
With eating disorders, electrolyte imbalances can occur, leading to abnormal heart rhythms. Option 1: Acne is a dermatologic disorder and not a complication of anorexia nervosa or bulimia. Options 3: Clients with anorexia nervosa and bulimia lose weight; they don't generally gain weight and progress to obesity. Option 4: Chlamydia is a sexually transmitted disease.
NP: Planning care
CN: Health promotion and maintenance
CNS: Prevention and early detection of disease
CL: Comprehension

344 A client is admitted to the hospital for a total hip replacement. During preoperative teaching, the nurse explains that the purpose of surgical skin preparation is to:
- ☐ 1. remove the dermis.
- ☐ 2. sterilize the skin.
- ☐ 3. clean the skin and inhibit bacterial growth.
- ☐ 4. increase the number of microorganisms.

CORRECT ANSWER: 3
The purpose of surgical skin preparation is to inhibit bacterial growth. Option 1: The dermis is the second layer of skin and isn't removed before surgery. Option 2: The skin can't be sterilized. Option 4: The goal is to decrease the number of microorganisms, not increase them.
NP: Evaluating care
CN: Safe, effective care environment
CNS: Safety and infection control
CL: Implementing care

345 A 71-year-old male client is told that he needs to increase his daily potassium intake. Which food should the nurse recommend?
- ☐ 1. Bananas
- ☐ 2. Oatmeal
- ☐ 3. Carrots
- ☐ 4. Corn chips

CORRECT ANSWER: 1
Bananas are high in potassium. Option 2: Oatmeal is high in fiber. Option 3: Carrots are high in beta-carotene. Option 4: Corn chips aren't high in potassium.
NP: Implementing care
CN: Health promotion and maintenance
CNS: Prevention and early detection of disease
CL: Comprehension

346 The nurse is caring for a client admitted with a possible myocardial infarction (MI). Which diagnostic test is used to rule out an MI?
☐ 1. Complete blood count
☐ 2. Cardiac biopsy
☐ 3. Arterial blood gas analysis
☐ 4. Cardiac enzyme analysis

CORRECT ANSWER: 4
Certain isoenzymes come only from myocardial cells and are released when the cells are damaged. Creatine kinase (CK) and its isoenzyme CK-MB are the least specific enzymes analyzed in acute MI. These cardiac enzymes should be tested in relation to the time of onset of chest discomfort or other symptoms to rule out MI. Options 1, 2, and 3: Blood counts, blood gases, and cardiac biopsies don't play large roles in ruling out an MI.
NP: Evaluating care
CN: Physiological adaptation
CNS: Reduction of risk potential
CL: Comprehension

347 A 70-year-old female client is diagnosed with heart failure. The nurse explains that the main goal of her treatment is to:
☐ 1. determine right ventricular function.
☐ 2. treat heart congestion.
☐ 3. decrease the workload of the right ventricle.
☐ 4. improve circulation to the coronary arteries.

CORRECT ANSWER: 4
The primary treatment goal for the client with heart failure is to improve circulation to the coronary arteries, which provide oxygen to the heart. Options 1, 2, and 3: Reaching this goal involves determining left ventricular function, reducing lung congestion, and decreasing the workload of the left ventricle.
NP: Implementing care
CN: Health promotion and maintenance
CNS: Prevention and early detection of disease
CL: Application

348 The nurse is caring for a 59-year-old male client diagnosed with myocardial infarction (MI). The purpose of giving nitrates to a client who has had an MI is to:
☐ 1. relieve pain.
☐ 2. dilate coronary arteries.
☐ 3. relieve headaches caused by other medications.
☐ 4. calm and relax the client.

CORRECT ANSWER: 2
Nitrates dilate the arteries, allowing oxygen to continue flowing to the heart. Option 1: Nitrates don't relieve pain. Option 3: Nitrates can cause headaches. Option 4: Nitrates don't calm or relax the client.
NP: Implementing care
CN: Physiological integrity
CNS: Pharmacological therapies
CL: Application

349 The nurse is taking a 49-year-old woman's health history when the client mentions that her heart sometimes seems to race. Which condition is a life-threatening cardiac rhythm?
☐ 1. Ventricular fibrillation
☐ 2. Ventricular tachycardia
☐ 3. Premature ventricular contractions
☐ 4. Premature atrial contractions

CORRECT ANSWER: 1
Ventricular fibrillation is a life-threatening arrhythmia. It occurs when the ventricle fibrillates, failing to fully contract and pump blood through the heart. Option 2: Ventricular tachycardia is a rapid ventricular beat and isn't life-threatening. Option 3: Premature ventricular contractions are early ventricular beats and aren't life-threatening. Option 4: Premature atrial contractions are premature atrial beats and aren't life-threatening.
NP: Evaluating care
CN: Health promotion and prevention
CNS: Prevention and early detection of disease
CL: Knowledge

350 The nurse palpates the pulse of a 41-year-old woman who is about to receive I.V. chemotherapy. The client's heart rate is 52 beats/minute. Which term describes this finding?
☐ 1. Complete heart block
☐ 2. Asystole
☐ 3. Tachycardia
☐ 4. Bradycardia

CORRECT ANSWER: 4
Bradycardia is a heart rate of less than 60 beats/minute. Option 1: Complete heart block can't be detected by palpating the pulse. Option 2: Asystole is the absence of heartbeats. Option 3: Tachycardia is a heart rate that's greater than 100 beats/minute.
NP: Evaluating care
CN: Health promotion and maintenance
CNS: Prevention and early detection of disease
CL: Knowledge

---

351 A 56-year-old woman is having a consultation about possible circulation problems. Which information should the nurse provide about varicosities?
☐ 1. They're located only in the calves of the lower extremities.
☐ 2. They become stronger as the walls of the vessels hold the blood.
☐ 3. They're caused by incompetent arteries.
☐ 4. They're veins that have become dilated and lost their elasticity.

CORRECT ANSWER: 4
Varicosities are veins that become dilated and lose their elasticity. Options 1 and 2: They can be located in the lower extremities, esophagus, or rectal area. Option 3: They're incompetent valves and veins, not arteries.
NP: Evaluating care
CN: Physiological integrity
CNS: Reduction of risk potential
CL: Application

---

352 A 27-year-old teacher who reports a number of GI-related symptoms is diagnosed with ulcerative colitis. The nurse explains that ulcerative colitis is:
☐ 1. an inflammatory disease of the colon and rectum.
☐ 2. an inflammatory disease of the GI tract from the mouth to the anus.
☐ 3. a disease that forms outpouches in the large colon.
☐ 4. an opening between two or more body structures or spaces.

CORRECT ANSWER: 1
Ulcerative colitis is an inflammatory disease that affects the mucosal lining of the colon and rectum. Option 2: Crohn's disease commonly affects the entire GI tract, from the mouth to the anus. Option 3: Diverticulitis causes outpouching in the large colon. Option 4: A fistula is an opening between two or more body structures.
NP: Implementing care
CN: Physiological integrity
CNS: Physiological adaptation
CL: Application

---

353 A 19-year-old male client comes to the clinic complaining of having painful urination for 4 days. The nurse documents this finding as:
☐ 1. hematuria.
☐ 2. oliguria.
☐ 3. dysuria.
☐ 4. polyuria.

CORRECT ANSWER: 3
Dysuria is painful urination. Option 1: Hematuria is blood in the urine. Option 2: Oliguria is decreased urine output. Option 4: Polyuria is increased urine output.
NP: Collecting data
CN: Health promotion and maintenance
CNS: Prevention and early detection of disease
CL: Application

---

354 The nurse is caring for a 15-year-old female who recently suffered a spinal cord injury from a fall during cheerleading practice. How often should this bedridden client be turned?
☐ 1. Once daily
☐ 2. Every 4 hours while awake
☐ 3. Every shift
☐ 4. Every 2 hours even if she's sleeping

CORRECT ANSWER: 4
Turning the client every 2 hours even if she's sleeping prevents skin breakdown and promotes circulation. Options 1, 2, and 3: Any turning routine that keeps the client in a position for more than 2 hours decreases circulation and leads to skin breakdown.
NP: Planning care
CN: Health promotion and maintenance
CNS: Prevention and early detection of disease
CL: Knowledge

355 A 33-year-old construction worker is brought to the emergency department after sustaining a severe blow to the head. What is the most important indicator of neurologic status change?
- ☐ 1. Vital signs
- ☐ 2. Motor function
- ☐ 3. Level of consciousness (LOC)
- ☐ 4. Pupil reaction

CORRECT ANSWER: 3
The client's LOC is the most obvious sign of a neurologic change. Options 1, 2, and 4: The client's vital signs, motor function, and pupil reaction may change as well, but these aren't as direct indicators as LOC.
NP: Evaluating care
CN: Physiological integrity
CNS: Physiological adaptation
CL: Comprehension

356 A 35-year-old male client who experienced a seizure while driving is admitted with a brain tumor. His intracranial pressure (ICP) is elevated. What intervention can the nurse do to prevent a further increase in ICP?
- ☐ 1. Put a radio next to the client's bed that plays his favorite music.
- ☐ 2. Encourage the client to bear down when having a bowel movement.
- ☐ 3. Administer antiemetics to prevent vomiting.
- ☐ 4. Encourage the client to do coughing and deep-breathing exercises while on bed rest.

CORRECT ANSWER: 3
Changes in the intrathoracic cavity during vomiting can cause an increase in ICP. Option 1: Keeping the client in a quiet area and making him comfortable would be more beneficial for lowering ICP. Options 2 and 4: Having the client bear down during bowel evacuation and doing coughing and deep-breathing exercises would increase ICP.
NP: Implementing care
CN: Physiological integrity
CNS: Reduction of risk potential
CL: Application

357 A 51-year-old male client is admitted with a brain tumor. He requires medication to decrease swelling and increase urine output. What medication will the physician most likely choose?
- ☐ 1. furosemide (Lasix)
- ☐ 2. dexamethasone (Decadron)
- ☐ 3. mannitol (Osmitrol)
- ☐ 4. phenytoin (Dilantin)

CORRECT ANSWER: 3
Mannitol is a hyperosmotic agent used to decrease cerebral edema and increase urine output. Option 1: Furosemide is a diuretic but it doesn't decrease cerebral edema. Option 2: Dexamethasone is an anti-inflammatory medication that decreases cerebral edema. Option 4: Phenytoin is an anticonvulsant medication.
NP: Evaluating care
CN: Physiological integrity
CNS: Pharmacological therapies
CL: Knowledge

358 The nurse is caring for a client with a brain tumor who hasn't responded well to conventional treatment for increased intracranial pressure (ICP). The physician has decided to initiate barbiturate therapy. The nurse recognizes that this:
- ☐ 1. treatment increases metabolic demands and protects the brain from further injury.
- ☐ 2. type of medication is given orally.
- ☐ 3. treatment requires monitoring of the client's ICP and serum barbiturate levels.
- ☐ 4. treatment rarely necessitates ventilator support.

CORRECT ANSWER: 3
Barbiturate therapy necessitates close monitoring because there is a possibility of electrocardiogram changes, respiratory problems, and changes in heart rate. Option 1: Barbiturate therapy decreases metabolic demands. Option 2: Barbiturate therapy is given I.V. Option 4: Barbiturate therapy is initiated to induce coma, thus necessitating ventilator support.
NP: Implementing care
CN: Physiological integrity
CNS: Physiological adaptation
CL: Knowledge

359 A client is admitted to the emergency department with a head injury and hyperthermia following an automobile accident. The nurse may observe all of the following except:
☐ 1. temperature of 105° F (40.6° C) or higher.
☐ 2. seizure activity.
☐ 3. increased urine output.
☐ 4. pale, cool skin.

CORRECT ANSWER: 3
The client may have a decreased urine output because of fluids lost with perspiration. Options 1, 2, and 4: The client's skin is most likely flushed and warm. Hyperthermia can cause temperature elevation, seizure activity due to swelling in the brain, and decreased level of consciousness. All of these changes are due to a malfunction in the hypothalamus.
NP: Evaluating care
CN: Physiological integrity
CNS: Physiological adaptation
CL: Comprehension

360 The nurse is caring for a 21-year-old man whose vision is impaired following corrective surgery for multiple fractures sustained in a motorcycle accident. Which is the most appropriate intervention the nurse can do when caring for a client with impaired sight?
☐ 1. Allow the client to walk around the room finding things on his own.
☐ 2. Take the client's arm and guide him in the direction he needs to go.
☐ 3. Rearrange items in different locations to provide more of a challenge.
☐ 4. Offer explanations to the client and tell him what to expect.

CORRECT ANSWER: 4
Offering the client an explanation and telling him what to expect will gain his confidence. Option 1: Provide the client with information about where things are located to promote confidence and safety. Option 2: Allow the client to hold your arm when guiding him. Option 3: Keep an item in the same location so the client knows its location and can get it himself.
NP: Planning care
CN: Safe, effective care environment
CNS: Safety and infection control
CL: Application

361 A 21-year-old client whose hearing is severely impaired is scheduled for surgery in 2 hours. The nurse is preparing to administer preoperative medication. Which is the best method of communicating with this client?
☐ 1. Speak loudly.
☐ 2. Speak slowly and don't overaccentuate words.
☐ 3. Attract the client's attention by tapping on her shoulder.
☐ 4. Use gestures.

CORRECT ANSWER: 2
The nurse should face the client and speak slowly so the client can detect what she's saying by reading lips. Option 1: Speaking loudly isn't the best method for communicating. Option 3: You can gently tap the client on the shoulder but you may startle her. Option 4: Using gestures won't necessarily improve the client's understanding.
NP: Planning care
CN: Safe, effective care environment
CNS: Safety and infection control
CL: Application

362 A male client is admitted with a severe migraine. The nurse has administered the prescribed pain medication to him. What is the next nursing intervention?
☐ 1. Provide a quiet, dark environment.
☐ 2. Teach exercise techniques.
☐ 3. Encourage the client to discuss details about his migraine.
☐ 4. Encourage the client to identify what precipitated the migraine.

CORRECT ANSWER: 1
After the medication has been given, it's important to decrease outside stimulus. Option 2: Teaching exercise techniques isn't appropriate at this time. Options 3 and 4: After the pain abates, encourage the client to discuss details about his migraine and what precipitated it.
NP: Implementing care
CN: Safe, effective care environment
CNS: Coordinated care
CL: Application

363 An 18-year-old college student is admitted and diagnosed with meningitis. While observing the client, what is a positive sign of meningeal irritation that the nurse should recognize?
- ☐ 1. Headache on one side of the head
- ☐ 2. Kernig's sign
- ☐ 3. Nausea
- ☐ 4. Pruritus

CORRECT ANSWER: 2

Kernig's sign is a classic sign of meningeal irritation. It's a contraction or pain in the hamstring muscle when the leg is extended as the hip is flexed. Option 1: A headache that affects one side of the head is a sign of a migraine headache. Options 3 and 4: Nausea and pruritus can be present with meningitis but aren't classic symptoms.

NP: Evaluating care
CN: Physiological integrity
CNS: Physiological adaptation
CL: Knowledge

---

364 A client is hospitalized after suffering a cerebrovascular accident. He exhibits left hemiplegia and homonymous hemianopsia. When planning his care, the nurse should:
- ☐ 1. approach him on the left side.
- ☐ 2. place his belongings on the affected side.
- ☐ 3. gradually teach him to compensate by scanning.
- ☐ 4. increase the stimulus in his surroundings.

CORRECT ANSWER: 3

Scanning, which teaches the client to slowly view things within his field of vision, enables the client to view his entire surroundings. Option 1: Approach the client on his unaffected side so he can see you. Option 2: Place his belongings on his unaffected side so that he can see them. Option 4: Reducing excessive stimuli will benefit this client.

NP: Planning care
CN: Physiological integrity
CNS: Physiological adaptation
CL: Application

---

365 A 61-year-old male client is diagnosed with Parkinson's disease. The physician prescribes levodopa. The client's wife asks the nurse what the medicine does. Which is the nurse's best response?
- ☐ 1. "Levodopa prevents anorexia, nausea, vomiting, and postural hypotension."
- ☐ 2. "Levodopa decreases a client's anxiety."
- ☐ 3. "Levodopa increases a client's sense of well-being."
- ☐ 4. "Levodopa relieves tremors and rigidity."

CORRECT ANSWER: 4

Levodopa increases the levels of dopamine in the brain, thus relieving tremors and rigidity. Option 1: Anorexia, vomiting, hypotension, hallucinations, and vivid dreams are potential adverse effects of levodopa. Precautions are taken when administering to clients with renal disease. Option 2: Levodopa doesn't decrease anxiety; it may actually increase anxiety. Option 3: Levodopa can cause vivid dreams rather than promote a feeling of well-being.

NP: Implementing care
CN: Physiological integrity
CNS: Physiological adaptation
CL: Knowledge

---

366 A 14-year-old male client is admitted with an exacerbation of multiple sclerosis (MS). What symptoms can the nurse expect to observe?
- ☐ 1. Varied and multiple symptoms depending on the site of the lesions
- ☐ 2. Photophobia with normal visual acuity
- ☐ 3. Improved motor function on one side
- ☐ 4. Rapid speech

CORRECT ANSWER: 1

Symptoms of MS vary depending on the sites of the lesions. Options 2, 3, and 4: The client's vision may be impaired, motor function is affected, and speech patterns tend to be slowed.

NP: Evaluating care
CN: Physiological integrity
CNS: Physiological adaptation
CL: Application

367 The nurse is caring for a 65-year-old man admitted with myasthenia gravis. Which surgical procedure is the physician most likely to consider as a mode of treatment?
- ☐ 1. Thyroidectomy
- ☐ 2. Parathyroidectomy
- ☐ 3. Splenectomy
- ☐ 4. Thymectomy

CORRECT ANSWER: 4
The thymus gland produces acetylcholine receptor antibodies, which have been linked to increasing symptoms of myasthenia gravis. Therefore, a thymectomy can cause remission of the disease, especially in clients with tumor or hyperplasia of the thymus gland. Options 1, 2, and 3: The thyroid gland, parathyroid gland, and spleen aren't linked to symptoms of myasthenia gravis. Therefore, surgery to remove the thyroid gland, parathyroid gland, or spleen isn't useful.
NP: Planning care
CN: Safe, effective care environment
CNS: Coordinated care
CL: Comprehension

368 The nurse is caring for a 69-year-old woman with myasthenia gravis. Which signs or symptoms might the nurse observe that are related to the disease?
- ☐ 1. Excessive salivation
- ☐ 2. Normal voice frequency
- ☐ 3. Pill-rolling tremor
- ☐ 4. Decreased muscle strength

CORRECT ANSWER: 4
Myasthenia gravis causes decreased muscle strength and weakness. Option 1: Adverse reactions to the drugs used to treat myasthenia gravis cause excessive salivation, but these symptoms aren't from the disorder itself. Option 2: The client often experiences hoarseness. Option 3: Pill-rolling tremors are indicative of Parkinson's disease.
NP: Evaluating care
CN: Physiological integrity
CNS: Physiological adaptation
CL: Comprehension

369 The physician has prescribed an anti-cholinesterase for a client with myasthenia gravis. Which nursing intervention is most appropriate with the administration of this type of medication?
- ☐ 1. Alter the times of administration each day.
- ☐ 2. Give the drug with milk and crackers.
- ☐ 3. Leave the medication with the client to take in private.
- ☐ 4. Don't give the drug with meals.

CORRECT ANSWER: 2
Giving an anticholinesterase with milk and crackers decreases the client's risk of GI upset. Option 1: Give the medication at the same time every day to maintain the drug level in the blood. Option 3: Stay with the client while he takes his medication so you can provide support and check the gag reflex. Option 4: The peak effect of the medication should coincide with meals; give it approximately 30 minutes before meals.
NP: Implementing care
CN: Physiological integrity
CNS: Pharmacological therapies
CL: Application

370 A client is experiencing a cholinergic crisis. What should the nurse have available for treatment?
- ☐ 1. tensilon and emergency equipment
- ☐ 2. atropine sulfate and emergency equipment
- ☐ 3. Additional anticholinergic medications and emergency equipment
- ☐ 4. Corticosteroids and emergency equipment

CORRECT ANSWER: 2
Atropine sulfate counteracts the effects of excessive amounts of anticholinesterase drugs. Option 1: Tensilon potentiates the symptoms of a cholinergic crisis. Option 3: Additional anticholinergic drugs also potentiate the cholinergic crisis. Option 4: Corticosteroids suppress the autoimmune response and don't reverse the effects of anticholinergics.
NP: Planning care
CN: Physiological integrity
CNS: Pharmacological therapies
CL: Application

371 A 53-year-old male is brought to the emergency department with a spinal cord injury stemming from a cliff-diving accident. The nurse knows that spinal shock:
☐ 1. can occur several days after the injury.
☐ 2. can occur several months after the injury.
☐ 3. can occur immediately.
☐ 4. won't occur if the spine is immobilized immediately after the injury.

CORRECT ANSWER: 3
Spinal or neurogenic shock is a sudden depression of the reflex activity in the spinal cord below the level of injury. Blood pressure and heart rate fall and the body parts below the level of the lesion are paralyzed and have no sensation. It can occur immediately upon injury to the cord or if the cord is transected and can last for 3 to 6 weeks. Options 1, 2, and 4: It doesn't occur several days or months after the injury and immobilizing the spine after the injury doesn't prevent it from occurring.
NP: Evaluating care
CN: Physiological integrity
CNS: Reduction of risk potential
CL: Comprehension

372 The nurse is caring for a 17-year-old female client who has an incomplete spinal cord injury at level C6. When mobilization is initiated, what equipment will the physician most likely use to stabilize the neck?
☐ 1. Cervical tongs
☐ 2. Stryker frame
☐ 3. Gardner-Wells tongs
☐ 4. Halo

CORRECT ANSWER: 4
A halo stabilizes the neck and permits early mobilization. Options 1 and 3: Cervical tongs and Gardner-Wells tongs have ropes running from the tongs to weights. These devices don't permit early mobilization. Option 2: The Stryker frame is a horizontal turning frame; it helps turn the client but isn't used for immobilization.
NP: Planning care
CN: Physiological integrity
CNS: Physiological adaptation
CL: Knowledge

373 A 19-year-old male client has just undergone a stapedectomy. Which postoperative instruction is most crucial for a good outcome?
☐ 1. Perform deep-breathing exercises every 4 hours.
☐ 2. Shampoo hair every 2 days.
☐ 3. Blow nose and cough daily.
☐ 4. Sneeze with an open mouth.

CORRECT ANSWER: 4
After stapedectomy (surgical replacement of the stapes to correct hearing loss), the nurse should instruct the client to sneeze with an open mouth to reduce pressure in the oropharyngeal area. Option 1: Deep-breathing exercises are recommended every 2 hours, not every 4 hours. Option 2: The client should avoid shampooing the hair until it's approved by the physician. Option 3: The client shouldn't blow his nose or cough because this could create added pressure on the surgical site.
NP: Planning care
CN: Physiological integrity
CNS: Reduction of risk potential
CL: Application

374 A 60-year-old man is admitted for eye surgery. The nursing plan of care indicates applying an eye shield at night. This is done to:
☐ 1. prevent bright light from shining in the affected eye.
☐ 2. decrease swelling.
☐ 3. prevent injury to the affected eye during sleep.
☐ 4. reduce pain.

CORRECT ANSWER: 3
An eye shield decreases the possibility of a foreign object injuring the affected eye. Option 1: The shield doesn't necessarily keep out light; many shields have tiny holes covering them, enabling light to come through. Options 2 and 4: It doesn't decrease swelling or eliminate pain.
NP: Planning care
CN: Physiological integrity
CNS: Reduction of risk potential
CL: Application

375 The nurse is instructing a client who recently had a pacemaker inserted. Which statement indicates that additional teaching is needed?
- ☐ 1. "I'll check my pulse daily for 1 minute."
- ☐ 2. "I'll wear loose-fitting clothing around the area of the pacemaker for comfort."
- ☐ 3. "If my pulse rate decreases, I'll write it in my ledger and tell my physician on the next visit."
- ☐ 4. "I'll make sure to carry an identification card or wear a bracelet with my pacemaker information on it."

CORRECT ANSWER: 3
The client should tell his physician immediately if his pulse rate decreases. Option 1: The client should check his pulse rate daily for 1 minute. Option 2: It's necessary to wear loose-fitting clothing around the area of the pacemaker for comfort. Option 4: The client should carry an identification card or wear a bracelet with the pacemaker information on it.
NP: Planning care
CN: Physiological integrity
CNS: Physiological adaptation
CL: Application

376 A 38-year-old woman is admitted with thrombophlebitis and is started on heparin therapy. The nursing plan of care calls for which medication as an antidote?
- ☐ 1. warfarin
- ☐ 2. protamine sulfate
- ☐ 3. Vitamin K
- ☐ 4. aspirin

CORRECT ANSWER: 2
Protamine sulfate counteracts the effects of heparin. Option 1: Warfarin (Coumadin) is another oral anticoagulant that blocks prothrombin syntheses by interfering with vitamin K and shouldn't be used concurrently. Option 3: Vitamin K counteracts the effects of warfarin. Option 4: Aspirin could increase bleeding.
NP: Planning care
CN: Physiological integrity
CNS: Pharmacological therapies
CL: Knowledge

377 A 70-year-old female cancer client with iron deficiency anemia is on iron replacement therapy. Which of the following statements indicates the client has a good understanding of her medication?
- ☐ 1. "I'll always take the iron supplement on an empty stomach."
- ☐ 2. "I'll take the iron supplement with orange juice."
- ☐ 3. "When I take liquid iron, I should swish it in my mouth before swallowing."
- ☐ 4. "Iron supplements might change my stools to a light color."

CORRECT ANSWER: 2
Taking iron with orange juice or ascorbic acid enhances iron absorption. Option 1: Taking iron after meals or a snack decreases GI upset. Option 3: Liquid iron can permanently stain the teeth. The client should use a straw to swallow the liquid. Option 4: Iron will turn the client's stools dark and tarry.
NP: Planning care
CN: Physiological integrity
CNS: Pharmacological therapies
CL: Knowledge

378 A 19-year-old I.V. heroine user is diagnosed with acquired immunodeficiency syndrome (AIDS). Which statement indicates that the client needs more teaching?
- ☐ 1. "The primary goal of my treatment is to treat opportunistic infections and provide supportive care."
- ☐ 2. "There is no cure for AIDS, but taking my medication will prevent it from spreading."
- ☐ 3. "AIDS is transmitted through sexual contact, contaminated blood, or blood products."
- ☐ 4. "AIDS may be transmitted from an infected woman to a child in utero."

CORRECT ANSWER: 2
Taking the medications as prescribed won't prevent the spread of this disease. Options 1, 3, and 4 are all correct statements that indicate the client's understanding about his disorder.
NP: Implementing care
CN: Physiological integrity
CNS: Pharmacological therapies
CL: Knowledge

379 A 20-year-old postoperative lung transplant client is undergoing insertion of a chest tube necessitated by pneumothorax. The nursing care in this case includes:
☐ 1. maintaining a chest tube that is attached to an underwater drainage system that allows the escape of air or fluid.
☐ 2. milking the chest tube every 4 hours.
☐ 3. emptying the drainage system every 8 hours.
☐ 4. positioning the client on the unaffected side or abdomen.

CORRECT ANSWER: 1
The underwater drainage system in a chest tube creates a seal, which prevents the reflux of air into the chest. The nurse needs to maintain the chest tube to ensure proper functioning. Option 2: The chest tube should be milked every 2 hours. Option 3: The closed-drainage system isn't emptied, but the amount of drainage is noted and documented on the output record. Option 4: The client's position should be changed frequently to promote comfort and drainage.
NP: Planning care
CN: Physiological integrity
CNS: Physiological adaptation
CL: Application

380 The nurse is caring for a client following chest tube insertion to relieve a pneumothorax. Which intervention is included in the plan of care?
☐ 1. Milk the chest tube and drainage tube every 8 hours.
☐ 2. Notify the physician if the drainage is blood-tinged.
☐ 3. Observe the fluid in the water seal drainage for rising on expiration and falling on inspiration.
☐ 4. Place petroleum gauze at the bedside for emergency purposes.

CORRECT ANSWER: 4
Petroleum gauze can be used to temporarily seal the chest tube site in an emergency. Option 1: Chest tubes and drainage tubes should be milked every 1 to 2 hours. Option 2: Drainage may be bloody or could be air. The nurse needs to document what she observes. Option 3: The fluid level within the water seal rises on inspiration and falls on expiration.
NP: Planning care
CN: Physiological integrity
CNS: Physiological adaptation
CL: Application

381 The nurse is suctioning the tracheostomy tube of a postoperative cancer client. Which situation indicates that the nurse isn't performing the procedure correctly?
☐ 1. The client is in semi-Fowler's or high Fowler's position.
☐ 2. The nurse uses sterile gloves and normal saline solution.
☐ 3. The nurse covers the thumb control when inserting the catheter.
☐ 4. The entire suctioning procedure takes less than 10 seconds.

CORRECT ANSWER: 3
The thumb control allows the catheter to suction. The nurse should suction when inserting the catheter. Options 1: The client should be in semi-Fowler's or high Fowler's position. Option 2: The nurse should use sterile gloves and normal saline solution. Option 4: The procedure shouldn't take longer than 10 seconds.
NP: Implementing care
CN: Safe, effective care environment
CNS: Safety and infection control
CL: Application

382 The nurse is caring for a client with possible bowel obstruction and has just inserted a nasogastric (NG) tube to relieve abdominal distention. Which method should be used to check the placement of the tube?
☐ 1. Checking aspirate with a Hemocult card
☐ 2. Testing to see if the client is able to speak
☐ 3. Checking the pH of fluid aspirated from the tube
☐ 4. Placing the end of the NG tube in water and watching for bubbles and rapid influx

CORRECT ANSWER: 3
Testing the gastric pH and injecting air through the tube and then ascultating for air are the recommended methods for determining correct tube placement. Normal gastric pH is 1.0 to 4.0. It's higher if the tube is in the intestine and even higher if it's in the lungs. Option 1: Testing of gastric pH is performed using a Gastrocult card, not a Hemocult card, which tests for the presence of blood. Option 2: If the client is unable to speak, the NG tube is in the larynx. Option 4: Don't use any liquid when initially checking the tube for fear of aspiration.
NP: Implementing care
CS: Physiological integrity
CNS: Physiological adaptation
CL: Application

383 A 61-year-old male client with a hiatal hernia is to be discharged home today. The nurse tells him to eat five to six small meals per day and sit in an upright position for at least 2 hours after eating. The rationale for these instructions is to:
☐ 1. enhance the weight reduction plan needed by the client.
☐ 2. promote changes in the client's diet.
☐ 3. minimize the use of antacids.
☐ 4. prevent gastric distention and acid reflux.

CORRECT ANSWER: 4
Eating smaller and more frequent meals allows for better digestion of foods and fewer GI complaints. Options 1, 2, and 3: Eating five to six smaller meals doesn't enhance weight reduction, promote changes in diet, or minimize the use of antacids.
NP: Implementing care
CN: Physiological integrity
CNS: Reduction of risk potential
CL: Application

384 A client is undergoing treatment for a gastric ulcer. The physician has recommended a medication that inhibits gastric secretion by inhibiting histamine. Which medication will the client most likely receive?
☐ 1. Milk of Magnesia
☐ 2. streptomycin
☐ 3. Amphojel
☐ 4. cimetidine (Tagamet)

CORRECT ANSWER: 4
Cimetidine is an histamine-2 receptor site antagonist that decreases the secretion of gastric juices. Option 1: Milk of Magnesia is a laxative in large doses but neutralizes the stomach in smaller doses. Option 2: Streptomycin is an antibiotic. Option 4: Amphojel neutralizes gastric acids and provides pain relief.
NP: Implementing care
CN: Physiological integrity
CNS: Physiological adaptation
CL: Knowledge

385 A 51-year-old female client with peptic ulcer disease hasn't responded to traditional medical management. The physician is planning to do a vagotomy. The nurse explains to the client that this is:
☐ 1. removal of the antrum of the stomach.
☐ 2. removal of 60% to 80% of the stomach.
☐ 3. severing the vagus nerve.
☐ 4. enlargement of the pyloric sphincter.

CORRECT ANSWER: 3
The vagus nerve receives the impulses from the brain to secrete hydrochloric acid. A vagotomy severs the vagus nerve, which decreases gastric acid by diminishing cholinergic stimulation to the parietal cells, making them less responsive to gastrin. Option 1: Removal of the antrum is an antrectomy. Option 2: Removal of 60% to 80% of the stomach is a gastrectomy. Option 4: Surgically enlarging the pyloric sphincter is a pyloroplasty.
NP: Evaluating care
CN: Physiological integrity
CNS: Physiological adaptation
CL: Knowledge

386 A 41-year-old man is admitted with absent bowel sounds, abdominal distention, rebound tenderness, and muscle rigidity. Which diagnosis does the nurse expect the client to receive?
☐ 1. Peritonitis
☐ 2. Diverticulitis
☐ 3. Dumping syndrome
☐ 4. Normal symptoms of diverticulitis

CORRECT ANSWER: 1
Absent bowel sounds, abdominal distention, rebound tenderness, and muscle rigidity are symptoms of peritonitis. Option 2: Diverticulitis is multiple diverticula of the colon. The major signs of diverticulitis are intervals of diarrhea, abrupt onset of crampy pain in the lower left quadrant of the abdomen, and a low-grade fever. Option 3: Dumping syndrome is rapid emptying of the stomach contents into the small intestine. It produces sweating and weakness after eating. Option 4: These are symptoms of peritonitis, not diverticulitis.
NP: Evaluating care
CN: Health promotion and maintenance
CNS: Prevention and early detection of disease
CL: Comprehension

387 The nurse is caring for a 61-year-old male client admitted with cirrhosis of the liver. His condition has become worse and he's confused. What most likely caused this neurologic change?
☐ 1. Normal ammonia levels
☐ 2. High ammonia levels
☐ 3. Thiamine deficiency
☐ 4. Normal thiamine levels

CORRECT ANSWER: 2
When the liver is unable to remove ammonia from the blood, the ammonia accumulates in the brain and causes neurologic changes. Option 1: Normal levels of ammonia would indicate that the liver is able to convert the ammonia to urea and not enter the bloodstream. Option 3: A deficiency in thiamine causes beriberi. Option 4: Normal levels of thiamine in the body promote nervous system functioning.
NP: Evaluating care
CN: Physiological integrity
CNS: Physiological adaptation
CL: Comprehension

388 A 28-year-old female client has an indwelling urinary catheter due to immobility following an automobile accident. Which nursing intervention will minimize the client's risk of infection?
☐ 1. Placing the drainage bag at the level of the bladder
☐ 2. Limiting fluid intake
☐ 3. Cleaning the perineal area from front to back
☐ 4. Securing the catheter tubing to the leg

CORRECT ANSWER: 3
Cleaning the perineal area from front to back wipes bacteria away from the more infection-prone genitourinary area. Option 1: The drainage bag should be placed below the bladder to aid drainage. Option 2: The intake of additional fluids promotes the flow of urine and decreases the bacteria count. Option 4: Securing the catheter tubing to the leg may prevent injury, but not infection.
NP: Implementing care
CN: Safe, effective care environment
CNS: Safety and infection control
CL: Application

389 The nurse is caring for a 21-year-old male college student following a kidney transplant. Which statement indicates that he needs additional teaching about his medications?
☐ 1. "I have to take anti-rejection medicines for 2 weeks."
☐ 2. "The cyclophosphamide (Cytoxan) could cause some of my hair to fall out."
☐ 3. "The corticosteroids could cause an upset stomach."
☐ 4. "The azathioprine (Imuran) could cause my blood count to drop."

CORRECT ANSWER: 1
The anti-rejection medication must be taken for the rest of the transplant recipient's life. Options 2, 3, and 4: These statements all indicate that the client understands possible adverse reactions to his medications.
NP: Evaluating care
CN: Physiological integrity
CNS: Physiological adaptation
CL: Analysis

390 The nurse is giving a client instructions on her new arteriovenous fistula. The nurse instructs the client not to sleep with her arm tucked under her on the affected side. What is the rationale for this?
☐ 1. It will cause an infection.
☐ 2. It will cause bleeding at the site.
☐ 3. It will prevent the nurse from infusing I.V. fluids through it.
☐ 4. There is a risk of compressing the vascular access.

CORRECT ANSWER: 4
Sleeping with the arm tucked under the affected side could compress the vascular access and close off the fistula, prohibiting its use. Option 1: Infections are caused by bacteria, not by lying on the affected side. Option 2: Lying on the fistula doesn't cause bleeding. Option 3: The fistula isn't used to infuse I.V. fluids.
NP: Implementing care
CN: Physiological integrity
CNS: Physiological adaptation
CL: Comprehension

391 A 68-year-old man is admitted with osteomyelitis after a hip replacement done 1 month ago. The nurse anticipates that osteomyelitis is treated by:
- ☐ 1. antineoplastics.
- ☐ 2. analgesics and rest.
- ☐ 3. using sterile technique.
- ☐ 4. drugs specific to the organism.

CORRECT ANSWER: 4
Osteomyelitis is an infection of the bone. It's treated with whatever drug is sensitive to the particular causative organism. Option 1: Antineoplastics aren't the correct drug choice for treating osteomyelitis; they're used to treat malignant disease, not infection. Option 2: Analgesics and rest help with pain but won't treat the infection. Option 3: Aseptic technique should be used for dressing changes.
NP: Implementing care
CN: Health promotion and maintenance
CNS: Prevention and early detection of disease
CL: Comprehension

392 The nurse is caring for a client who received a kidney transplant 2 days ago. The nurse sees the following information on the client's chart: anuria, blood urea nitrogen (BUN) 55 mg, and creatinine 4.3 mg. What does this indicate?
- ☐ 1. Normal levels in a postoperative transplant client
- ☐ 2. Renal failure
- ☐ 3. Signs of a malignancy
- ☐ 4. Need for a diuretic

CORRECT ANSWER: 2
The absence of urine and high levels of BUN and creatinine indicate that the kidneys aren't functioning. Option 1: A normal BUN level is 7 to 25 mg and the normal creatinine level is 0.6 to 1.5 mg. Option 3: This assessment doesn't confirm a malignancy. Option 4: There isn't a need for a diuretic.
NP: Evaluating care
CN: Physiological integrity
CNS: Physiological adaptation
CL: Knowledge

393 The nurse is caring for a 51-year-old firefighter scheduled to receive a kidney transplant. The physician has started him on tacrolimus (Prograf). The nurse explains that this medication:
- ☐ 1. prevents kidney rejection.
- ☐ 2. prevents infection.
- ☐ 3. prevents bleeding.
- ☐ 4. prevents pain.

CORRECT ANSWER: 1
Tacrolimus is an immunosuppressive agent given to prevent rejection of the transplanted organ. Options 2, 3, and 4: Tacrolimus doesn't prevent infection, bleeding, or pain.
NP: Implementing care
CN: Physiological integrity
CNS: Pharmacological therapies
CL: Application

394 The nurse is instructing a 31-year-old woman diagnosed with renal calculi. The physician has chosen lithotripsy treatment for the client. The nurse explains that:
- ☐ 1. if the client has a pacemaker, he can't receive shock wave lithotripsy.
- ☐ 2. if the calculi are in the lower ureter, percutaneous lithotripsy is used.
- ☐ 3. there should be no urinary drainage from the percutaneous lithotripsy incision.
- ☐ 4. there should be no pain due to extracorporeal shock wave lithotripsy.

CORRECT ANSWER: 1
Clients with pacemakers aren't candidates for shock wave lithotripsy. Option 2: Calculi in the lower ureters can be removed by cystoscope. Option 3: For percutaneous lithotripsy, there may be urinary drainage from the incision. Option 4: Shock wave lithotripsy fragments the calculi so it can be excreted with the urine, which causes some pain.
NP: Planning care
CN: Physiological integrity
CNS: Physiological adaptation
CL: Application

395 A client is admitted with acute lymphoblastic leukemia. He's scheduled to have a bone marrow transplant in which he will receive his own harvested bone marrow. What type of transplant does this describe?

☐ 1. Allogeneic transplant
☐ 2. Autologous transplant
☐ 3. Solid organ transplant
☐ 4. Syngeneic transplant

CORRECT ANSWER: 2

An autologous transplant is the use of the client's own bone marrow. Option 1: An allogeneic bone marrow transplant is from another donor. Option 3: A solid organ transplant is the transplant of an organ, such as the heart, lung, or kidney. Option 4: A syngeneic transplant is a transplant between twins.

NP: Implementing care
CN: Physiological integrity
CNS: Physiological adaptation
CL: Knowledge

---

396 A 13-year-old girl is donating bone marrow for her brother's bone marrow transplant. To prepare the boy's sister for bone marrow aspiration, which area does the nurse expose?

☐ 1. The iliac crest
☐ 2. Any long bone
☐ 3. Any short bone
☐ 4. The occipital bone

CORRECT ANSWER: 1

Exposing the iliac crest allows the physician to use multiple sites for bone marrow aspiration. Options 2, 3, and 4: These areas aren't good choices.

NP: Planning care
CN: Safe, effective care environment
CNS: Coordinated care
CL: Application

---

397 An 81-year-old male client is admitted with right-sided heart failure. Which of the following signs and symptoms is the nurse most likely to assess?

☐ 1. Dyspnea and tachycardia
☐ 2. Muscle weakness and tiredness
☐ 3. Dependent pitting edema and jugular vein distention
☐ 4. Cyanosis and rales

CORRECT ANSWER: 3

The client's heart is unable to pump blood into the pulmonary system, causing systemic venous congestion. This causes pitting edema and elevates the jugular vein pressure. Option 1: Dyspnea and tachycardia are seen in left-sided heart failure. Option 2: Because of increased congestion in the interstitial tissues, muscles become weak and tired. Option 4: Cyanosis and rales are also seen in left-sided heart failure.

NP: Implementing care
CN: Physiological integrity
CNS: Physiological adaptation
CL: Application

Maternal-Neonatal Nursing

1 While assessing a client in her 24th week of pregnancy, the nurse learns that the client has been experiencing signs and symptoms indicative of pregnancy-induced hypertension, or preeclampsia. Which sign or symptom helps differentiate preeclampsia from eclampsia?
☐ 1. Seizures
☐ 2. Headaches
☐ 3. Blurred vision
☐ 4. Weight gain

CORRECT ANSWER: 1
The primary difference between preeclampsia and eclampsia is the occurrence of seizures, which occur when the client becomes eclamptic. Headaches (option 2), blurred vision (option 3), weight gain (option 4), increased blood pressure, and edema of the hands and feet are all indicative of preeclampsia.
NP: Collecting data
CN: Physiological integrity
CNS: Physiological adaptation
CL: Comprehension

2 A diabetic client delivers a full-term neonate who weighs 4.6 kg (10 lb, 2 oz). While caring for the large-for-gestational-age (LGA) neonate, the nurse is careful to palpate the clavicles because:
☐ 1. neonates of diabetic mothers have brittle bones.
☐ 2. clavicles are commonly absent in neonates of diabetic mothers.
☐ 3. one of the clavicles may have been broken during delivery.
☐ 4. LGA neonates have glucose deposits on their clavicles.

CORRECT ANSWER: 3
Because of the neonate's large size, clavicular fractures are common during delivery. The nurse should assess all LGA neonates for this occurrence. Options 1, 2, and 4 aren't true.
NP: Collecting data
CN: Physiological integrity
CNS: Physiological adaptation
CL: Application

3 A neonate who is 10 hours old appears exceptionally irritable; he cries easily and startles when touched. The physician orders a drug screen test, which indicates that the neonate is positive for cocaine. Which nursing action would best help to soothe this neonate?
☐ 1. Leaving the light beside the bassinet on at night
☐ 2. Wrapping the neonate snugly in a blanket
☐ 3. Providing multisensory stimulation while the neonate is awake
☐ 4. Giving the neonate a warm bath

CORRECT ANSWER: 2
A cocaine-addicted neonate typically experiences withdrawal 8 to 10 hours after birth; signs and symptoms include constant crying, jitteriness, poor feeding, emesis, respiratory distress, and seizures. To minimize or prevent these signs and symptoms, sensory stimulation is kept to a minimum. The practice of tightly wrapping, or swaddling, a neonate provides a safe, secure environment and maintains body warmth, both of which are soothing. Options 1 and 3: A neonate who tests positive for drugs is typically kept in a quiet, dimly lit environment. Option 4: A bath would necessitate the removal of clothing and exposing the neonate to changes in temperature, both of which are too stimulating.
NP: Implementing care
CN: Physiological integrity
CNS: Basic care and comfort
CL: Application

4 When caring for a neonate receiving phototherapy, the nurse should remember to:
☐ 1. decrease the amount of formula.
☐ 2. dress the neonate warmly.
☐ 3. massage the neonate's skin with lotion.
☐ 4. reposition the neonate frequently.

CORRECT ANSWER: 4
Phototherapy works by the chemical interaction between the light source and the bilirubin in the neonate's skin. Therefore, the larger the skin area exposed to light, the more effective the treatment. Changing the neonate's position frequently ensures maximum exposure. Option 1: Because the neonate will lose water through the skin as a result of evaporation, the amount of formula or water added to the formula may need to be increased to keep the neonate adequately hydrated. Option 2: The neonate is typically undressed to ensure maximum skin exposure. However, the eyes are covered to protect them from the light source and an abbreviated diaper may be used to prevent soiling. Option 3: The skin should be clean and patted dry. Use of lotions would interfere with the phototherapy.
NP: Implementing care
CN: Physiological integrity
CNS: Physiological adaptation
CL: Application

---

5 A client who is into her 32nd week of pregnancy is having contractions. The physician prescribes terbutaline (Brethine), which helps to:
☐ 1. stabilize the blood pressure.
☐ 2. relax smooth muscle.
☐ 3. control bleeding.
☐ 4. stimulate contractions.

CORRECT ANSWER: 2
Terbutaline, a selective beta$_2$-adrenergic agonist, relaxes smooth muscles of the bronchi and uterus. It's commonly used for bronchospasm and premature labor. This drug doesn't stabilize blood pressure (option 1) and has no effect on bleeding (option 3). Terbutaline is given to slow contractions, not stimulate them (option 4).
NP: Implementing care
CN: Physiological integrity
CNS: Pharmacological therapies
CL: Comprehension

---

6 During a pregnant client's initial visit to the facility, the physician diagnoses gonorrhea. Which fact about gonorrhea should the nurse explain to the client?
☐ 1. Her partner won't need to be treated.
☐ 2. The disease will cause no problems for her neonate.
☐ 3. Unless she's treated, her neonate can become infected during delivery.
☐ 4. Unless she's treated, her neonate can have severe congenital defects.

CORRECT ANSWER: 3
During delivery, the neonate may contract the infection, which causes blindness (ophthalmia neonatorum). If the infection is detected early in prenatal care, the client can take medication to successfully treat gonorrhea. Some females *may* have a white or yellow discharge (yellow is most common); some *may not* notice any change in vaginal discharge. Males typically experience burning on urination and a purulent discharge. Because gonorrhea is sexually transmitted, it's important for all sexual partners to be tested and treated as appropriate (option 1). Option 2 is inaccurate. Option 4 is incorrect because gonorrhea doesn't cause congenital defects.
NP: Implementing care
CN: Physiological integrity
CNS: Reduction of risk potential
CL: Comprehension

7 In the delivery room, the nurse positions a client for insertion of an indwelling urinary catheter and notices a glistening white umbilical cord protruding from the client's vagina. What should be the nurse's first action?
- ☐ 1. Return to the nurse's station and call the physician.
- ☐ 2. Start oxygen by mask at 6 to 10 L, then take vital signs.
- ☐ 3. Place a clean towel over the umbilical cord, then wet the cord with sterile saline solution.
- ☐ 4. Apply manual pressure to the presenting part and place the client in the knee-chest position.

CORRECT ANSWER: 4
A prolapsed umbilical cord causes cord compression, compromising fetal blood flow and causing anoxia. Nursing intervention is directed at relieving the pressure on the cord. This is accomplished by placing the client in the knee-chest position, which enables the presenting part to fall away from the cord. Option 1: Because this is a medical emergency, the nurse shouldn't leave the client's side. Only after priorities are met should the nurse call the physician. Option 2 may be done after the cord compression is relieved. Oxygen is typically used if the fetal monitor shows evidence of variable decelerations indicative of hypoxia. Option 3: The cord should be protected from drying with sterile saline compresses but only after the client has been repositioned.
NP: Implementing care
CN: Physiological integrity
CNS: Reduction of risk potential
CL: Application

8 What is a major complication of a fetus in a breech presentation?
- ☐ 1. Premature labor
- ☐ 2. Uterine atony
- ☐ 3. Prolapsed umbilical cord
- ☐ 4. Uterine inversion

CORRECT ANSWER: 3
A prolapsed umbilical cord is more likely to occur with a breech presentation than with a cephalic presentation because a breech presentation doesn't engage the cervix as snugly as does a cephalic presentation and causes early rupture of membranes. Premature labor (option 1) doesn't usually result from breech presentation. Uterine atony (option 2) isn't caused by difficulty with fetal position, but rather by the force of uterine contractions. Uterine inversion (option 4) occurs after delivery, when traction is applied to the umbilical cord to remove the placenta.
NP: Collecting data
CN: Physiological integrity
CNS: Physiological adaptation
CL: Comprehension

9 During labor involving a breech presentation, the nurse should anticipate:
- ☐ 1. a greater amount of bloody show.
- ☐ 2. slower than normal labor progress.
- ☐ 3. more intense labor contractions.
- ☐ 4. a precipitous delivery.

CORRECT ANSWER: 2
Because the presenting part doesn't fit the cervix snugly in a breech presentation, dysfunctional labor may result. A breech presentation wouldn't account for a greater amount of bloody show (option 1). Fetal positioning wouldn't affect uterine contractions (option 3). The delivery of a neonate in a breech presentation is more likely to be prolonged, not swift (option 4).
NP: Planning care
CN: Physiological integrity
CNS: Physiological adaptation
CL: Comprehension

10 A diabetic client delivers a 5.4 kg (12 lb) neonate. In addition to the usual neonatal assessment, the nurse should:
☐ 1. watch for signs of bleeding.
☐ 2. assess the neonate's visual acuity.
☐ 3. check the neonate's blood glucose level.
☐ 4. watch for signs of infection.

CORRECT ANSWER: 3
When the mother's diabetes is poorly controlled, the neonate may weigh over 4.5 kg (10 lb) and be classified as a large-for-gestational-age (LGA) neonate. Such neonates are at higher risk for hypoglycemia. Therefore, the nurse should assess the neonate's blood glucose level. Bleeding (option 1) wouldn't be expected with an LGA neonate. Visual acuity (option 2) is difficult to assess in a neonate, so it should be checked when the infant is older. An LGA neonate isn't at higher risk for infection than other neonates (option 4).
NP: Collecting data
CN: Physiological integrity
CNS: Physiological adaptation
CL: Application

11 Which technique is best to use when bathing a 5-hour-old girl?
☐ 1. Place her on a table covered with blankets and give her a sponge bath.
☐ 2. Bathe her in a tub of warm water.
☐ 3. Keep her under a radiant warmer and give a sponge bath.
☐ 4. Wash only her hands and head because her condition isn't stable enough for her to have a complete bath.

CORRECT ANSWER: 3
During the first several hours after delivery, a neonate's thermal regulatory system is adapting to extra-uterine life. Core temperature must be maintained and oxygen consumption minimized. Conduction, convection, evaporation, or radiation may produce heat loss. The neonate produces heat through increased metabolic activity, increased muscle activity, and brown-fat metabolism — all of which increase oxygen consumption, glucose use, and caloric expenditure. Brown-fat metabolism releases fatty acids into circulation, which in abundance can produce metabolic acidosis. When bathing a neonate under a radiant warmer, the external heat decreases the chances for cold stress by decreasing the amount of internal mechanisms the neonate must use to stay warm. Bathing a neonate on a table (option 1), where she's exposed to air drafts and cooler air currents, can set her up for cold stress. A neonate can loose up to 100 calories/minute from evaporative cooling. Bathing the neonate in a tub (option 2) and then removing her increases her heat loss and metabolism. Washing only the hands and head (option 4) would chill the neonate and reduce thermoregulation because most heat is lost through the head, which is one-quarter of the neonate's body surface.
NP: Implementing care
CN: Physiological integrity
CNS: Physiological adaptation
CL: Application

12 A 5-day-old boy is admitted to the pediatric unit for hyperbilirubinemia. He's placed under phototherapy lights. What is the most likely cause of the hyperbilirubinemia?
- ☐ 1. The mother's breast milk
- ☐ 2. ABO blood incompatibility
- ☐ 3. Unconjugated bilirubin in the neonate's system
- ☐ 4. A problem with the neonate's liver

CORRECT ANSWER: 3

Physiologic jaundice occurs during the transitional state of bilirubin metabolism as the neonate develops mechanisms to replace the placental clearance of bilirubin. The effects of this process usually peak 3 days after delivery. The neonate can become quite jaundiced and have bilirubin concentrations high enough to treat with phototherapy. Option 2: Jaundice caused by ABO incompatibility is usually noted within 24 to 48 hours after delivery and requires immediate intervention. Options 1 and 4: Breast milk and the liver aren't involved in hyperbilirubinemia.

NP: Collecting data
CN: Physiological integrity
CNS: Physiological adaptation
CL: Comprehension

---

13 A 2-hour-old girl is jittery and somewhat irritable, but her vital signs are stable. Which nursing action is most appropriate?
- ☐ 1. Perform a heelstick to test her blood glucose level.
- ☐ 2. Do nothing because this response is the result of an immature central nervous system (CNS).
- ☐ 3. Increase the temperature of the radiant warmer.
- ☐ 4. Perform a heelstick to test her hematocrit.

CORRECT ANSWER: 1

The nurse should perform a heelstick to check for hypoglycemia, which can cause jittery movements in a neonate. Option 2: The neonate's immature CNS may cause hypoglycemia, so it should be ruled out because it can cause neonatal depression and potential complications if not corrected. Consequently, doing nothing is incorrect. Option 3: Jitteriness isn't a sign of hypothermia because neonates don't have the ability to shiver when cold. Option 4: A hematocrit test is inappropriate for this sign.

NP: Collecting data
CN: Physiological integrity
CNS: Physiological adaptation
CL: Application

---

14 A female neonate has a blood glucose level of 20 mg/dl as determined by blood from a heelstick. The nurse's initial action should be to:
- ☐ 1. arrange for an I.V. line of dextrose 10% in water at a rate of 10 ml/hour.
- ☐ 2. check the venous blood glucose level to verify the result.
- ☐ 3. feed her sterile water and repeat the test in 30 minutes.
- ☐ 4. feed her a high-caloric formula and repeat the test in 30 minutes.

CORRECT ANSWER: 4

Sometimes, a neonate's initial blood glucose level will be under 30 mg/dl. In such instances, it's necessary to feed the neonate a formula containing 20 calories/oz and retest the blood glucose level about 30 minutes later to determine if the level has increased. If the level fails to rise, the physician may order further treatment, which may include I.V. therapy (option 1). Checking the venous blood glucose level (option 2) is unnecessary because a heelstick sample that has hemolyzed is more likely to give a blood glucose value greater than what is accurate; therefore, it's safe to assume that the neonate's blood glucose level is low and treatment is warranted. Sterile water (option 3) has no caloric value and doesn't alter the glucose level.

NP: Implementing care
CN: Physiological integrity
CNS: Physiological adaptation
CL: Application

15 The nurse performs a heelstick hematocrit test on a 4-hour-old male neonate. The result is 63%. What does this finding indicate?
☐ 1. Serious anemia
☐ 2. Nothing because this is normal for a neonate
☐ 3. Possible risk of hyperbilirubinemia
☐ 4. Necessity to repeat the test using venous blood

CORRECT ANSWER: 2
A hematocrit of 45% to 65% is normal in a neonate because of increased blood supply during intrauterine life. Option 1: A hematocrit of 63% doesn't indicate serious anemia because the value is within the normal hematocrit range for a neonate. Option 3: Although all neonates have the potential to develop hyperbilirubinemia, a hematocrit of 63% is inconclusive for this finding. Option 4: If the heelstick blood test shows a hematocrit greater than 65%, a venous blood sample is obtained for testing because hemolysis of the heelstick sample can show a false reading. A hematocrit greater than 65% requires treatment after the physician has been notified.
NP: Collecting data
CN: Health promotion and maintenance
CNS: Prevention and early detection of disease
CL: Comprehension

16 Which finding in a pregnant client's history places her at risk for toxoplasmosis?
☐ 1. She swims regularly in a community pool.
☐ 2. She's responsible for emptying her cat's litter box.
☐ 3. She occasionally eats raw clams and oysters.
☐ 4. She works in a factory that manufactures plastic toys.

CORRECT ANSWER: 2
The parasitic disease toxoplasmosis is commonly transmitted to pregnant women who engage in such activities as handling cat feces and eating or handling raw meat. Options 1, 3, and 4 are all unrelated to toxoplasmosis.
NP: Collecting data
CN: Health promotion and maintenance
CNS: Prevention and early detection of disease
CL: Comprehension

17 A primigravida says to the nurse, "The physician told me that my hemoglobin level is 11 grams. But before I was pregnant, it was 12 grams." Which response by the nurse is appropriate?
☐ 1. "Have you had any recent bleeding episodes?"
☐ 2. "Are you tired after walking a short distance?"
☐ 3. "Your hemoglobin level was high before pregnancy."
☐ 4. "During pregnancy, a decrease in your hemoglobin level is normal."

CORRECT ANSWER: 4
The hemoglobin level usually decreases during pregnancy because of the increase in fluid content. Options 1 and 2: There is no need to question the client about bleeding or signs of anemia because this is a normal finding. Option 3: In females, 12 g/dl is within the normal range for a hemoglobin level.
NP: Implementing care
CN: Health promotion and maintenance
CNS: Prevention and early detection of disease
CL: Application

18 A 28-year-old primigravida who is in her first trimester of pregnancy says to the nurse, "I was so anxious to be pregnant and now that I am, I'm not so sure I want to be pregnant." The nurse would respond appropriately based on an understanding of which true statement?
☐ 1. Having mixed feelings in the first trimester increases the chances of poor postpartum bonding.
☐ 2. Having mixed feelings about pregnancy is normal in the first trimester.
☐ 3. Women who are uncertain about wanting to be pregnant should be told of the options available to them.
☐ 4. Women who are uncertain about wanting to be pregnant need counseling to enable them to deal with their femininity.

CORRECT ANSWER: 2
Ambivalence, or having mixed feelings, is a normal reaction in the first trimester of pregnancy as a woman attempts to adjust to her new role. Options 1, 3, and 4 are incorrect.
NP: Implementing care
CN: Psychosocial integrity
CNS: Coping and adaptation
CL: Analysis

19 The nurse provides information about preventing heartburn to a primigravida who is in her third trimester of pregnancy. The nurse knows that the client needs further teaching if she makes which comment?
☐ 1. "I can sometimes take a little milk 20 minutes before eating."
☐ 2. "I'll stop eating cucumbers and radishes."
☐ 3. "I should lie flat in bed for 15 minutes after I eat."
☐ 4. "I should eat a lot of little meals throughout the day."

CORRECT ANSWER: 3
Lying flat immediately after eating is likely to cause stomach acid reflux and increase the chance of heartburn. Ingesting fats, such as milk (option 1), inhibits and neutralizes the secretion of stomach acids and would be appropriate. This client should avoid gas-forming foods, such as cucumbers and radishes (option 2). Frequent small meals (option 4) are recommended to prevent heartburn.
NP: Evaluating care
CN: Health promotion and maintenance
CNS: Prevention and early detection of disease
CL: Analysis

20 A primigravida is in labor and her cervix is dilated 8 cm. The client's husband says to the nurse, "Things were going fine, but now I can't seem to do anything right. She just yelled at me and told me to leave her alone." Which action should the nurse take?
☐ 1. Explain to the husband that his wife's behavior is normal for a woman in the transition phase of labor.
☐ 2. Find out exactly what the husband did to upset his wife.
☐ 3. Suggest that the husband sit in the waiting room until it's time for the delivery.
☐ 4. Ask the husband when he and his wife last had a verbal disagreement.

CORRECT ANSWER: 1
During transition, the phase of labor during which the cervix dilates to 7 to 10 cm, a client is likely to become irritable and not want to be touched. Such a client is extremely uncomfortable and needs to be assured that labor is coming to an end. The husband requires assistance to help his wife during this difficult period. Options 2, 3, and 4 do nothing to help the client or the husband.
NP: Implementing care
CN: Psychosocial integrity
CNS: Coping and adaptation
CL: Application

21 A primigravida is admitted to the labor room, where the attending nurse will time her contractions. The nurse should time them from:
☐ 1. the beginning of one contraction to the beginning of the next contraction.
☐ 2. the beginning of one contraction to the end of that contraction.
☐ 3. the end of one contraction to the end of the next contraction.
☐ 4. the end of one contraction to the beginning of the next contraction.

CORRECT ANSWER: 2
The duration of a contraction is measured from the time the uterus begins to contract until it relaxes. Option 1 disrupts the timing of the frequency of contractions. Options 3 and 4 fail to accurately time uterine contractions.
NP: Collecting data
CN: Health promotion and maintenance
CNS: Prevention and early detection of disease
CL: Comprehension

22 The nurse is examining a client in her 20th week of pregnancy. At about this point in the pregnancy, the nurse would expect the client to report:
☐ 1. fetal movement.
☐ 2. urinary frequency.
☐ 3. Braxton Hicks contractions.
☐ 4. thick, white vaginal discharge.

CORRECT ANSWER: 1
Quickening, the feeling of fetal movement, usually occurs between the 16th and 20th weeks of pregnancy. Urinary frequency (option 2) is common during the 1st and last weeks of pregnancy. Braxton Hicks contractions (option 3) usually occur near the end of the third trimester of pregnancy. A thick, white vaginal discharge (option 4) is abnormal and should be reported; it may indicate a fungal infection.
NP: Collecting data
CN: Health promotion and maintenance
CNS: Prevention and early detection of disease
CL: Application

23 A client is admitted to the facility in active labor. On admission, the fetal heart rate was 138 beats/minute. An hour later, the nurse finds the fetal heart rate to be 150 beats/minute. Based on this finding, which measure should be included in the client's plan of care?
- ☐ 1. Prepare for insertion of an internal fetal monitor.
- ☐ 2. Continue to monitor the fetal heart rate.
- ☐ 3. Prepare to administer oxygen to the client.
- ☐ 4. Compare this fetal heart rate with the prenatal findings.

CORRECT ANSWER: 2
A normal fetal heart rate is between 120 and 160 beats/minute. During labor, fluctuations in the heart rate are considered normal. Options 1, 3, and 4 are unnecessary.
NP: Planning care
CN: Health promotion and maintenance
CNS: Prevention and early detection of disease
CL: Application

24 A 3-day-old boy is scheduled for circumcision without anesthesia. Which measure should be included in the infant's postcircumcision plan of care?
- ☐ 1. Chart the time of the infant's voiding.
- ☐ 2. Keep the infant's penis exposed to air.
- ☐ 3. Feed the infant only clear fluids for the first 12 hours.
- ☐ 4. Place a small ice cap on the infant's penis.

CORRECT ANSWER: 1
After a circumcision, urine retention may occur. Option 2: A petroleum dressing is commonly applied to the penis, then the infant is diapered. Option 3: Because no anesthetic was given, feeding restrictions are unnecessary. Option 4: Although the penis should be inspected for swelling and bleeding, further care is unnecessary.
NP: Planning care
CN: Safe, effective care environment
CNS: Safety and infection control
CL: Application

25 The nurse is caring for a full-term neonate. Which finding is considered abnormal?
- ☐ 1. Respiratory rate of 52 breaths/minute
- ☐ 2. Small pinpoint white dots on the nose
- ☐ 3. Strabismus
- ☐ 4. Two veins and one artery in the umbilical cord

CORRECT ANSWER: 4
The umbilical cord normally contains two arteries and one vein. Option 1: A normal respiratory rate for a neonate is between 30 and 80 breaths/minute. Option 2: Small white dots on the nose, which are known as milia, are normal. Option 3: Strabismus is normal in the first month of life.
NP: Collecting data
CN: Health promotion and maintenance
CNS: Growth and development through the life span
CL: Comprehension

26 A primiparous woman who delivered a boy is talking with the nurse. Which statement by the mother may indicate that she's having difficulty bonding with and attaching to her infant?
- ☐ 1. "The baby looks just like my brother."
- ☐ 2. "I really wanted a girl."
- ☐ 3. "He's the first boy grandchild."
- ☐ 4. "My husband will be so good with him."

CORRECT ANSWER: 2
Any remark that indicates dissatisfaction with the infant may indicate a problem with attachment or bonding. Options 1, 3, and 4 are all viewed as positive signs of bonding and attachment.
NP: Collecting data
CN: Health promotion and maintenance
CNS: Growth and development through the life span
CL: Analysis

27 The nurse is providing instructions about breast-feeding to a new mother the day after delivery. Which statement indicates that the client understands the instructions?
- [ ] 1. "I'll call the clinic if the baby's stool becomes soft and yellow."
- [ ] 2. "If the baby isn't sucking well, I'll try placing my nipple under the baby's tongue."
- [ ] 3. "I expect the baby to have six to eight wet diapers per day if he's getting enough milk."
- [ ] 4. "I won't feed the baby more than six times per day."

CORRECT ANSWER: 3
A sign of adequate hydration in a neonate is six to eight wet diapers per day. Option 1: A breast-feeding neonate usually has soft, yellow stools; there would be no reason to call the clinic. Option 2: The nipple should always be placed above the neonate's tongue to allow for proper sucking and swallowing. Option 4: Infants should be fed on demand. In the beginning, this may be every 2 to 3 hours (8 to 10 times per day).
NP: Evaluating care
CN: Health promotion and maintenance
CNS: Prevention and early detection of disease
CL: Analysis

28 A primigravida who is in her 38th week of gestation has been instructed to call the clinic if danger signs or symptoms occur. Which statement indicates that she knows what to report?
- [ ] 1. "I'll call the clinic if I have blurring of vision."
- [ ] 2. "I'll call the clinic if I have shortness of breath when I walk up steps."
- [ ] 3. "I'll call the clinic if I notice my feet swelling at the end of the day."
- [ ] 4. "I'll call the clinic if I have a sudden burst of energy."

CORRECT ANSWER: 1
Blurred vision is a symptom of pregnancy-induced hypertension and should be reported to the physician. Shortness of breath (option 2) and foot swelling (option 3) are normal findings at the end of the third trimester. A sudden burst of energy (option 4) is a sign of impending labor; this client is far enough along in her pregnancy that delivery would be safe.
NP: Evaluating care
CN: Health promotion and maintenance
CNS: Prevention and early detection of disease
CL: Application

29 The nurse has been conducting a class on the types of breathing exercises recommended during labor. The nurse knows that a client has an understanding of breathing exercises if she makes which comment?
- [ ] 1. "I shouldn't begin my breathing exercises until I'm uncomfortable with my contractions."
- [ ] 2. "If taking six to nine breaths doesn't work, I'll begin quicker, shallow breathing."
- [ ] 3. "Anytime I feel the urge to push, I'll continue breathing and call the nurse immediately."
- [ ] 4. "I'll probably have to use my pant-blow breathing when I'm almost fully dilated."

CORRECT ANSWER: 3
When the client feels the urge to push during labor, it's important for the cervix to be fully dilated before she can begin bearing down. Therefore, she should continue her breathing until she is told she can push — when the cervix is dilated. Option 1: Some clients may choose to begin exercises when uncomfortable. Options 2 and 4 demonstrate an incorrect understanding of the proper technique for performing breathing exercises.
NP: Evaluating care
CN: Health promotion and maintenance
CNS: Growth and development through the life span
CL: Application

30 The nurse assesses a neonate delivered at 28 weeks' gestation. Which finding would the nurse expect to observe?
- [ ] 1. The skin is pale, and no vessels show through it.
- [ ] 2. Creases appear on the anterior two-thirds of the sole.
- [ ] 3. The pinna of the ear is soft and flat and stays folded.
- [ ] 4. The neonate has 7 to 10 mm of breast tissue.

CORRECT ANSWER: 3
The ear has a soft pinna that is flat and stays folded. Options 1 and 4 are characteristic of a neonate at 40 weeks' gestation. Option 2 is characteristic of a neonate at 36 weeks' gestation.
NP: Collecting data
CN: Health promotion and maintenance
CNS: Growth and development through the life span
CL: Knowledge

31 The purpose of administering vitamin K to a neonate is to:
- ☐ 1. decrease the risk of developing jaundice.
- ☐ 2. decrease the risk of developing pernicious anemia.
- ☐ 3. increase the absorption of iron.
- ☐ 4. increase the prothrombin time.

CORRECT ANSWER: 4
Vitamin K is administered to decrease the risk of hemorrhage due to the neonate's low prothrombin time at birth. Options 1, 2, and 3 aren't valid reasons for administering vitamin K.
NP: Planning care
CN: Health promotion and maintenance
CNS: Prevention and early detection of disease
CL: Comprehension

32 A client who was just informed that she's 8 weeks pregnant makes all of the following statements to the nurse. Which statement reflects a behavior that could be dangerous to the fetus?
- ☐ 1. "I usually jog indoors twice per week."
- ☐ 2. "I generally have wine with dinner."
- ☐ 3. "I belong to a bowling league that bowls once per week."
- ☐ 4. "I drink two cups of coffee per day."

CORRECT ANSWER: 2
Alcohol is considered a teratogen. Because no specific amount has been determined as safe during pregnancy, all pregnant women are advised to abstain from alcohol. The activities discussed in options 1, 3, and 4 are considered safe as long as the pregnancy is uneventful.
NP: Collecting data
CN: Health promotion and maintenance
CNS: Prevention and early detection of disease
CL: Application

33 The nurse provides information about various contraceptives to a postpartum client. The nurse knows that the client needs further instruction if she makes which statement?
- ☐ 1. "To best protect me from herpes, my husband should use a latex condom."
- ☐ 2. "I can expect some breast tenderness if I decide to use the pill."
- ☐ 3. "If I choose the rhythm method, I must first determine when I ovulate."
- ☐ 4. "It's OK for me to remove my diaphragm 1 hour after intercourse."

CORRECT ANSWER: 4
A diaphragm should be left in place for at least 8 hours after intercourse. The statements discussed in options 1, 2, and 3 are all true.
NP: Evaluating care
CN: Health promotion and maintenance
CNS: Prevention and early detection of disease
CL: Application

34 A 28-year-old client has been visiting the fertility clinic because she's having trouble becoming pregnant. The nurse teaches her how to determine the time of ovulation by tracking her temperature. The nurse knows that the client understands the instructions because she correctly states that her temperature will:
- ☐ 1. rise and then sharply drop at the time of ovulation.
- ☐ 2. rise 2 days after her menses and remain elevated until after ovulation.
- ☐ 3. drop at the time of ovulation.
- ☐ 4. drop just before it rises at the time of ovulation.

CORRECT ANSWER: 4
Menstruating women typically experience a change in body temperature at about the time of ovulation. The temperature remains high in the postovulation phase, then drops just before it rises again at the time of ovulation. Options 1, 2, and 3 are incorrect.
NP: Evaluating care
CN: Health promotion and maintenance
CNS: Prevention and early detection of disease
CL: Comprehension

35 A client who is 34 weeks pregnant complains to the nurse that she's having muscle cramps in her calf. After reporting the complaint to the physician, which instruction should the nurse give the client when the pain occurs?
☐ 1. "Stand up."
☐ 2. "Apply cold compresses to the affected leg."
☐ 3. "Flex the knee of the affected leg."
☐ 4. "Wrap the leg with an elastic bandage."

CORRECT ANSWER: 1
A leg cramp can usually be relieved by standing up or extending the cramped leg. Applying cold to the leg (option 2) may aggravate the cramp. Flexing the knee (option 3) or wrapping the leg (option 4) wouldn't relieve the leg cramp.
NP: Implementing care
CN: Physiological integrity
CNS: Basic care and comfort
CL: Application

36 A multiparous client in her 40th week of gestation is admitted to the facility because of severe pregnancy-induced hypertension. She's being treated with magnesium sulfate. The purpose of this medication is to:
☐ 1. decrease the respiratory rate.
☐ 2. relax the uterine muscle.
☐ 3. increase placental profusion.
☐ 4. prevent seizures.

CORRECT ANSWER: 4
Magnesium sulfate, given parentally, is a central nervous system depressant that can prevent seizures in a client with severe pregnancy-induced hypertension. None of the actions described in options 1, 2, or 3 are associated with magnesium sulfate.
NP: Implementing care
CN: Physiological integrity
CNS: Pharmacological therapies
CL: Comprehension

37 A multiparous client delivered a stillborn full-term infant 2 hours ago. The woman says to the nurse, "I'd really like to hold the baby." Which response by the nurse would be appropriate?
☐ 1. "Can you tell me why you want to hold the baby?"
☐ 2. "I'll make arrangements for you to hold the baby."
☐ 3. "Why not wait until your family comes before you hold the baby?"
☐ 4. "I think you should speak with a member of the clergy."

CORRECT ANSWER: 2
Allowing the mother to see and hold her stillborn child when she requests to do so helps her to deal with her loss and begin grieving. Option 1 is intrusive and interferes with this normal grieving process. Options 3 and 4 deny the mother's wish and prevent her from dealing with her present feelings.
NP: Implementing care
CN: Psychosocial integrity
CNS: Coping and adaptation
CL: Application

38 The nurse observes a 24-hour-old neonate who was delivered at 38 weeks' gestation. Which observation should be reported immediately?
☐ 1. The neonate makes random movements while sleeping.
☐ 2. The neonate has nasal flaring.
☐ 3. The neonate has a greenish black and tarry stool.
☐ 4. The neonate's head is turned to one side and the leg and arm on that side are extended.

CORRECT ANSWER: 2
Because a neonate breathes through his nose, not his mouth, nasal flaring is a sign of respiratory distress. Because his nervous system is immature, a neonate frequently moves in his sleep (option 1). Meconium, the stool described in option 3, is passed during the first 24 hours after delivery. Option 4 describes the tonic neck reflex, a normal neonatal response.
NP: Collecting data
CN: Physiological integrity
CNS: Physiological adaptation
CL: Application

39 A primigravida in active labor is receiving an epidural anesthetic. Which action should the nurse take?
☐ 1. Encourage the client to cough and breathe deeply between contractions.
☐ 2. Check the client's urine for acetone.
☐ 3. Monitor the client's blood pressure.
☐ 4. Keep the foot of the bed slightly elevated.

CORRECT ANSWER: 3
When a client in labor receives an epidural anesthetic, it's important to monitor for any sign of hypertension by checking the heart rate and blood pressure and evaluating her contractions. Option 1 isn't done for a client receiving an epidural anesthetic. Option 2: There is no reason that acetone would be present in this client's urine. Option 4: Such a client would be placed with the head of the bed elevated.
NP: Implementing care
CN: Safe, effective care environment
CNS: Safety and infection control
CL: Application

40 The physician tells a multigravida who is in active labor that, because of fetal distress, he may need to perform a cesarean delivery. The client is upset and expresses concern for her fetus. Which nursing measure would be most helpful in this situation?
☐ 1. Explain to the client that being fearful may impede the progress of her labor.
☐ 2. Remind the client that she has other children at home.
☐ 3. Provide the client with accurate information about the condition of her fetus.
☐ 4. Reassure the client that the outcome of the pregnancy will be positive.

CORRECT ANSWER: 3
Offering truthful information about the fetus's condition and the progress of her labor would be most helpful to the client at this time. Telling the client not to worry (option 1) isn't a helpful response. Asking the client to focus on other issues at this time (option 2) is inappropriate. Offering unfounded or false reassurances (option 4) is also inappropriate.
NP: Implementing care
CN: Psychosocial integrity
CNS: Coping and adaptation
CL: Application

41 A primigravida with a history of cardiac problems is admitted to the facility in the beginning stages of labor. Despite her cardiac condition, the client has tolerated her pregnancy well. Which nursing action should be included in the client's plan of care during labor?
☐ 1. Assess the client for signs of abruptio placentae.
☐ 2. Assess the client frequently for signs of dyspnea.
☐ 3. Keep the lights in the room dimmed.
☐ 4. Check the client's urine for signs of cardiac problems.

CORRECT ANSWER: 2
Labor and delivery tend to place extra demands on the heart. A pregnant client with known cardiac problems should be observed for signs of cardiac distress, including dyspnea and increased heart rate. Options 1 and 3 are incorrect because the client has no signs of abruptio placentae, which would warrant further assessment, or of preeclampsia, which would warrant dimming the lights. Option 4: Urine wouldn't indicate signs of cardiac problems.
NP: Planning care
CN: Physiological integrity
CNS: Physiological adaptation
CL: Application

42 A 26-year-old client with a 10-year history of diabetes mellitus is in her 8th week of pregnancy. To assist in planning the client's care, the nurse should know that, in general, a client's insulin need decreases at the beginning of pregnancy and:
☐ 1. decreases drastically later in pregnancy.
☐ 2. remains decreased but stable in the second and third trimesters.
☐ 3. increases in the second trimester and decreases in the third trimester.
☐ 4. increases later in pregnancy.

CORRECT ANSWER: 4
Although insulin need may fluctuate, it typically decreases until about the 18th week, then increases until the end of the pregnancy. Options 1, 2, and 3 are incorrect.
NP: Planning care
CN: Health promotion and maintenance
CNS: Prevention and early detection of disease
CL: Comprehension

43 A nurse demonstrates the proper way to give a neonate a sponge bath to a group of new mothers. After the demonstration, the nurse observes a mother bathing her 2-day-old girl. The nurse knows the mother needs further instruction if the mother:
☐ 1. uses a cotton-tipped applicator to clean inside the neonate's ears.
☐ 2. washes the genital area from front to back.
☐ 3. uses a cotton ball to apply a little alcohol to the base of the umbilical cord.
☐ 4. dresses the neonate in a shirt before washing the legs and buttocks.

CORRECT ANSWER: 1
Only the external ear should be cleaned; nothing should be placed inside the ear canal. The genital area is washed from the cleanest area to the dirtiest area, so the behavior in option 2 is correct. Applying alcohol to the base of the umbilical cord (option 3) helps to keep the area clean and dry. Option 4 is done to prevent the neonate from becoming chilled during the bath.
NP: Evaluating care
CN: Health promotion and maintenance
CNS: Prevention and early detection of disease
CL: Application

44 A multiparous client who delivered 12 hours ago plans to breast-feed her neonate. When the nurse brings the neonate, who is awake and alert, to the mother's room, the mother is asleep. Which action should the nurse take?
☐ 1. Provide the infant with a clear fluid feeding.
☐ 2. Return the infant to the nursery and wait until the mother wakes to feed the infant.
☐ 3. Report this situation to the head nurse.
☐ 4. Wake the mother and allow her to feed the infant.

CORRECT ANSWER: 4
Neonates should breast-feed when they're awake and alert. In the beginning, this is especially important to ensure that the neonate adapts well to breast-feeding and obtains colostrum, the rich antibody-containing breast milk. More vigorous sucking, while the neonate is alert, also stimulates the production of breast milk. Clients who elect to breast-feed should be encouraged to nap between feedings. Options 1, 2, and 3 are improper actions for the nurse to take.
NP: Implementing care
CN: Health promotion and maintenance
CNS: Growth and development through the life span
CL: Application

45 A husband accompanies his wife, a primigravida in her 20th week of pregnancy, to the prenatal clinic. He asks the nurse when he and his wife will have to stop having sexual intercourse. The nurse should base her response on the knowledge that sexual intercourse is generally permitted:
☐ 1. until ballottement occurs.
☐ 2. throughout the entire pregnancy.
☐ 3. for the first 36 weeks of pregnancy.
☐ 4. until lightening occurs.

CORRECT ANSWER: 2
A woman can continue having sexual intercourse throughout her pregnancy as long as she remains comfortable and has no contraindications, such as premature labor and bleeding. Options 1, 3, and 4 aren't reasons to cease intercourse.
NP: Implementing care
CN: Health promotion and maintenance
CNS: Growth and development through the life span
CL: Comprehension

46 During a routine visit to the clinic, a client tells the nurse that she thinks she may be pregnant. The physician orders a pregnancy test. The nurse should know that the purpose of this test is to determine which change in the client's hormone level?
☐ 1. Increase in human chorionic gonadotropin (HCG)
☐ 2. Decrease in HCG
☐ 3. Increase in luteinizing hormone (LH)
☐ 4. Decrease in LH

CORRECT ANSWER: 1
HCG increases in a woman's blood and urine to fairly large concentrations until the 15th week of pregnancy. Options 2, 3, and 4 aren't indicative of pregnancy.
NP: Collecting data
CN: Health promotion and maintenance
CNS: Prevention and early detection of disease
CL: Comprehension

47 A primigravida in her 42nd week of gestation is undergoing induced labor. An I.V. infusion of oxytocin (Pitocin) is started. Which sign or symptom would indicate that the client is experiencing an adverse reaction to the oxytocin?
☐ 1. Hypotension
☐ 2. Proteinuria
☐ 3. Uterine contractions lasting 90 seconds
☐ 4. Epigastric pain

CORRECT ANSWER: 3
Oxytocin is used to stimulate uterine contractions, thereby precipitating labor. However, contractions lasting 90 seconds could cause fetal distress. Hypertension, not hypotension (option 1), is an adverse effect of oxytocin. Proteinuria (option 2) and epigastric pain (option 4) aren't associated with oxytocin use.
NP: Evaluating care
CN: Physiological integrity
CNS: Pharmacological therapies
CL: Comprehension

48 A primigravida who is 30 weeks pregnant is admitted to the facility in labor. She's started on ritodrine hydrochloride (Yutopar) to arrest her labor. The nurse should observe the client for adverse reactions to this drug, which include:
☐ 1. chest pain.
☐ 2. bradycardia.
☐ 3. hyperglycemia.
☐ 4. diplopia.

CORRECT ANSWER: 1
Adverse effects of ritodrine hydrochloride include chest pain, tachycardia, and temporary hypoglycemia. Options 2, 3, and 4 aren't associated with this drug.
NP: Evaluating care
CN: Physiological integrity
CNS: Pharmacological therapies
CL: Comprehension

49 The nurse is instructing a 25-year-old client who thinks she may be pregnant. Which instruction should the nurse provide to ensure an accurate pregnancy test?
☐ 1. Collect a urine specimen after eating breakfast in the morning and just before coming to the clinic.
☐ 2. Using the clean-catch method, collect a specimen at the first voiding of the day, before eating or drinking .
☐ 3. Collect the last-voided urine of the day and place it in the refrigerator until your clinic appointment.
☐ 4. Collect the second-voided specimen of the day after drinking two glasses of water.

CORRECT ANSWER: 2
A client's first-voided urine specimen, collected in the morning before eating or drinking, is more concentrated and contains a greater amount of human chorionic gonadotropin, which allows more accurate testing. The clean-catch method prevents excess debris from getting in the urine. Options 1 and 4: The client shouldn't eat or drink before collecting the morning urine specimen. Option 3: Urine specimens shouldn't be kept overnight; a fresh urine specimen is required.
NP: Implementing care
CN: Health promotion and maintenance
CNS: Prevention and early detection of disease
CL: Application

50 The nurse in a family practice facility is assessing a client who is at 30 weeks' gestation. The nurse hears a fetal heart rate (FHR) of 88 beats/minute. What should the nurse do next?
☐ 1. Notify the physician immediately.
☐ 2. Permit the mother to hear the heartbeat.
☐ 3. Assess the client's radial pulse.
☐ 4. Recognize that the rate is within the normal limits and document the rate.

CORRECT ANSWER: 3
A normal FHR is 120 to 160 beats/minute. The 88-beat/minute rate the nurse is hearing could actually belong to the client (heard through the uterine blood vessels), so the nurse should assess the radial pulse for comparison. Option 1: If the FHR is confirmed to be 88 beats/minute, the nurse should notify the physician immediately. Option 2: After a full assessment is made, the client may be allowed to hear the heartbeat. Option 4: An FHR of 88 beats/minute is below the normal heart rate and other action needs to be taken.
NP: Collecting data
CN: Health promotion and maintenance
CNS: Prevention and early detection of disease
CL: Application

51 A 31-year-old client is admitted to the nursing unit with the diagnosis of placenta previa. Which sign or symptom isn't seen with placenta previa?
☐ 1. Bright red, painless vaginal bleeding
☐ 2. Separation of the placenta as the cervix ripens
☐ 3. Implantation of the placenta in the lower uterine segment
☐ 4. Severe pelvic pain

CORRECT ANSWER: 4
With placenta previa, the placenta covers all or part of the cervical opening. Placenta previa normally involves painless bleeding. Severe pelvic pain is associated with abruptio placentae, not placenta previa. Options 1 and 2: Bright red, painless vaginal bleeding and separation of the placenta are seen with placenta previa during labor. Option 3: Implantation of the placenta in the lower uterine segment is associated with placenta previa.
NP: Collecting data
CN: Health promotion and maintenance
CNS: Prevention and early detection of disease
CL: Comprehension

52 An obstetric client in her first pregnancy asks the nurse when she should expect to feel the first fetal movements. The nurse tells her that they usually take place between:
☐ 1. 2 and 6 gestational weeks.
☐ 2. 4 and 10 gestational weeks.
☐ 3. 6 and 12 gestational weeks.
☐ 4. 16 and 20 gestational weeks.

CORRECT ANSWER: 4
Most pregnant women, including primigravidas, feel fetal movement (quickening) between the 16th and 20th gestational weeks, when the fetus becomes more active. Options 1, 2, and 3: Pregnant women generally don't feel fetal movement before the 13th week.
NP: Implementing care
CN: Health promotion and maintenance
CNS: Growth and development through the life span
CL: Comprehension

53 The nurse is teaching a new mother about breast-feeding. Which pituitary hormone stimulates the secretion of milk from the mammary glands?
☐ 1. Prolactin
☐ 2. Estrogen
☐ 3. Progesterone
☐ 4. Oxytocin

CORRECT ANSWER: 1
Prolactin is an anterior pituitary hormone that stimulates mammary gland secretion. Options 2 and 3: Estrogen and progesterone are ovarian hormones. Option 4: Oxytocin is a posterior pituitary hormone that stimulates the uterus to contract and causes the letdown reflex.
NP: Implementing care
CN: Health promotion and maintenance
CNS: Growth and development through the life span
CL: Knowledge

54 A 22-year-old primigravida complains to the nurse that she has been feeling very tired and sick to her stomach, especially in the morning. What is the nurse's best response?
☐ 1. "This is common during early pregnancy; don't worry about it."
☐ 2. "This is common during early pregnancy because of all the changes going on in your body."
☐ 3. "This is common during early pregnancy because of all the changes going on in your body. Can you tell me more about how you feel in the morning?"
☐ 4. "You should ask the physician about that."

CORRECT ANSWER: 3
Option 3 is an open-ended question, which encourages more communication and allows the client to describe her sensations. Option 1: This response doesn't encourage further communication and can minimize the client's feelings. Option 2: This response is true, but it limits communication. Option 4: This response can be stressful for the client because she may worry that something is wrong with her or the pregnancy.
NP: Collecting data
CN: Health promotion and maintenance
CNS: Growth and development through the life span
CL: Comprehension

55 A 27-year-old primigravida asks the nurse what signs and symptoms indicate that labor will begin soon. Which sign or symptom should the nurse describe?
- ☐ 1. Quickening
- ☐ 2. Bloody show
- ☐ 3. Period of lethargy and fatigue
- ☐ 4. Weight gain of 1 to 3 lb (0.5 to 1.5 kg)

CORRECT ANSWER: 2

An early sign of labor is the passage of the mucus plug or a bloody show as the cervix ripens. Option 1: Quickening is the perception of fetal movement at 16 to 20 weeks' gestation. Option 3: Another early symptom of labor is a burst of energy. Option 4: A weight loss of 1 to 3 lb over 2 to 3 weeks, rather than a weight gain, is an early sign of labor.
NP: Implementing care
CN: Health promotion and maintenance
CNS: Growth and development through the life span
CL: Comprehension

56 The nurse is instructing a 21-year-old primigravida. What is the definitive sign indicating that true labor has begun?
- ☐ 1. Lightening
- ☐ 2. Passage of the mucus plug
- ☐ 3. Rupture of amniotic membranes
- ☐ 4. Regular, progressive uterine contractions that increase in intensity with activity

CORRECT ANSWER: 4

Progressive uterine contractions are the definitive sign of true labor. Options 1 and 2: Lightening (a feeling of decreased abdominal distention) and passage of the mucus plug are early indications that the onset of labor is about to begin. Option 3: The rupture of amniotic membranes usually occurs during labor.
NP: Implementing care
CN: Health promotion and maintenance
CNS: Growth and development through the life span
CL: Comprehension

57 A full-term pregnant woman is admitted to the facility with a diagnosis of abruptio placentae. Which assessment finding isn't related to abruptio placentae?
- ☐ 1. Tender, boardlike uterus
- ☐ 2. Signs of shock
- ☐ 3. Hypertension
- ☐ 4. Painful vaginal bleeding

CORRECT ANSWER: 3

Decreasing blood pressure, not hypertension, is a sign of shock that occurs with abruptio placentae. Options 1, 2, and 4: A tender and boardlike uterus, signs of shock, and painful vaginal bleeding are all signs and symptoms of abruptio placentae.
NP: Collecting data
CN: Physiological integrity
CNS: Physiological adaptation
CL   Comprehension

58 The nurse is caring for a client in labor who just had spontaneous rupture of the amniotic membranes. What should the nurse do first?
- ☐ 1. Assess the fetal heart rate (FHR).
- ☐ 2. Perform a vaginal examination.
- ☐ 3. Assess the client's vital signs.
- ☐ 4. Inspect the characteristics of the amniotic fluid.

CORRECT ANSWER: 1

Changes in the FHR can indicate if the ruptured amniotic membranes are causing fetal distress. Options 2, 3, and 4: Performing a vaginal examination, assessing the client's vital signs, and inspecting the amniotic fluid are important measures and should be done after the FHR is assessed.
NP: Evaluating care
CN: Health promotion and maintenance
CNS: Growth and development through the life span
CL: Analysis

59 The nurse is performing a postpartum check on a 40-year-old client. Which nursing measure is appropriate?
- ☐ 1. Place the client in a supine position with her arms overhead for the examination of her breasts and fundus.
- ☐ 2. Instruct the client to empty her bladder before the examination.
- ☐ 3. Wear sterile gloves when assessing the pad and perineum.
- ☐ 4. Perform the examination as quickly as possible.

CORRECT ANSWER: 2
An empty bladder facilitates the examination of the fundus. Option 1: The client should be in a supine position with her arms at her sides and knees bent. The arms-overhead position is unnecessary. Option 3: Clean gloves should be used when assessing the perineum. Sterile gloves aren't necessary. Option 4: The postpartum examination shouldn't be done quickly. The nurse can take this time to teach the client about the changes in her body after delivery.
NP: Collecting data
CN: Health promotion and maintenance
CNS: Growth and development through the life span
CL: Application

60 The nurse is caring for an Rh-negative postpartum client; the physician orders RhoGAM administration. How many hours after the delivery can the RhoGAM be administered?
- ☐ 1. No longer than 12 hours
- ☐ 2. No longer than 24 hours
- ☐ 3. No longer than 48 hours
- ☐ 4. No longer than 72 hours

CORRECT ANSWER: 4
RhoGAM can be given shortly after delivery, but the latest that RhoGAM can be effectively given is 72 hours postpartum. Options 1, 2, and 3: RhoGAM can be given 12, 24, and 48 hours after delivery.
NP: Implementing care
CN: Physiological integrity
CNS: Pharmacological therapies
CL: Comprehension

61 The nurse is evaluating a postpartum client for factors that increase the risk of postpartum hemorrhage. Which postpartum client is at low risk for postpartum hemorrhage?
- ☐ 1. A multiparous client who experienced a precipitous labor and birth
- ☐ 2. A primiparous client who gave birth to a 3-kg (6 lb, 10 oz) neonate
- ☐ 3. A multiparous client who gave birth to her seventh child
- ☐ 4. A primiparous client who continues to receive an infusion of magnesium sulfate for preeclampsia

CORRECT ANSWER: 2
Giving birth to a 3-kg neonate is an expected outcome of pregnancy, so this primiparous client is at low risk for postpartum hemorrhage. Options 1, 3, and 4: A multiparous client who has a history of precipitous labor and birth, a multiparous client who has given birth to her seventh child, and a primiparous client with preeclampsia who is receiving magnesium sulfate are all at risk for postpartum hemorrhage.
NP: Evaluating care
CN: Health promotion and maintenance
CNS: Growth and development through the life span
CL: Comprehension

62 A nurse is teaching a childbirth education class. Birth occurs at which stage of labor?
- ☐ 1. First stage of labor
- ☐ 2. Second stage of labor
- ☐ 3. Third stage of labor
- ☐ 4. Fourth stage of labor

CORRECT ANSWER: 2
The second stage of labor begins with complete dilation (10 cm) and ends with the birth of the infant. Option 1: The first stage of labor is the stage of dilation, which is divided into three distinct phases: latent, active, and transition. Option 3: The third stage of labor begins after the birth of the infant and ends with the expulsion of the placenta. Option 4: The fourth stage of labor is the first 4 hours after placental expulsion, in which the client's body begins the recovery process.
NP: Planning care
CN: Physiological integrity
CNS: Basic care and comfort
CL: Knowledge

63 The pediatric nurse is caring for infants in a busy nursery. When weighing a neonate, the nurse should:
☐ 1. leave the diaper on for comfort.
☐ 2. place a sterile scale paper on the scale for infection control.
☐ 3. keep a hand on the neonate's abdomen for safety.
☐ 4. weigh the neonate at the same time each day for accuracy.

CORRECT ANSWER: 4
A client of any age should be weighed at the same time each day, using the same technique and wearing the same clothes. Option 1: A neonate should be weighed undressed. Option 2: Clean scale paper should be used when weighing the neonate. Sterile scale paper is unnecessary. Option 3: The nurse should keep a hand above, not on, the abdomen when weighing the neonate.
NP: Collecting data
CN: Health promotion and maintenance
CNS: Growth and development through the life span
CL: Application

64 The nurse is caring for a 36-year-old client in the delivery room. When examining the umbilical cord immediately after birth, what does the nurse expect to observe?
☐ 1. Two veins
☐ 2. One artery
☐ 3. Whitish gray coloration
☐ 4. Slight odor

CORRECT ANSWER: 3
The umbilical cord is whitish gray in color. Options 1 and 2: The umbilical cord contains two arteries and one vein. Option 4: The umbilical cord should have no odor.
NP: Collecting data
CN: Health promotion and maintenance
CNS: Growth and development through the life span
CL: Knowledge

65 The nurse is instructing a first-time mother before discharge. The nurse knows that the breast-feeding mother needs further instruction if she:
☐ 1. leans forward to bring the breast toward the baby.
☐ 2. holds the breast with her four fingers along the bottom and thumb at top.
☐ 3. stimulates the rooting reflex, then inserts the nipple and areola into the neonate's open mouth.
☐ 4. puts her finger into the neonate's mouth before removing the breast.

CORRECT ANSWER: 1
Instruct the mother to bring the neonate to the breast, not the breast to the neonate. Options 2, 3, and 4 are correct breast-feeding methods.
NP: Evaluating care
CN: Health promotion and maintenance
CNS: Growth and development through the life span
CL: Application

66 The nurse is instructing 29-year-old new parents who are trying to decide whether to have their son circumcised. Which is the best response to assist them in their decision?
☐ 1. "I had my son circumcised and I'm glad it was done."
☐ 2. "Circumcision is a difficult decision, but your physician knows best; it's better to have the baby circumcised now instead of later."
☐ 3. "Here are several pamphlets that relate the pros and cons about circumcision; read them and I'll return later and answer any questions you have."
☐ 4. "Circumcision prevents cancer and sexually transmitted diseases; it's easier to keep the baby clean. I definitely would have my son circumcised."

CORRECT ANSWER: 3
By giving written information to the parents, the nurse is allowing them to make an informed and educated decision. Options 1, 2, and 4 are forms of nontherapeutic communication and impose the nurse's opinions.
NP: Implementing care
CN: Psychosocial integrity
CNS: Coping and adaptation
CL: Application

67 A woman who is 32 weeks pregnant is brought into the emergency department after an automobile crash. She's bleeding vaginally, and fetal assessment reveals moderate distress. What should the nurse do first to reduce stress on the fetus?
☐ 1. Make sure that her I.V. fluids are being administered at a keep-vein-open rate.
☐ 2. Administer oxygen (O₂) by face mask at 6 to 10 L/minute.
☐ 3. Elevate the head of the bed to semi-Fowler's position.
☐ 4. Set up for an emergency cesarean delivery.

CORRECT ANSWER: 2
Providing O_2 to the mother increases the amount of O_2 circulating to the fetus, no matter how much blood is lost. Option 1: I.V. fluids administered at a keep-vein-open rate may increase uteroplacental perfusion but won't provide immediate direct care to the fetus. Option 3: Elevating the head of the bed is contraindicated until the cervical spine is cleared. Option 4: Although a cesarean birth may be an option if the stress on the fetus isn't alleviated, administering oxygen provides a more immediate and direct effect on the fetus and should be initiated first.
NP: Implementing care
CN: Physiological integrity
CNS: Reduction of risk potential
CL: Application

68 The nurse is caring for a client who is receiving oxytocin (Pitocin) to induce labor. While administering the oxytocin, it's most important for the nurse to monitor the:
☐ 1. fetal heart rate.
☐ 2. urine output.
☐ 3. maternal blood glucose level.
☐ 4. central venous pressure.

CORRECT ANSWER: 1
Oxytocin produces uterine contractions, which can cause fetal anoxia. The nurse should monitor the fetal heart rate and notify the physician of any changes. Options 2, 3, and 4: Urine output, maternal blood glucose level, and central venous pressure aren't related to the administration of oxytocin.
NP: Collecting data
CN: Physiological integrity
CNS: Pharmacological therapies
CL: Application

69 The nurse is caring for a 38-year-old pregnant woman in the first trimester who requires a transabdominal ultrasound. Which instructions should the nurse include?
☐ 1. Come to the office first for a contrast dye injection.
☐ 2. Take nothing by mouth (NPO) after 6 a.m. on the morning of the test.
☐ 3. Drink 1 to 2 qt (1 to 2 L) of water and don't urinate before the test.
☐ 4. No special instructions are needed before the ultrasound.

CORRECT ANSWER: 3
During the first trimester, the bladder needs to be full in order to push the uterus higher into the abdomen to obtain a clearer image. Options 1 and 2: The client doesn't need contrast dye or NPO instructions. Option 4: The client does need special instructions before undergoing an ultrasound.
NP: Implementing care
CN: Health promotion and maintenance
CNS: Growth and development through the life span
CL: Application

70 A primigravida at 40 weeks' gestation arrives in the labor room with ruptured amniotic membranes. Her cervix is 3 cm dilated and 100% effaced. Her contractions are occurring every 10 minutes. In the plan of care for this client, what should the nurse include?
☐ 1. Send the client home with instructions to return when her contractions increase to every 5 minutes.
☐ 2. Allow the client to walk around the nursing unit as long as the presenting part is engaged.
☐ 3. Assess fetal heart rate and maternal status every 5 minutes.
☐ 4. Place the client on a fetal monitor to assess the fetus.

CORRECT ANSWER: 2
Allowing the client to walk around aids contractions and dilation of the cervix; however, the presenting part must be engaged, without a risk of prolapsed umbilical cord. Option 1: Because the amniotic membranes have ruptured, sending the client home is contraindicated. Options 3 and 4: Constant or frequent monitoring isn't necessary at this early stage of labor.
NP: Planning care
CN: Health promotion and maintenance
CNS: Growth and development through the life span
CL: Application

71 The nurse is instructing a 19-year-old first-time mother before discharge. The mother demonstrates that she understands proper umbilical cord care for her neonate when she:
- ☐ 1. reads a booklet on neonate cord care.
- ☐ 2. states that bacitracin (Baciguent) ointment should be applied three times per day.
- ☐ 3. watches a video on neonate cord care.
- ☐ 4. cleans the cord and surrounding area with an alcohol swab.

CORRECT ANSWER: 4
The mother should understand how to care for her neonate before discharge. Umbilical cord care includes cleaning the cord stump three times per day with alcohol until the cord falls off in 1 to 2 weeks. Options 1 and 3: Reading a book or watching a video doesn't demonstrate understanding or knowledge. Repeat demonstrations should be used to confirm understanding. Option 2: No preparation other than alcohol should be used for cord care.
NP: Evaluating care
CN: Health promotion and maintenance
CNS: Growth and development through the life span
CL: Application

72 A nurse is teaching a prenatal class about immediate neonatal care after delivery. Which medication is given to the neonate to prevent hemorrhagic disease?
- ☐ 1. Vitamin K
- ☐ 2. heparin sodium (Hep-Lock)
- ☐ 3. Iron
- ☐ 4. warfarin sodium (Coumadin)

CORRECT ANSWER: 1
Neonates have coagulation deficiencies because of a lack of vitamin K in the intestines. Vitamin K helps the liver synthesize clotting factors II, VII, IX, and X. Options 2 and 4: Heparin and warfarin are given as anticoagulants, not as antihemorrhagics. Option 3: Iron is stored in the fetal liver; hemoglobin binds to iron and carries oxygen and isn't necessary to give to the neonate.
NP: Implementing care
CN: Health promotion and maintenance
CNS: Growth and development through the life span
CL: Knowledge

73 The nurse is caring for a 25-year-old client who has missed two of her regular menstrual periods. Her physician confirms an early, intrauterine pregnancy. This is the client's first pregnancy. To determine her expected due date, which fact is most important?
- ☐ 1. The date of her first menstrual cycle
- ☐ 2. The date of last intercourse
- ☐ 3. The age of menarche
- ☐ 4. The dates of her last normal menstrual period

CORRECT ANSWER: 4
The first day of the client's last normal menstrual period is used to calculate her expected due date. Options 1, 2, and 3: The other answers provide needed information as part of the client's general health history but wouldn't help determine her expected due date.
NP: Collecting data
CN: Health promotion and maintenance
CNS: Growth and development through the life span
CL: Comprehension

74 A 32-year-old client is admitted to the nursing unit for treatment of severe preeclampsia. Which finding is unusual for this condition?
- ☐ 1. Blood pressure of 168/108 mm Hg while the client is on bed rest
- ☐ 2. Proteinuria of 3+ in two urine samples collected 4 hours apart
- ☐ 3. Generalized edema, especially of the hands and face
- ☐ 4. Seizures or coma before the onset of labor

CORRECT ANSWER: 4
Seizures and coma are associated with an eclamptic condition. Options 1, 2, and 3: High blood pressure, proteinuria, and generalized edema are usual findings with severe preeclampsia.
NP: Collecting data
CN: Physiological integrity
CNS: Physiological adaptation
CL: Comprehension

75 The nurse is caring for a woman admitted to the facility in active labor. Which information is most important for the nurse to assess to avoid respiratory complications during labor and delivery?
- ☐ 1. Family history of lung disease
- ☐ 2. Food allergies
- ☐ 3. Whether the client smokes
- ☐ 4. When the client last ate

CORRECT ANSWER: 4
Aspiration is a respiratory complication that the nurse needs to watch for, especially if the client requires anesthesia. Options 1, 2, and 3: A family history of lung disease, food allergies, or smoking has no direct effect on respiratory complications during the labor process.
NP: Collecting data
CN: Physiological integrity
CNS: Physiological adaptation
CL: Application

---

76 The nurse is caring for a 33-year-old client who is in labor and 8 cm dilated. While giving support during this phase of labor, the nurse should:
- ☐ 1. offer her a back rub during contractions.
- ☐ 2. leave her alone.
- ☐ 3. offer her liquids.
- ☐ 4. place warm blankets over her.

CORRECT ANSWER: 1
The pain of the contractions can be reduced by rubbing the client's back during the contractions. Options 2 and 3: The client is in the transition phase of labor and shouldn't be left alone or offered liquids. Option 4: Women in labor generally feel hot due to increased metabolic changes, so a blanket isn't needed.
NP: Implementing care
CN: Physiological integrity
CNS: Physiological adaptation
CL: Application

---

77 The nurse is instructing a 28-year-old first-time mother before discharge. What is the best indication that the breast-fed baby is digesting the breast milk properly?
- ☐ 1. The baby passes dark green, pasty stools.
- ☐ 2. The baby passes soft, golden yellow stools.
- ☐ 3. The baby sleeps through the night after each feeding.
- ☐ 4. The baby doesn't experience colic.

CORRECT ANSWER: 2
A breast-fed baby has 6 to 10 small, loose, golden yellow stools per day. Option 1: A formula-fed baby has dark green, pasty stools. Option 3: After feeding, a satisfied, well-fed baby sleeps for a few hours, not necessarily through the night. Option 4: Any baby can have colic.
NP: Evaluating care
CN: Health promotion and maintenance
CNS: Growth and development through the life span
CL: Comprehension

---

78 Five minutes after birth, a baby girl is crying vigorously and moving all extremities. Her hands and feet are still slightly cyanotic, and her heart rate is 136 beats/minute. Which Apgar score should the nurse record?
- ☐ 1. 7
- ☐ 2. 8
- ☐ 3. 9
- ☐ 4. 10

CORRECT ANSWER: 3
The total Apgar score is 9. Slight cyanosis (acrocyanosis) is normal in a neonate for the first 24 hours; the Apgar score for this is 1. Crying vigorously (indicative of a 2-point respiratory score as well as a 2-point reflex score on Apgar), moving all extremities, and having a heart rate of 136 beats/minute are normal signs and should be rated 2 each. Options 1, 2, and 4 are incorrect scores.
NP: Collecting data
CN: Health promotion and maintenance
CNS: Growth and development through the life span
CL: Application

79 The nurse is talking to a pregnant client in the facility. The client says she has swelling in her feet and ankles. Which recommendation would be most appropriate for the nurse to make?
- ☐ 1. Limit fluid intake.
- ☐ 2. Buy walking shoes.
- ☐ 3. Sit and elevate the feet twice daily.
- ☐ 4. Start taking a diuretic as needed daily.

CORRECT ANSWER: 3
Sitting down and putting her feet up at least once daily will promote venous return and, therefore, decrease edema. Limiting fluid intake (option 1) isn't recommended unless there are additional medical complications such as heart failure. Buying walking shoes (option 2) won't necessarily decrease edema. Diuretics (option 4) aren't recommended during pregnancy because it's important to maintain an adequate circulatory volume.
NP: Planning care
CN: Physiological integrity
CNS: Basic care and comfort
CL: Application

---

80 The nurse is instructing a 22-year-old client in a family-planning facility. The client states, "I just can't believe that I'm going to have a baby." Which response by the nurse is best?
- ☐ 1. "Your pregnancy has been confirmed so you shouldn't have any doubts now."
- ☐ 2. "Would you like me to make an appointment with the mental health nurse for pregnancy counseling?"
- ☐ 3. "These feelings are normal for first-time mothers; tell me how you feel."
- ☐ 4. "I can give you some pamphlets on pregnancy and childbirth."

CORRECT ANSWER: 3
Acknowledging the client's feelings and allowing her to discuss them opens communication between nurse and client. Options 1 and 4: Telling the client that she should have no doubts or simply handing her pamphlets on pregnancy and childbirth would shut down any chance of good communication between nurse and client. Option 2: There is no indication that a mental health consultation is needed.
NP: Implementing care
CN: Health promotion and maintenance
CNS: Growth and development through the life span
CL: Application

---

81 While conducting a childbirth class, the nurse is reviewing the anatomy and physiology of pregnancy and fetal development. Which statement about the umbilical cord is correct?
- ☐ 1. The umbilical cord contains one vein and one artery.
- ☐ 2. The umbilical cord contains two veins and two arteries.
- ☐ 3. The umbilical cord contains one vein and two arteries.
- ☐ 4. The umbilical cord contains two veins and one artery.

CORRECT ANSWER: 3
The umbilical cord normally contains one vein and two arteries. Nutrients and oxygen are carried to the fetal circulation through the umbilical vein to the fetus. Oxygen-poor blood is carried back to the placenta by the two umbilical arteries. Options 1, 2, and 4 are false statements.
NP: Planning care
CN: Health promotion and maintenance
CNS: Growth and development through the life span
CL: Knowledge

---

82 The nurse educator is conducting a presentation about conception to practical nursing students. A student asks, "How many days after conception does the fertilized ovum implant in the uterine wall?" The nurse educator's best response is that the process normally takes:
- ☐ 1. 3 days.
- ☐ 2. 7 days.
- ☐ 3. 15 days.
- ☐ 4. 24 days.

CORRECT ANSWER: 2
The fertilized ovum stays in the fallopian tube for about 3 days and in the uterus for about 4 days before it implants into the uterine wall, so there are 7 days between conception and implantation. Options 1, 3, and 4 are incorrect.
NP: Implementing care
CN: Health promotion and maintenance
CNS: Growth and development through the life span
CL: Knowledge

83 The nurse is caring for a primigravida admitted to the facility at 12 weeks' gestation. She has abdominal cramping and bright red vaginal spotting. Her cervix isn't dilated. Which diagnosis is most likely?
☐ 1. Incomplete abortion
☐ 2. Missed abortion
☐ 3. Inevitable abortion
☐ 4. Threatened abortion

CORRECT ANSWER: 4
During a threatened abortion, the client experiences vaginal bleeding or spotting; the cervix isn't dilated, and abdominal pain may be present. Option 1: In an incomplete abortion, some of the products of conception are expelled from the uterus; usually, the placenta remains. Option 2: In a missed abortion, the fetus dies, but the products of conception aren't expelled from the uterus. Uterine growth ceases, the cervix is closed, and no bleeding occurs, but there may be a brownish discharge. Option 3: In an inevitable abortion, the client experiences more bleeding and increased cramping; the cervix dilates and the loss of the pregnancy can't be prevented.
NP: Collecting data
CN: Physiological integrity
CNS: Physiological adaptation
CL: Comprehension

84 A 28-year-old primiparous woman is admitted to the facility. She had a spontaneous abortion and underwent dilatation and curettage. The nurse finds the client crying and clearly upset. Which nursing diagnosis is most important for the client at this time?
☐ 1. *Deficient knowledge related to the lost pregnancy*
☐ 2. *Powerlessness related to loss and grief*
☐ 3. *Anxiety related to self-esteem*
☐ 4. *Acute pain related to surgical procedure*

CORRECT ANSWER: 2
Crying and feeling upset are related to the client's feelings of powerlessness over the loss of her pregnancy. Options 1 and 3: The client's current behavior probably isn't related to deficient knowledge or anxiety but is related more to the feeling of hopelessness and powerlessness in being able to control what happened to her. Option 4: The client may be experiencing pain, but *Powerlessness* is the most important nursing diagnosis at this time.
NP: Collecting data
CN: Psychosocial integrity
CNS: Coping and adaptation
CL: Application

85 A 17-year-old client visits the prenatal clinic where she has been receiving care for her pregnancy. She's at 30 weeks' gestation and is experiencing early signs of pregnancy-induced hypertension. Which data indicates mild pregnancy-induced hypertension?
☐ 1. Urine output of less than 400 ml/24 hours
☐ 2. Proteinuria of more than 5 g/24 hours
☐ 3. Swelling of face, fingers, hands, and ankles
☐ 4. Blood pressure of 166/112 mm Hg on two occasions

CORRECT ANSWER: 3
Generalized edema—especially in the face, fingers, hands, and ankles—is a common sign of mild pregnancy-induced hypertension. Options 1, 2, and 4: Urine output of less than 400 ml/24 hours, proteinuria of more than 5 g/24 hours, and blood pressure of 166/112 mm Hg on two occasions are signs of severe pregnancy-induced hypertension.
NP: Collecting data
CN: Physiological integrity
CNS: Physiological adaptation
CL: Comprehension

86 A nurse is teaching a prepared childbirth class. Which activity is inappropriate to include in the class?
☐ 1. Practicing bearing-down exercises
☐ 2. Relaxing and deep breathing to music
☐ 3. Taking a tour of the labor areas of the facility
☐ 4. Discussing nutritional needs

CORRECT ANSWER: 1
Bearing-down exercises should be avoided to prevent accidental premature rupture of the membranes, which could result from the force of bearing down. Options 2, 3, and 4: Components of prepared childbirth classes should include positioning, relaxation, and deep-breathing exercises. Discussion of choices the mother needs to make during the childbearing experience—such as nutrition, rest, exercise, lifestyle, selection of a pediatrician, and options for promoting comfort during labor—should also be included.
NP: Implementing care
CN: Health promotion and maintenance
CNS: Growth and development through the life span
CL: Knowledge

---

87 A 38-year-old client is admitted with a suspected ectopic pregnancy. While interviewing the client, the nurse needs to assess whether the client:
☐ 1. recently had intercourse.
☐ 2. is taking birth control pills.
☐ 3. knows when her last menstrual period began.
☐ 4. has been pregnant before.

CORRECT ANSWER: 3
The most important information is the 1st day of the client's last menstrual period. This will aid in the diagnosis of ectopic pregnancy. Options 1, 2, and 4: The nurse needs to learn whether the client recently had intercourse, is taking birth control pills, or has been pregnant before, but these aren't the primary concerns in diagnosing this client's suspected problem.
NP: Collecting data
CN: Physiological integrity
CNS: Reduction of risk potential
CL: Application

---

88 A nurse working in the nursery observes that a neonate has circumoral cyanosis. This is indicated by:
☐ 1. bluish discoloration of the hands and feet.
☐ 2. bluish discoloration around the mouth.
☐ 3. mottled skin with bluish discoloration of the hands and feet.
☐ 4. bluish discoloration of the skin varying in size of area covered that is usually found on the lower back.

CORRECT ANSWER: 2
Circumoral cyanosis is bluish discoloration around the mouth. Option 1: Acrocyanosis is localized bluish discoloration of the hands and feet. Option 3: Vasomotor instability causes mottled skin with bluish discoloration of the hands. Option 4: Bluish discoloration on the trunk, usually on the lower back, is called mongolian spots.
NP: Implementing care
CN: Health promotion and maintenance
CNS: Growth and development through the life span
CL: Application

---

89 A 29-year-old primigravida delivers a viable male neonate who is given an Apgar score of 8. The nurse concludes that the neonate's physical condition is:
☐ 1. good.
☐ 2. fair.
☐ 3. poor.
☐ 4. critical.

CORRECT ANSWER: 1
The Apgar system rates the neonate's heart rate, respiratory effort, muscle tone, reflex irritability, and color at 1 minute after birth and again at 5 minutes. Each assessment is worth 0 to 2 points, with a maximum total of 10. The higher the score, the better the neonate's condition. Options 2, 3, and 4: A score of 6 to 7 indicates fair physical condition. A score of 4 to 5 indicates poor physical condition. A score of 0 to 3 indicates critical condition.
NP: Collecting data
CN: Health promotion and maintenance
CNS: Prevention and early detection of disease
CL: Application

90 A 30-year-old primigravida at 38 weeks' gestation is admitted to the obstetric nursing unit in active labor. The client's husband is coaching her with breathing and relaxation techniques they learned in childbirth classes. When the client reaches the transition stage, she screams out, "I can't do this anymore!" What is an appropriate suggestion for the nurse to give to the husband?
- ☐ 1. Ask his wife if she wants analgesia.
- ☐ 2. Leave the room until his wife gets control of herself.
- ☐ 3. Tell his wife that she's doing well and it will be over soon.
- ☐ 4. Talk to his wife while maintaining eye contact and breathing with her.

CORRECT ANSWER: 4
The transition of labor is taught in childbirth classes. The husband needs to reinforce the teaching during this phase of labor by maintaining eye contact and helping his wife to concentrate on each contraction as it comes. Option 1: During the transition phase, offering analgesia is inappropriate because delivery is imminent and respiration can be depressed in the fetus. Option 2: The husband needs to stay and support his wife, especially now. Option 3: Telling the client that she's doing well and that it will be over soon may be helpful but isn't as important as maintaining eye contact and breathing with her during this difficult stage of labor.
NP: Implementing care
CN: Physiological integrity
CNS: Reduction of risk potential
CL: Application

91 The nurse is caring for a 34-year-old client who just delivered her second child. The physician orders oxytocin (Pitocin) I.V. following delivery of the placenta. Which sign or symptom indicates that the placenta is about to be delivered?
- ☐ 1. The abdominal wall relaxes markedly.
- ☐ 2. The client complains of back pain.
- ☐ 3. The umbilical cord lengthens outside the vagina.
- ☐ 4. The uterus falls below the symphysis pubis.

CORRECT ANSWER: 3
The most reliable sign that the placenta has detached from the uterine wall is the umbilical cord lengthening outside the uterus. Options 1 and 2: The abdominal wall doesn't relax and the client doesn't complain of back pain when the placenta is about to be delivered. Option 4: The uterine fundus rises in the uterus and the uterus becomes globular, which is noticeable on the abdominal wall.
NP: Collecting data
CN: Physiological integrity
CNS: Reduction of risk potential
CL: Comprehension

92 The nurse is caring for a 24-year-old first-time mother who just delivered a male neonate. While the client holds the infant, she begins to cry. The nurse concludes that the client is:
- ☐ 1. likely to have trouble bonding with the neonate.
- ☐ 2. disappointed in the baby's sex.
- ☐ 3. grieving over the loss of the pregnancy.
- ☐ 4. experiencing a normal response to the birth.

CORRECT ANSWER: 4
Childbirth is a very emotional experience for most mothers. Tears of happiness are a normal response. Options 1, 2, and 3: Crying is a normal response and doesn't indicate a bonding problem, disappointment in the baby's sex, or grieving over the loss of the pregnancy.
NP: Collecting data
CN: Health promotion and maintenance
CNS: Growth and development through the life span
CL: Application

93 The nurse is caring for a 28-year-old first-time mother who just delivered a full-term female neonate. The client asks the nurse when she can begin to breast-feed her baby. The nurse tells the client that breast-feeding can begin:
- ☐ 1. immediately after birth.
- ☐ 2. in about 2 hours, after the baby is bathed.
- ☐ 3. in about 8 hours, after the baby has had some rest.
- ☐ 4. after the baby's first bottle-feeding.

CORRECT ANSWER: 1
The American Academy of Pediatrics recommends beginning breast-feeding as soon as possible after delivery. Option 2: A bath isn't needed to begin breast-feeding. Option 3: The baby is active and alert at this time and doesn't need to rest. Option 4: If a baby is going to be breast-fed, a bottle shouldn't be given.
NP: Implementing care
CN: Health promotion and maintenance
CNS: Growth and development through the life span
CL: Application

94 A 26-year-old primigravida is admitted to the obstetric nursing unit. The nurse notes on the chart that the client is 3 cm dilated. The client asks if she must remain in bed. What is the nurse's best response?
- ☐ 1. "It's best to stay in bed to help prevent the cord from prolapsing."
- ☐ 2. "You may get up to go to the bathroom, but otherwise you should remain in bed."
- ☐ 3. "It's best to remain in bed and lie on your left side for better oxygen supply to the baby."
- ☐ 4. "You may walk around, but notify me immediately if the amniotic membranes rupture."

CORRECT ANSWER: 4
Most physicians recommend walking around in the early stages of labor if there are no complications. After the amniotic membranes rupture, the client should remain in bed. Option 1: In primigravidas, engagement usually occurs 2 weeks before the onset of labor, thus reducing the risk of a prolapsed cord. Option 2: Because the client's amniotic membranes haven't yet ruptured, she doesn't have to remain in bed. Option 3: If the client must stay in bed for some reason—for instance, if her membranes have ruptured—then having her lie on her left side is the best option.
NP: Implementing care
CN: Physiological integrity
CNS: Reduction of risk potential
CL: Analysis

---

95 The nurse is caring for a 27-year-old primigravida in the obstetric nursing unit. The client has the urge to push, but on examination the nurse notes that she isn't completely dilated. What is the nurse's best action at this time?
- ☐ 1. Administer a prescribed sedative.
- ☐ 2. Let the client push.
- ☐ 3. Position the client for pushing.
- ☐ 4. Suggest the client use a pant-blow breathing pattern.

CORRECT ANSWER: 4
The pant-blow breathing pattern will help the client to overcome the urge to push. Option 1: Sedatives aren't recommended at this time because they would prolong the labor process. Options 2 and 3: Pushing before the cervix is completely dilated tends to make labor more difficult.
NP: Implementing care
CN: Health promotion and maintenance
CNS: Growth and development through the life span
CL: Application

---

96 A 31-year-old primigravida in the obstetric nursing unit is in the transition stage of labor. During this stage, the nurse's primary action is to provide:
- ☐ 1. encouragement and support.
- ☐ 2. extra fluids.
- ☐ 3. extra blankets.
- ☐ 4. distraction from the pain.

CORRECT ANSWER: 1
The transitional phase of labor can be very difficult and painful, especially when the contractions become stronger. The nurse's primary responsibility is to provide encouragement and support during this time. Option 2: There is no indication that extra fluids should be given. Option 3: Extra blankets aren't required because most women feel hot during labor because of metabolic changes. Option 4: Providing distraction from the pain is a secondary nursing concern.
NP: Implementing care
CN: Health promotion and maintenance
CNS: Growth and development through the life span
CL: Application

---

97 A 37-year-old multigravida has been admitted to the obstetric nursing unit in active labor. The client calls out to the nurse, "The baby is coming!" What should the nurse do next?
- ☐ 1. Time the contractions.
- ☐ 2. Inspect the perineum.
- ☐ 3. Contact the physician.
- ☐ 4. Assess the fetal heart rate (FHR).

CORRECT ANSWER: 2
The nurse should inspect the client's perineum for crowning at this time. Most multigravidous clients are aware of the baby's movement in the vaginal canal and may feel the "baby coming." This should never be disputed with the client. Options 1, 3, and 4: Timing contractions, contacting the physician, and assessing the FHR rate (which is done continuously during labor) aren't the nurse's primary responses at this time.
NP: Implementing care
CN: Health promotion and maintenance
CNS: Growth and development through the life span
CL: Application

98 A 27-year-old primigravida in the obstetric nursing unit is in active labor. Which response best helps the client remain calm and cooperative during the delivery?

- ☐ 1. "The baby is coming; I'll explain everything and guide you as we go along."
- ☐ 2. "Even though the baby is coming, the physician will be here soon."
- ☐ 3. "Do you want me to call your husband?"
- ☐ 4. "The baby is coming; just relax and everything will be fine."

CORRECT ANSWER: 1
The client must remain calm during the sudden delivery. Giving explanations and guiding the client will assist her to remain calm. Options 2, 3, and 4: The remaining responses aren't supportive answers during a sudden delivery.
NP: Implementing care
CN: Psychosocial integrity
CNS: Coping and adaptation
CL: Application

99 The nurse is caring for a 27-year-old primigravida in active labor. What should the nurse do as the baby's head is being delivered?

- ☐ 1. Apply gentle traction on the baby's anterior shoulder.
- ☐ 2. Apply gentle pressure on the client's uterine fundus with one hand.
- ☐ 3. Tell the client to push forcefully.
- ☐ 4. Check for the umbilical cord around the baby's neck.

CORRECT ANSWER: 4
The nurse should always check for an umbilical cord around the baby's neck after the head is delivered. If the cord is found to be tight around the baby's neck, the cord should be double clamped and cut to facilitate the delivery. If it isn't tight, the nurse should try to ease the cord over the baby's head and proceed with assisting with the delivery. Options 1, 2, and 3: Applying pressure or traction or having the client push isn't indicated.
NP: Implementing care
CN: Physiological integrity
CNS: Reduction of risk potential
CL: Application

100 The nurse is caring for a 21-year-old first-time mother whose female neonate is in good condition after delivery. What should the nurse do next after suctioning the infant's airway?

- ☐ 1. Perform cardiac massage.
- ☐ 2. Assist with intubation.
- ☐ 3. Ensure adequate warmth.
- ☐ 4. Administer oxygen therapy.

CORRECT ANSWER: 3
A neonate in good condition needs to be kept warm. All assessments can be done while keeping the neonate warm. Options 1, 2, and 4: A neonate in good condition doesn't require cardiac massage, intubation, or oxygen therapy.
NP: Implementing care
CN: Physiological integrity
CNS: Reduction of risk potential
CL: Application

101 The nurse is caring for a new mother and her infant in the client's room. When the bassinet is accidentally bumped, the neonate throws out its arms, opens its hands, and begins to cry. The nurse explains to the mother that this is the:

- ☐ 1. Moro reflex.
- ☐ 2. grasping reflex.
- ☐ 3. tonic neck reflex.
- ☐ 4. rooting reflex.

CORRECT ANSWER: 1
The Moro or startle reflex is present in neonates and disappears in about 3 months. Option 2: The grasping reflex occurs when the neonate grasps at objects placed near the hand. Option 3: The tonic neck reflex is noted when the neonate is supine and turns the head to one side. Option 4: The rooting reflex is present when the neonate turns the head and opens the mouth to the side on which the cheek is stroked in preparation for nursing. Head turning to the side causes the extremities on that side to straighten and on the opposite side to flex.
NP: Implementing care
CN: Health promotion and maintenance
CNS: Growth and development through the life span
CL: Comprehension

102 The nurse is caring for a first-time mother about 5 hours after a spontaneous vaginal delivery under local anesthesia. The client states that she needs to void. What should the nurse do?
- ☐ 1. Catheterize the client.
- ☐ 2. Offer the client a bedpan.
- ☐ 3. Check her bladder for distention.
- ☐ 4. Assist the client to the bathroom.

CORRECT ANSWER: 4
About 4 hours after a spontaneous vaginal delivery under local anesthesia, the client may begin to walk around with the assistance of the nurse, especially to the bathroom. Option 1: Catheterization is a last resort. Option 2: There is no need for a bedpan. Option 3: If the client has to void, her bladder may be distended, but there is no need to check it if the client has the urge to void.
NP: Implementing care
CN: Physiological integrity
CNS: Basic care and comfort
CL: Application

103 The nurse is teaching a 16-year-old primipara before her discharge. The client asks the nurse how often she should hold her baby to avoid "spoiling him." The nurse's best response is to teach the new mother to hold her baby:
- ☐ 1. only when feeding him.
- ☐ 2. as much as possible.
- ☐ 3. only when he's fussy.
- ☐ 4. occasionally.

CORRECT ANSWER: 2
Holding and caressing the baby helps him to develop trust in his caregivers. Stimulation is important and should be encouraged. Holding a baby doesn't "spoil" him. Options 1, 3, and 4: Holding a baby only when feeding him, when he's fussy, or occasionally doesn't promote maternal-infant bonding and doesn't help the baby develop trust in his caregivers.
NP: Implementing care
CN: Health promotion and maintenance
CNS: Growth and development through the life span
CL: Application

104 A 16-year-old primipara changes her baby's diaper for the first time while the nurse evaluates her mothering skills. When caring for an adolescent mother, the nurse should focus on the client's need for:
- ☐ 1. her mother to assist her.
- ☐ 2. special psychological counseling.
- ☐ 3. prolonged verbal instructions.
- ☐ 4. praise and encouragement.

CORRECT ANSWER: 4
An adolescent mother needs praise and encouragement about her mothering skills to improve her confidence and self-esteem. Option 1: The nurse can teach the client without the client's mother present. Option 2: Special psychological counseling isn't indicated for this client. Option 3: Prolonged verbal instructions would overwhelm the adolescent mother.
NP: Collecting data
CN: Health promotion and maintenance
CNS: Growth and development through the life span
CL: Application

105 A 19-year-old primipara has delivered a viable male neonate who has a strong sucking reflex. The client has decided to breast-feed and her husband supports her decision. The client tells the nurse, "I'm going to need a lot of help with breast-feeding because I've never done this before." While assessing the client, the nurse should:
- ☐ 1. evaluate the literature on breast-feeding that the client has read.
- ☐ 2. determine the client's level of motivation to breast-feed.
- ☐ 3. assess the client's nutritional status.
- ☐ 4. perform a physical examination of the client's breasts.

CORRECT ANSWER: 2
Willingness and motivation to breast-feed are important for successful breast-feeding. Having the husband's support is also important. Option 1: Evaluating the client's literature wouldn't ensure the success of breast-feeding. Option 3: If the client's nutrition is poor, the nurse can teach the client how to improve her diet but this wouldn't necessarily ensure successful breast-feeding. Option 4: Examining the client's breasts isn't necessary.
NP: Collecting data
CN: Health promotion and maintenance
CNS: Growth and development through the life span
CL: Application

106 The nurse is teaching a 24-year-old primipara before discharge with her infant. What's the correct sleeping position for the baby?
☐ 1. On the right side
☐ 2. On the left side
☐ 3. Prone, with the head elevated
☐ 4. Supine, without the head elevated

CORRECT ANSWER: 4
The American Academy of Pediatrics recommends that babies be placed flat on their backs when sleeping. Options 1, 2, and 3: On the right side, on the left side, and prone with the head elevated aren't appropriate positions for babies to sleep.
NP: Implementing care
CN: Physiological integrity
CNS: Reduction of risk potential
CL: Application

107 A 24-year-old primipara required a cesarean delivery because of cephalopelvic disproportion. The client has been ordered a full liquid diet as tolerated following the delivery. Before providing a full liquid dinner, the nurse should assess the client's:
☐ 1. breath sounds.
☐ 2. ability to walk.
☐ 3. bowel sounds.
☐ 4. degree of pain.

CORRECT ANSWER: 3
The nurse should assess for the presence of bowel sounds before serving the client a full liquid dinner. Bowel sounds indicate that normal peristalsis is present and that GI function has returned. Options 1, 2, and 4: The client's breath sounds, ability to walk, and degree of pain are checked in an assessment, but not before serving the client a liquid meal.
NP: Implementing care
CN: Physiological integrity
CNS: Basic care and comfort
CL: Application

108 A 41-year-old multiparous client delivers her fourth child prematurely, and the neonate is stillborn. The client asks to see her baby. Which response by the nurse is most appropriate?
☐ 1. Allow her to see and hold her baby as desired to aid in the grieving process.
☐ 2. Allow her to see her baby only if it's physically normal.
☐ 3. Don't allow her to see her baby, because this may precipitate postpartum depression.
☐ 4. Don't allow her to see her baby, because it's the nurse's responsibility to protect the client from unnecessary trauma.

CORRECT ANSWER: 1
The client has the right to see her baby. Options 2, 3, and 4: The other responses aren't appropriate, because seeing and holding her baby's body, regardless of the baby's physical condition, aids the client in the grieving process.
NP: Implementing care
CN: Psychosocial integrity
CNS: Coping and adaptation
CL: Application

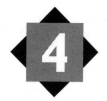

Pediatric Nursing

1 A nanny is taught to administer digoxin (Lanoxin) to a 6-month-old infant at home. Which statement by the nanny indicates the need for additional teaching?
☐ 1. "I'll count the baby's pulse before every dose."
☐ 2. "I'll make sure the pulse is regular before I give the drug."
☐ 3. "I'll measure the dose carefully."
☐ 4. "I'll withhold the medication if the pulse is below 60."

CORRECT ANSWER: 4
A pulse rate under 60 beats/minute is an indication for withholding digoxin from an adult. Withholding digoxin from an infant is appropriate if the infant's pulse is under 90 beats/minute. Option 1: The pulse rate must be counted before each dose of digoxin is given to an infant. Option 2: An irregular pulse may be a sign of digoxin toxicity; if this occurs, the physician should be consulted before the drug is given. Option 3: The dose must be measured carefully to decrease any risk of toxicity.
NP: Evaluating care
CN: Physiological integrity
CNS: Pharmacological therapies
CL: Application

2 A 12-year-old client with cystic fibrosis reports that he has been taking his pancrelipase (Pancrease) as prescribed. Which statement indicates that the child understands when this medication must be taken?
☐ 1. "I always take it whenever I have a meal or snack."
☐ 2. "I take it even if I'm in a rush and skip breakfast."
☐ 3. "I take it only if I feel like I need it."
☐ 4. "I always take my doses 12 hours apart, at 7:00 a.m. and 7:00 p.m."

CORRECT ANSWER: 1
Cystic fibrosis prevents essential pancreatic enzymes from reaching the duodenum. This causes marked impairment of the digestion and absorption of nutrients. Oral administration of pancreatic enzymes that are taken at every meal or snack offsets this physiologic dysfunction. Options 2, 3, and 4: This medication has the same action as naturally produced pancreatic enzymes and should therefore be taken with each meal or snack.
NP: Evaluating care
CN: Physiological integrity
CNS: Pharmacological therapies
CL: Comprehension

3 The nurse is caring for a 17-year-old girl who is receiving total parenteral nutrition (TPN). The nurse understands that this solution is given:
☐ 1. directly into a superficial vein.
☐ 2. directly into the superior vena cava.
☐ 3. through a gastrostomy tube.
☐ 4. orally as part of the prescribed diet.

CORRECT ANSWER: 2
TPN is given through a catheter passed directly into the superior vena cava by way of the jugular or subclavian vein. A cellulose membrane filter is used to filter out bacteria. Options 1, 3, and 4: These routes are never used for TPN.
NP: Implementing care
CN: Physiological integrity
CNS: Pharmacological therapies
CL: Comprehension

4 The nurse is trying to weigh a 3-year-old child who is irritable and refuses to stand on the scale. What is the best way to obtain an accurate weight?
☐ 1. Ask the mother to approximate the weight.
☐ 2. Ask the mother to hold the child and record the combined weights.
☐ 3. Weigh the mother and child and subtract the mother's weight from the combined weight.
☐ 4. Obtain the admission weight and add 2 oz per day.

CORRECT ANSWER: 3
Subtracting the mother's weight from the combined weight will yield the child's accurate weight. Options 1 and 4: Weight is an important parameter used in calculating drug doses based on kilograms per body weight. It also provides the most accurate information about a client's fluid balance. For these reasons, it should never be approximated. Option 2: Combining the weights would be inaccurate.
NP: Collecting data
CN: Health promotion and maintenance
CNS: Growth and development through the life span
CL: Application

5 The physician prescribes an I.M. injection for a 15-month-old infant. Which injection site is recommended?
☐ 1. Vastus lateralis
☐ 2. Deltoid
☐ 3. Dorsogluteal
☐ 4. Ventrogluteal

CORRECT ANSWER: 1
The vastus lateralis, the largest muscle mass in small children, is used for I.M. injections. Option 2: The deltoid is avoided in children under age 6; it's used for small-volume injections only. Options 3 and 4: Gluteal sites aren't used unless a child has been walking for 2 years.
NP: Planning care
CN: Physiological integrity
CNS: Pharmacological therapies
CL: Application

6 Which statement by a caregiver indicates that a 10-month-old infant is at high risk for iron deficiency anemia?
☐ 1. "The baby is sleeping through the night without a bottle."
☐ 2. "The baby drinks about five 8-oz bottles of milk per day."
☐ 3. "The baby likes egg yolk in his cereal."
☐ 4. "The baby dislikes some vegetables, especially carrots."

CORRECT ANSWER: 2
The recommended intake of milk, which doesn't contain iron, is 24 oz per day; 40 oz per day exceeds the recommended allotment and may reduce iron intake from solid food sources, risking iron deficiency anemia. Option 1: This is an anticipated behavior at this age. Option 3: Egg yolk is a good source of iron and would minimize any risk factor related to nutritional anemia. Option 4: Because only dark green, leafy vegetables are good sources of iron, this wouldn't be significant.
NP: Collecting data
CN: Physiological integrity
CNS: Basic care and comfort
CL: Analysis

7 Which action by the nurse is most effective in preventing postoperative atelectasis in a child who has just undergone surgery?
☐ 1. Support the incision with a pillow.
☐ 2. Change the client's position every 6 hours.
☐ 3. Teach the child how to deep breathe and cough.
☐ 4. Elevate the head of the bed 45 degrees.

CORRECT ANSWER: 3
Atelectasis, the collapse of the alveoli, can occur when postoperative secretions accumulate. Deep breathing and coughing promote lung expansion, thereby mobilizing secretions. Supporting the incision (option 1) may be helpful and should be incorporated into the plan of care, but it doesn't actively promote lung expansion. The child's position should be changed more frequently than every 6 hours (option 2). Elevating the head of the bed (option 4) wouldn't be important in promoting lung expansion.
NP: Implementing care
CN: Physiological integrity
CNS: Basic care and comfort
CL: Application

8 A 9-year-old child is admitted to the hospital with an infectious disease. Which action is consistent with standard precautions?
- ☐ 1. Capping all needle after use
- ☐ 2. Substituting glove wearing for hand washing
- ☐ 3. Using mouth-to-mouth breathing for pulmonary resuscitation
- ☐ 4. Using puncture-resistant containers for sharp objects

CORRECT ANSWER: 4
Only the use of a puncture-proof container for sharp objects is an application of standard precautions. Option 1: Used needles are never recapped; this would risk a contaminated puncture wound. Option 2: Hand washing is the most important barrier against the transmission of disease. Gloves don't replace this basic and effective means of preventing cross-contamination. Option 3: When implementing standard precautions, disposable ventilation devices — not mouth-to-mouth breathing — are used.
NP: Implementing care
CN: Safe, effective care environment
CNS: Safety and infection control
CL: Application

9 The nurse teaches a diabetic client about NPH and regular insulin. Which statement indicates that the client understands the instructions?
- ☐ 1. "I'll draw up the NPH insulin first."
- ☐ 2. "I must keep insulin in the refrigerator."
- ☐ 3. "I'll draw up the regular insulin first."
- ☐ 4. "Exercise will slow the absorption of my insulin."

CORRECT ANSWER: 3
The recommended technique is to draw up the regular insulin before the NPH. Option 1: NPH insulin shouldn't be drawn up first. Option 2: Insulin may be stored at room temperature, below 85° F (29.4° C). Option 4: Exercising muscles used for injection increases the absorption of insulin. For this reason, the client should avoid excessive exercise at insulin's peak action time or should use an alternate site, such as the abdomen, for injection.
NP: Evaluation
CN: Health promotion and maintenance
CNS: Prevention and early detection of disease
CL: Application

10 When attempting to dislodge a foreign object from an infant's airway, the rescuer should initiate five back blows followed by:
- ☐ 1. a blind sweep of the airway.
- ☐ 2. five abdominal thrusts.
- ☐ 3. five chest thrusts.
- ☐ 4. five ventilations.

CORRECT ANSWER: 3
To dislodge a foreign object, the rescuer should support the infant's head, keeping it lower than the trunk; turn the infant, placing him supine on the rescuer's thigh; and then administer five quick thrusts, in rapid succession, in the same location as external chest compressions used in cardiopulmonary resuscitation. Back blows and chest compressions are continued until the object is dislodged. Option 1: A blind sweep of the airway is never performed on children. Option 2: Abdominal thrusts are recommended for children over age 1. Option 4: Ventilations would be useless because the airway is obstructed.
NP: Implementing care
CN: Physiological integrity
CNS: Reduction of risk potential
CL: Comprehension

11 A 13-year-old client with asthma has been taking 5 mg of prednisone (Deltasone) daily for the past 6 months. Which finding would indicate a serious complication of this steroid therapy?
- ☐ 1. Weight gain of 1 lb (.5 kg)
- ☐ 2. Full face
- ☐ 3. Edema over the sacral area
- ☐ 4. Melena

CORRECT ANSWER: 4
Melena (blood in the stool) is an indication of peptic ulceration and GI bleeding, a serious sequela of steroid therapy. Options 1, 2, and 3 are anticipated adverse effects of long-term prednisone use. These signs are associated with Cushing's syndrome.
NP: Collecting data
CN: Physiological integrity
CNS: Pharmacological therapies
CL: Comprehension

12 A 4-year-old boy falls from his bed and sustains a ¹/₃" (1-cm) laceration of the forehead, which is bleeding profusely. The child is sitting on the floor crying. What should the nurse do first?
☐ 1. Lay him on the floor and determine the extent of his injuries.
☐ 2. Return him to bed and call the physician.
☐ 3. Apply pressure to the laceration and summon help.
☐ 4. Record his pulse and blood pressure.

CORRECT ANSWER: 3
Because the child is conscious, the first priority is to apply pressure to the head wound and stop the active bleeding. Options 1, 2, and 4 are appropriate actions and should be taken after the bleeding is controlled.
NP: Implementing care
CN: Physiological integrity
CNS: Reduction of risk potential
CL: Application

---

13 A 3-year-old child has nephrotic syndrome. As the amount of protein loss in the urine decreases, what response would the nurse expect?
☐ 1. Increased weight gain
☐ 2. Increased hyperlipidemia
☐ 3. Decreased edema
☐ 4. Decreased appetite

CORRECT ANSWER: 3
The loss of protein in the urine results in decreased osmotic pressure in the vascular system, causing a fluid shift to the extravascular compartments and producing edema. As the proteinuria decreases, the edema decreases. Option 1 is consistent with proteinuria and a fluid shift from the vascular to the interstitial spaces. Options 2 and 4: Hyperlipidemia and anorexia are associated with nephrotic syndrome but decrease as the disease resolves.
NP: Evaluating care
CN: Physiological integrity
CNS: Reduction of risk potential
CL: Comprehension

---

14 A client with thoracic water-seal drainage is on the elevator. The transport aide has placed the drainage system on the stretcher. What action should a nurse on the elevator take?
☐ 1. Assist the aide in placing the drainage system lower than the client's chest.
☐ 2. Report the incident to the registered nurse when she returns to the unit.
☐ 3. Clamp the drainage tubing with a hemostat.
☐ 4. Immediately take the client's respiratory and pulse rates.

CORRECT ANSWER: 1
The drainage device must be kept below the level of the chest to maintain straight gravity drainage. Placing it on the stretcher may cause a backflow of drainage into the thoracic cavity, which could collapse the partially expanded lung. Option 2: Reporting the incident is indicated, but the immediate safety of the client takes priority. Option 3: Clamping the tubing would place the client at risk for a tension pneumothorax. Option 4: After the drainage system has been properly repositioned, the client's respiratory and pulse rates may be taken.
NP: Implementing care
CN: Physiological integrity
CNS: Basic care and comfort
CL: Application

---

15 Which statement by a child with glomerulonephritis would require the nurse's immediate attention?
☐ 1. "I don't want anything for lunch except milk."
☐ 2. "The pictures in my book look all blurry."
☐ 3. "I don't want to stay in bed all the time."
☐ 4. "I want to go to the playroom like everybody else."

CORRECT ANSWER: 2
With glomerulonephritis, blurred vision is a possible sign of hypertension, which must be anticipated and identified early. While blood pressure measurements are taken every 4 to 6 hours, blurred vision would be an indication to take the blood pressure immediately. Option 1: Anorexia is an anticipated clinical manifestation of glomerulonephritis. Options 3 and 4: These statements are most probably indications of recovery. Lethargy is associated with the acute stage of this illness.
NP: Collecting data
CN: Physiological integrity
CNS: Physiological adaptation
CL: Application

16 An 8-year-old boy is being prepared for an electroencephalogram (EEG). Which statement indicates that he requires further explanation?
☐ 1. "I think I'll have pancakes for breakfast."
☐ 2. "I'm going to bring my book to read during the test."
☐ 3. "I'll be very still while they're doing the test."
☐ 4. "The test won't hurt. I'm not afraid."

CORRECT ANSWER: 2
During an EEG, the client must lie perfectly still. The activity associated with reading wouldn't be allowed. Option 1: No dietary restrictions are necessary before an EEG. Option 3 indicates the client's willingness to cooperate during the test. Option 4: This is a simple procedure that doesn't cause pain.
NP: Evaluating care
CN: Physiological integrity
CNS: Reduction of risk potential
CL: Application

17 A 9-year-old with sickle cell anemia is prepared for discharge. Which statement by the child's mother indicates that she needs more teaching?
☐ 1. "Whenever he gets a fever, I'll give him Tylenol, make him drink lots of water, and call the physician."
☐ 2. "He and his brother joined the chess club at school. He'll need to stay later on 2 days, but he enjoys it."
☐ 3. "Whenever he has a little contusion, I'll put cold packs right on the injury."
☐ 4. "During the summer, we keep a little chart on the refrigerator door just to make sure he drinks enough."

CORRECT ANSWER: 3
The local application of cold enhances vasoconstriction and may contribute to sickling. This is contraindicated. Option 1: Fever is a known cause of sickle cell crisis. Acetaminophen (Tylenol) given to reduce the fever and fluids given to prevent dehydration are appropriate until medical advice can be obtained. Option 2: Chess is a quiet, age-appropriate diversion that doesn't place the child at risk. Option 4: Monitoring hydration in the summer months minimizes the risk of dehydration, a common cause of sickle cell crisis.
NP: Evaluating care
CN: Health promotion and maintenance
CNS: Prevention and early detection of disease
CL: Analysis

18 Self-management of diabetes is established as a major goal for a 12-year-old diabetic client. The nurse realizes that a milestone has been reached when the child identifies the clinical signs of hypoglycemia, or "insulin reaction," as:
☐ 1. flushed skin, lethargy, and thirst.
☐ 2. pallor, diaphoresis, and increased heart rate.
☐ 3. nausea, mental confusion, and fruity breath odor.
☐ 4. vomiting, abdominal pain, and polyuria.

CORRECT ANSWER: 2
Pallor, diaphoresis, and increased heart rate are signs of hypoglycemia, which occurs with too much insulin. Options 1, 3, and 4: Flushed skin, lethargy, thirst, nausea, fruity breath odor, mental confusion, vomiting, abdominal pain, and polyuria are all signs of hyperglycemia.
NP: Collecting data
CN: Physiological integrity
CNS: Reduction of risk potential
CL: Application

19 Which statement by the parent of a 4-week-old infant is most consistent with a history of pyloric stenosis?
☐ 1. "The baby couldn't keep formula down from the day he was born."
☐ 2. "The baby started vomiting about 2 weeks after he was born."
☐ 3. "The baby has gained ½ lb (0.2 kg) per week since he was born."
☐ 4. "The baby never seems hungry."

CORRECT ANSWER: 2
Symptoms of pyloric stenosis typically don't appear until an infant is 2 or 3 weeks old. By this age, progressive hypertrophy of the circular muscles of the pylorus have delayed the passage of food from the pylorus to the duodenum. Option 1: Vomiting since birth isn't consistent with pyloric stenosis because symptoms don't occur during the first 2 to 3 weeks. Options 3 and 4: An infant with pyloric stenosis has a history of poor weight gain and is always hungry. The infant will eagerly feed again after vomiting.
NP: Collecting data
CN: Physiological integrity
CNS: Basic care and comfort
CL: Analysis

20 A 6-month-old infant with tetralogy of Fallot suddenly becomes acutely cyanotic and hyperpneic. What should the nurse do first?
- ☐ 1. Administer emergency oxygen.
- ☐ 2. Check and record the apical pulse.
- ☐ 3. Place the infant in semi-Fowler's position.
- ☐ 4. Place the infant in a knee-chest position.

CORRECT ANSWER: 4

The infant should be placed in the knee-chest position to increase venous return to the heart. Hypercyanotic spells are caused by sudden infundibular spasm, which decreases pulmonary blood flow and increases right-to-left shunting in the child with tetralogy. Options 1 and 3: Oxygen would be indicated after the child has been placed in the knee-chest position. Once measures have been taken to relieve the hypercyanotic spell, the next step is to record the pulse rate; however, option 2 wouldn't relieve the symptoms. If no action is taken, the child may experience severe cerebral hypoxia.

NP: Implementing care
CN: Physiological integrity
CNS: Basic care and comfort
CL: Application

---

21 Which nursing diagnosis should receive the nurse's highest priority when caring for a child with pneumonia?
- ☐ 1. *Interrupted family processes*
- ☐ 2. *Risk for deficient fluid volume*
- ☐ 3. *Risk for impaired parent–child attachment*
- ☐ 4. *Ineffective breathing pattern*

CORRECT ANSWER: 4

The highest priority is given to airway function and integrity. Option 2: Deficient fluid volume is a major consideration but doesn't take priority over ineffective breathing pattern. Options 1 and 3 would be incorporated to complete the plan of care for this client.

NP: Planning care
CN: Physiological integrity
CNS: Basic care and comfort
CL: Application

---

22 Which statement by a client with insulin-dependent diabetes best describes a cause of hypoglycemia?
- ☐ 1. "I didn't have time to eat breakfast after I took my insulin."
- ☐ 2. "I forgot to take my insulin this morning."
- ☐ 3. "There was a birthday party and I ate more than I should have."
- ☐ 4. "I took less insulin today because I had a bad tooth infection."

CORRECT ANSWER: 1

The onset of regular insulin is between 30 minutes and 1 hour. Skipping breakfast would precipitate a hypoglycemic reaction. The actions described in options 2 and 3 would result in hyperglycemia — not hypoglycemia. Option 4: An acute infection would increase the blood glucose level; therefore, the client would need to increase insulin requirements.

NP: Collecting data
CN: Health promotion and maintenance
CNS: Prevention and early detection of disease
CL: Application

---

23 The parents of a 9-year-old boy with leukemia have decided to tell him that he has "a little problem with his blood, like anemia." This approach will probably:
- ☐ 1. protect the child from anxiety.
- ☐ 2. assist the child to express his fears more readily.
- ☐ 3. enable the parents to be more supportive of the child.
- ☐ 4. waste energy that is needed to live with a serious illness.

CORRECT ANSWER: 4

Energy is wasted in maintaining a deceit. This energy should be applied to the real problem of living with a life-threatening illness. Also, the deceit leaves the child to suffer alone, unable to express fears and sadness or even to say good-bye. Options 1 and 2: School-age children are often aware of the seriousness of their illness. Being unable to express their fears contributes to their anxiety. Option 3: This type of parental support is based on concealment, not sharing, and won't be supportive for the child.

NP: Planning care
CN: Psychosocial integrity
CNS: Coping and adaptation
CL: Application

24 A 2-year-old girl is clutching a worn carriage blanket. She refuses to let go of it. The nurse understands that this behavior is:
- ☐ 1. an indication of poor maternal bonding.
- ☐ 2. a sign of extreme insecurity.
- ☐ 3. an indication of regression.
- ☐ 4. typical of this age-group.

CORRECT ANSWER: 4

A transitional object, such as a familiar blanket, provides security for a child, especially one who is separated from her parents and dealing with new stressors or fatigue. Options 1, 2, and 3: This behavior isn't an indication of poor bonding, regression, or insecurity.

NP: Evaluating care
CN: Health promotion and maintenance
CNS: Growth and development through the life span
CL: Comprehension

---

25 A nurse is administering medications. Which action indicates that the nurse has safely identified the correct pediatric client?
- ☐ 1. Calling the client's name
- ☐ 2. Checking the room number
- ☐ 3. Reading the identification band
- ☐ 4. Reading the name on the crib

CORRECT ANSWER: 3

Correct identification of a client can be made only by using the identification band. Options 1, 2, and 4: All other methods can contribute to medication errors and are unsafe.

NP: Implementing care
CN: Safe, effective care environment
CNS: Safety and infection control
CL: Application

---

26 A toddler has sustained a minor head injury. Which statement by the caregiver should be brought to the physician's attention?
- ☐ 1. "I only gave him ginger ale to drink."
- ☐ 2. "I put ice on the bump."
- ☐ 3. "I gave him Tylenol; that is why he's sleepy."
- ☐ 4. "I washed the abrasion with soap and water."

CORRECT ANSWER: 3

Administration of an analgesic, such as acetaminophen (Tylenol), may be contraindicated with a head injury because such drugs may cause drowsiness and mask changes in level of consciousness. The nurse should report this information to the physician and be prepared for further neurologic evaluations. Options 1 and 4: Giving ginger ale and washing the abrasion with soap and water wouldn't be contraindicated and don't need to be reported. Option 2: Application of cold would promote vasoconstriction and decrease local edema.

NP: Collecting data
CN: Basic care and comfort
CNS: Physiological integrity
CL: Analysis

---

27 Which statement by the mother of an 18-month-old toddler indicates a typical feeding response at this age?
- ☐ 1. "His appetite is so inconsistent from one day to the next."
- ☐ 2. "He eats everything I give him."
- ☐ 3. "His favorite foods are casseroles."
- ☐ 4. "He eats as much as his 5-year-old sister."

CORRECT ANSWER: 1

A toddler at this age typically manifests a decreased appetite known as physiologic anorexia and experiences a slower growth rate. Option 2: Toddlers typically become fussy eaters with strong taste preferences; few eat "everything." Option 3: Casseroles aren't usually favorites with this age-group. Option 4: This behavior wouldn't be consistent with the physiologic anorexia anticipated at this age.

NP: Collecting data
CN: Health promotion and maintenance
CNS: Growth and development through the life span
CL: Comprehension

28 Which action indicates that a nurse is using an acceptable technique when administering a Z-track injection?
- ☐ 1. The nurse selects a ⁵/₈" needle.
- ☐ 2. The nurse inserts the needle at a 40-degree angle.
- ☐ 3. The nurse pulls the skin laterally 1" (2.5 cm) before injecting.
- ☐ 4. The nurse compresses the muscle tissue firmly before injecting.

CORRECT ANSWER: 3
Z-track administration is used for medications that irritate subcutaneous tissue. Pulling the skin laterally creates a zigzag track for medication injection. Options 1, 2, and 4 don't create the zigzag track.
NP: Implementing care
CN: Physiological integrity
CNS: Pharmacological therapies
CL: Application

29 Which action confirms that a nasogastric (NG) tube is properly positioned in a client's stomach?
- ☐ 1. Inverting the tube into a glass of water and observing for bubbling
- ☐ 2. Instilling 10 ml of air into the tube and listening with a stethoscope for air entering the stomach
- ☐ 3. Clamping the tube for 10 minutes and listening with a stethoscope for increased peristalsis
- ☐ 4. Instilling 30 ml of normal saline solution and observing the client's response

CORRECT ANSWER: 2
The "whooshing" sound of air entering the stomach confirms that the NG tube is in the stomach. To further verify positioning, the pH of the gastric aspirate should be checked. The pH of gastric aspirate is approximately 3.0 (acidic), whereas the pH of respiratory aspirate is 7.0 or greater (alkalotic). Option 1 would be done to verify that an NG tube is in the respiratory tract. Option 3 provides no information on the location of the tube. Option 4 is dangerous. If the tube is in the respiratory tract, this action will cause coughing, choking and, possibly, cyanosis.
NP: Collecting data
CN: Physiological integrity
CNS: Reduction of risk potential
CL: Application

30 When is the best time to obtain a sputum specimen for culture and sensitivity testing from a 12-year-old child?
- ☐ 1. 7 a.m.
- ☐ 2. 11 a.m.
- ☐ 3. 3 p.m.
- ☐ 4. 8 p.m.

CORRECT ANSWER: 1
A sputum specimen is best obtained early in the morning because a higher volume of secretions is likely to have accumulated throughout the night. Options 2, 3, and 4: These times aren't optimal for obtaining the specimen.
NP: Implementing care
CN: Physiological integrity
CNS: Reduction of risk potential
CL: Comprehension

31 Which observation indicates a malfunction of a thoracic water-seal drainage system?
- ☐ 1. Continuous bubbling of the suction chamber
- ☐ 2. Continuous bubbling in the water-seal chamber
- ☐ 3. Fluctuation of the water level in the water-seal chamber
- ☐ 4. Airtight connections in the system

CORRECT ANSWER: 2
Constant bubbling in the water-seal chamber indicates an air leak in the system. Option 1: Constant bubbling is anticipated in the suction-control chamber. Option 3: Fluctuation is anticipated in the water-seal chamber until the lung is expanded. Option 4: Airtight connections are necessary; they aren't malfunctions.
NP: Collecting data
CN: Physiological integrity
CNS: Reduction of risk potential
CL: Application

32 A nurse who has been assigned complete care of a client in isolation is removing isolation garments. Which garment should be removed first?
☐ 1. Cap
☐ 2. Gown
☐ 3. Mask
☐ 4. Gloves

CORRECT ANSWER: 4
Garments of greater contamination are always removed first. Gloves should be removed before using the hands to touch or remove other isolation garments. Options 1, 2, and 3: These garments should be removed following glove removal.
NP: Implementing care
CN: Safe, effective care environment
CNS: Safety and infection control
CL: Application

---

33 A 7-month-old infant has acquired all of the following skills. Which skill was probably acquired last?
☐ 1. Reaching for a rattle
☐ 2. Moving hands to mouth
☐ 3. Pulling up to a sitting position
☐ 4. Transferring a clothes pin from one hand to another

CORRECT ANSWER: 4
Transferring objects is commonly the last skill acquired by a 7-month-old infant. Options 1 and 2: Reaching for objects and moving hands to the mouth are accomplished at 3 months. Option 3: Typically, an infant can pull up to a sitting position at 6 months.
NP: Collecting data
CN: Health promotion and maintenance
CNS: Growth and development through the life span
CL: Comprehension

---

34 The nurse assesses a 1-month-old infant with hydrocephalus for signs of increased intracranial pressure (ICP). Which statement by the infant's mother is most significant?
☐ 1. "The baby is so tired that I couldn't even keep him awake long enough to feed him."
☐ 2. "You really have to support his head when you pick him up."
☐ 3. "The monitor says his pulse is 110 beats/minute."
☐ 4. "I'm feeding the baby every 3 hours because he seems so hungry."

CORRECT ANSWER: 1
This statement may indicate increased lethargy, a sign of increased ICP. The infant should be evaluated for other signs to determine if ICP is actually present. Other signs include bulging fontanels, tenseness, irritability, and a change in level of consciousness or feeding behavior (such as vomiting). Option 2: Head lag is expected in a 1-month-old infant. Option 3: A heart rate of 110 beats/minute is normal for an infant of this age. Bradycardia would be more indicative of increased ICP. Option 4: Vomiting, not a strong sucking reflex, would be a sign of increased ICP.
NP: Collecting data
CN: Physiological integrity
CNS: Physiological adaptation
CL: Analysis

---

35 A pediatric client is receiving an I.V. infusion. At 7:00 a.m., 230 ml of fluid was in the 500-ml infusion bag. At 10:00 a.m., the infusion was discontinued and 130 ml of fluid remained in the bag. How much fluid should the nurse record as absorbed on the client's intake and output record?
☐ 1. 100 ml
☐ 2. 130 ml
☐ 3. 330 ml
☐ 4. 500 ml

CORRECT ANSWER: 1
To determine the correct amount of fluid absorbed, the nurse would subtract 130 ml (the amount left in the bag) from the 230 ml (the amount of fluid at the start of the infusion). This yields a difference of 100 ml, which should be recorded as "intake" under the column marked "absorbed." Options 2, 3, and 4: These options are incorrect.
NP: Implementing care
CN: Physiological integrity
CNS: Basic care and comfort
CL: Application

36 A 4-month-old girl is admitted to the hospital with gastroenteritis and profuse diarrhea. Which symptom is most indicative of a diarrhea stool?
☐ 1. Meconium
☐ 2. Clay-colored stools
☐ 3. Watery, green stools
☐ 4. Loose, tarry stools

CORRECT ANSWER: 3
Watery stools indicate diarrhea. Green stools indicate bile content with rapid transit through the GI tract such as occurs in diarrhea. Option 1: Meconium is the green-black stool seen in the first few days of life. Option 2: Clay-colored stools indicate a lack of bile in the stool and are characteristic of liver diseases. Option 4: Loose, tarry stools indicate GI bleeding; diarrhea may or may not be present.
NP: Evaluating care
CN: Physiological integrity
CNS: Basic care and comfort
CL: Application

37 Which assessment finding would indicate that an infant is retaining excessive fluid?
☐ 1. Weight loss and temperature increase
☐ 2. Tachycardia and puffy eyelids
☐ 3. Tenting of abdominal skin
☐ 4. Depressed fontanels

CORRECT ANSWER: 2
The heart rate elevates to increase cardiac output and compensate for excessive fluid volume. An increased heart rate also increases kidney perfusion and thus increases urine output. With fluid retention in infants, edema frequently occurs in the periorbital area. Options 1, 3, and 4 are all signs of dehydration.
NP: Collecting data
CN: Physiological integrity
CNS: Basic care and comfort
CL: Application

38 A 2-month-old girl is hospitalized with vomiting and diarrhea. Which assessment information is most critical in evaluating this child for dehydration?
☐ 1. Appearance of fontanels
☐ 2. Daily temperature
☐ 3. Abdominal girth measurement
☐ 4. Daily weight

CORRECT ANSWER: 4
Daily weight is the best measure of the degree of dehydration. Option 1: Bulging fontanels would indicate overhydration. Option 2: Temperature measurement is important but can't gauge the degree of dehydration. Option 3: Abdominal girth measurement is used to assess abdominal distention related to GI function or dysfunction.
NP: Evaluating care
CN: Health promotion and maintenance
CNS: Prevention and early detection of disease
CL: Application

39 Which method of recording output is most accurate and should be part of a 2-month-old girl's nursing care plan?
☐ 1. Counting and recording the number of soiled diapers each day
☐ 2. Measuring and recording the weight of soiled diapers minus the weight of dry diapers
☐ 3. Recording the time, color, and amount of each void
☐ 4. Saving the last three urine specimens for comparison

CORRECT ANSWER: 2
Because 1 g equals 1 ml, keeping track of the weight of all soiled diapers is as accurate as measuring the volume of urine output. Option 1: The number of voids is a less accurate measure of urine output. Option 3 is used after surgery of the urinary tract to assess the clearing of blood as well as urinary tract function. Option 4 is done in conjunction with option 3 to visually compare changes in color of urine.
NP: Implementing care
CN: Physiological integrity
CNS: Basic care and comfort
CL: Application

40 Which developmental milestone would the nurse expect an 11-month-old infant to have achieved?
☐ 1. Sitting independently
☐ 2. Walking independently
☐ 3. Building a tower of four cubes
☐ 4. Turning a doorknob

CORRECT ANSWER: 1
Infants typically sit independently, without support, by age 8 months. Option 2: Walking independently may be accomplished as late as age 15 months and still be within the normal range. Few infants walk independently by age 11 months. Option 3: Building a tower of three or four blocks is a milestone of an 18-month-old infant. Option 4: Turning a doorknob is a milestone of a 24-month-old child.
NP: Evaluating care
CN: Health promotion and maintenance
CNS: Growth and development through the life span
CL: Application

41 If a child with tetralogy of Fallot has a hyper-cyanotic ("blue" or "tet") spell, which action should the nurse take?
☐ 1. Place the child in a prone position.
☐ 2. Administer I.V. push morphine.
☐ 3. Place the child in a knee-chest position.
☐ 4. Administer 40% oxygen by mask.

CORRECT ANSWER: 3
A knee-chest position increases venous return and blood pressure in the heart, forcing blood through the pulmonary artery and into the lungs. Option 1: A prone position doesn't provide the leg flexion necessary to ensure venous return and may hinder respirations. Option 2: Administration of I.V. push medication doesn't fall within the scope of practice for a practical nurse. Option 4: The child would be given 100% oxygen to rapidly increase oxygenation.
NP: Implementing care
CN: Physiological integrity
CNS: Basic care and comfort
CL: Application

42 During assessment of a child who has undergone cardiac catheterization, the nurse notes bleeding from the percutaneous femoral catheterization site. Which action should be taken first?
☐ 1. Apply direct, continuous pressure.
☐ 2. Assess the pulse and blood pressure.
☐ 3. Seek the assistance of a registered nurse.
☐ 4. Check the pedal pulse in the affected leg.

CORRECT ANSWER: 1
Bleeding from a major vessel must be stopped immediately to prevent massive hemorrhage. Option 2: Vital signs would be taken after bleeding control measures are instituted. Option 3: Calling for help is important, but pressure on the site must be applied and maintained while help is being found. Option 4: Pedal pulses would be checked after bleeding is controlled.
NP: Implementing care
CN: Physiological integrity
CNS: Reduction of risk potential
CL: Application

43 A 3-year-old client has a high red blood cell count and polycythemia. In planning care, the nurse would anticipate which goal to help prevent blood clot formation?
☐ 1. The child won't have signs of dehydration.
☐ 2. The child won't have signs of dyspnea.
☐ 3. The child will be pain-free.
☐ 4. The child will attain the 40th percentile of weight for her age.

CORRECT ANSWER: 1
When dehydration occurs, blood is thicker and more prone to clotting. Option 2: Dyspnea would be a sign of hypoxia. Option 3: Pain wouldn't cause an embolus. Option 4: Optional weight would be an indicator of nutritional status and not a risk for embolism.
NP: Planning care
CN: Physiological integrity
CNS: Reduction of risk potential
CL: Application

44 A 10-month-old boy with bacterial meningitis was started on antibiotic therapy today. Which nursing action is especially important in this situation?
☐ 1. Wearing a mask while providing care
☐ 2. Flexing the child's neck every 4 hours to maintain range of motion
☐ 3. Administering oral gentamicin (Garamycin)
☐ 4. Encouraging the child to drink 3,000 ml of fluid per day

CORRECT ANSWER: 1
With bacterial meningitis, respiratory isolation must be maintained for at least 24 hours after beginning antibiotic therapy. Wearing a mask is an important part of respiratory isolation. Option 2: Moving the child's head would cause pain because his meninges are inflamed. Option 3: Gentamicin is never administered orally. Option 4: This amount of fluid would cause overhydration in a 10-month-old infant and place him at risk for increased intracranial pressure.
NP: Implementing care
CN: Safe, effective care environment
CNS: Safety and infection control
CL: Application

45 Which nursing action should be included in the plan of care to promote comfort in a 4-year-old child hospitalized with meningitis?
☐ 1. Avoid making noise when in the child's room.
☐ 2. Rock the child frequently.
☐ 3. Have the child's 2-year-old brother stay in the room.
☐ 4. Keep the lights on brightly so that he can see his mother.

CORRECT ANSWER: 1
Meningeal irritation may cause seizures and heightens a child's sensitivity to all stimuli, including noise, lights, movement, and touch. Options 2, 3, and 4 all are incorrect because, in each case, stimulation would be increased.
NP: Planning care
CN: Physiological integrity
CNS: Basic care and comfort
CL: Application

46 Which nursing diagnosis would the nurse expect to find on the plan of care of a 10-month-old infant to promote coping during hospitalization?
☐ 1. *Toileting self-care deficit related to the child's age*
☐ 2. *Powerlessness related to hospital environment*
☐ 3. *Deficient diversional activity related to hospital environment*
☐ 4. *Anxiety related to separation from parents*

CORRECT ANSWER: 4
Attachment is critical in infancy, and prolonged separation has been well documented as a risk factor that compromises normal infant development. Option 1: Toilet training wouldn't be an issue for a 10-month-old. Option 2: Powerlessness is a concern after the toddler stage, when a child develops autonomy and independence. Option 3: Diversion won't be an issue until the acute phase of the illness has passed. Providing diversion for infants is easily accomplished by the use of age-appropriate toys and play activities.
NP: Planning care
CN: Psychosocial integrity
CNS: Coping and adaptation
CL: Application

47 An 18-month-old boy is being evaluated at the clinic. In reviewing his chart, the nurse notices that he has missed many appointments and, consequently, his immunizations aren't up-to-date. While discussing communicable diseases and the importance of immunizations with his mother, the nurse explains that meningitis can be prevented with:
☐ 1. corticosteroid therapy.
☐ 2. tetanus toxoid vaccination.
☐ 3. tine testing.
☐ 4. *Haemophilus influenzae* vaccination.

CORRECT ANSWER: 4
H. influenzae vaccination is recommended for all children as a preventive measure for meningitis. Option 1: Corticosteroids such as prednisone weaken the immune system and increase susceptibility to infectious disease. Option 2: Tetanus toxoid vaccination provides immunity against tetanus or "lockjaw." Option 3: A tine test is a screening measure for tuberculosis.
NP: Implementing care
CN: Health promotion and maintenance
CNS: Prevention and early detection of disease
CL: Application

48 Which nursing action would relieve respiratory distress and dyspnea in a 2-year-old boy with laryngotracheobronchitis?
☐ 1. Stimulating the child to keep him awake
☐ 2. Providing an atmosphere of high humidity
☐ 3. Offering frequent oral feedings
☐ 4. Administering frequent sedatives

CORRECT ANSWER: 2
High humidity reduces mucosal edema and prevents drying of secretions, thus helping to maintain an open airway. Option 1: Keeping the child calm, not stimulated, helps to reduce oxygen need. Option 3: Oral feedings may need to be withheld in a child experiencing respiratory distress because eating may interfere with his ability to breathe. Option 4: Sedation is generally contraindicated because it may cause respiratory depression and mask anxiety, a sign of respiratory distress.
NP: Implementing care
CN: Physiological integrity
CNS: Physiological adaptation
CL: Application

49 When assessing a child for increased laryngotracheal edema and early signs of impending airway obstruction, the nurse should observe for which of the following warning signs?
☐ 1. Decreased heart and respiratory rates and a high peak flow rate
☐ 2. Increased heart and respiratory rates, retractions, and restlessness
☐ 3. Decreased blood pressure
☐ 4. Increased temperature

CORRECT ANSWER: 2
These signs are all classic indicators of hypoxia. The heart and respiratory rates increase to enable increased oxygenation. Accessory breathing muscles are used, causing retractions in substernal, suprasternal, and intercostal areas. Reduced oxygen to the brain causes restlessness initially and altered level of consciousness later. Option 1: A decrease in heart and respiratory rates would be a late ominous sign of decompensation. Peak flow rate is a test used in asthma. A decrease, not increase, in peak flow is diagnostic of disease. Option 3: A drop in blood pressure would be a late sign of hypoxia. Option 4: An increase in temperature is more indicative of infection or inflammation than respiratory distress.
NP: Collecting data
CN: Physiological integrity
CNS: Physiological adaptation
CL: Application

50 A child who has taken an overdose of acetaminophen arrives in the emergency department. Which equipment should be prepared to treat the acetaminophen overdose?
☐ 1. Hyperbaric oxygen chamber
☐ 2. Tetanus toxoid injection
☐ 3. Gastric lavage equipment
☐ 4. Chelating agents

CORRECT ANSWER: 3
Treatment for acetaminophen overdose includes administration of activated charcoal to absorb the acetaminophen, gastric lavage to wash the charcoal out of the stomach, and then oral administration of acetylcysteine (Mucomyst) to replenish liver stores of glutathione. The charcoal inactivates the acetylcysteine if both are in the stomach. Option 1: A hyperbaric oxygen chamber may be used to treat carbon monoxide poisoning and is available only at large medical centers. Option 2: Tetanus toxoid is an immunization given if a laceration or puncture wound occurs with a dirty object or if the client's immunization status warrants a booster. Option 4: Chelating agents are used in the treatment of lead poisoning.
NP: Planning care
CN: Physiological integrity
CNS: Physiological adaptation
CL: Application

51 Which assessment should the nurse complete first after a child with suspected acetaminophen poisoning has been admitted to the emergency department?
☐ 1. Heart rate
☐ 2. Respiratory rate
☐ 3. Airway evaluation
☐ 4. Pupil evaluation

CORRECT ANSWER: 3
Emergency protocol always follows the ABCs of assessment: airway, breathing, and circulation, in that order. If the mechanism of injury suggests a possible spinal injury, the nurse should protect the cervical spine when performing an airway assessment. Options 1 and 2: Checking the heart rate and respiratory rate are also part of emergency management. However, these assessments may be delayed until the presence of an open airway, breathing, and circulation are established. Option 4: Assessing pupillary reactions is a later assessment, depending on the child's level of consciousness and the type of poison ingested.
NP: Collecting data
CN: Physiological integrity
CNS: Physiological adaptation
CL: Application

52 Which nursing diagnosis would the nurse include in the plan of care to help prevent the recurrence of acetaminophen poisoning in a child?
☐ 1. *Ineffective health maintenance*
☐ 2. *Deficient knowledge (parent)*
☐ 3. *Risk for trauma*
☐ 4. *Risk for aspiration*

CORRECT ANSWER: 2
Parent teaching is the key to preventing childhood poisoning. The diagnoses in options 1, 3, and 4 don't apply to poison prevention.
NP: Planning care
CN: Health promotion and maintenance
CNS: Prevention and early detection of disease
CL: Application

53 A 4-year-old boy is hospitalized to rule out acute lymphocytic leukemia. Which reaction to hospitalization is a typical response of a preschool child?
☐ 1. Having a temper tantrum
☐ 2. Believing that he's being hospitalized because he broke his older brother's model airplane
☐ 3. Feeling afraid of not being accepted by his friends because he's sick and has to go to the hospital
☐ 4. Understanding the significance of his hospitalization

CORRECT ANSWER: 2
Preschoolers frequently think illness and hospitalization are punishment for misdeeds. Option 1: Temper tantrums are more typical of toddlers; however, preschoolers may regress and have tantrums during hospitalization. Option 3: School-age and older children commonly fear a lack of acceptance when they become ill. Option 4: Adolescents, not younger children, can understand the significance of hospitalization on a concrete and philosophical level.
NP: Evaluating care
CN: Psychosocial integrity
CNS: Coping and adaptation
CL: Application

54 A 4-year-old boy is diagnosed as having acute lymphocytic leukemia. His white blood cell (WBC) count, especially the neutrophil count, is low. Which nursing action would be best for this child?
☐ 1. Protect the child from falls because of his increased risk of bleeding.
☐ 2. Protect the child from infections because his resistance to infection is decreased.
☐ 3. Provide rest periods because the oxygen-carrying capacity of the child's blood is diminished.
☐ 4. Treat constipation, which frequently accompanies a decrease in WBCs.

CORRECT ANSWER: 2
One of the complications of both acute lymphocytic leukemia and its treatment is a decreased WBC count, specifically a decreased absolute neutrophil count. Because neutrophils are the body's first line of defense against infection, the child must be protected from infection. Option 1: Bleeding is a risk factor if platelets or other coagulation factors are decreased. Option 3: A decreased hemoglobin level, hematocrit or both would reduce the oxygen-carrying capacity of the child's blood. Option 4: Constipation isn't related to the WBC count.
NP: Implementing care
CN: Safe, effective care environment
CNS: Safety and infection control
CL: Application

55 A child with nephrotic syndrome develops generalized edema as a result of his nephrosis. Which goal would be included in the plan of care to prevent complications of edema?
☐ 1. Continually support the scrotum.
☐ 2. Change the child's position every 2 hours.
☐ 3. The child's skin will remain intact during hospitalization.
☐ 4. Maintain continuous bed rest.

CORRECT ANSWER: 3
This is the only option written as a goal. Options 1, 2, and 4 are interventions recommended to maintain skin integrity.
NP: Planning care
CN: Physiological integrity
CNS: Basic care and comfort
CL: Application

---

56 When evaluating a client with acute glomerulonephritis, the nurse would look for which finding as the best indicator of recovery?
☐ 1. +3 glucose in the urine
☐ 2. Urine negative for acetone
☐ 3. +3 urine albumin
☐ 4. No protein in the urine

CORRECT ANSWER: 4
Excessive proteinuria is a major indicator of nephrosis. The proteinuria may be due to a change in the basement membrane of the glomeruli, which allows protein to spill into the urine. Symptoms of nephrosis are related to the degree of proteinuria. Option 1: The spillage of glucose into the urine is related to stress or diabetes mellitus. Option 2: Acetone is a ketone that is elevated in diabetic ketoacidosis. Option 3: Albumin levels greater than 0 indicate that this protein is being excreted into urine, an indication of active nephrosis — not of recovery.
NP: Evaluating care
CN: Physiological integrity
CNS: Basic care and comfort
CL: Application

---

57 The physician prescribes prednisone (Deltasone) for a client with nephrosis. Which statement by the client's mother indicates that she understands how to care for him while he's receiving this drug?
☐ 1. "If I forget to give him a dose, I'll give him a double dose the next time."
☐ 2. "I'll feed him a low-protein, high-sodium diet."
☐ 3. "I'll call his physician if he has swelling or weight gain."
☐ 4. "It's okay for him to play with his cousin who has chickenpox."

CORRECT ANSWER: 3
Prednisone's adverse effects include fluid retention and weight gain as a result of sodium retention. Both should be reported to the physician. Because weight gain and fluid retention are also signs of a relapse of the nephrosis, the client should be reevaluated. Option 1: Prednisone is an adrenal steroid and should be given exactly as prescribed. Missed doses may result in signs of adrenal insufficiency, including low blood pressure. Doubling the dose may cause hypertension. Option 2: A diet high in protein, calcium, and potassium is suggested for clients on long-term steroid therapy. A low-sodium diet is suggested because salt and water retention are adverse effects of prednisone. Option 4: Prednisone causes immunosuppression, thus exposure to contagious diseases must be avoided.
NP: Evaluating care
CN: Health promotion and maintenance
CNS: Prevention and early detection of disease
CL: Application

58 A 10-year-old boy develops rheumatic fever after a group A beta-hemolytic streptococcal throat infection. He's scheduled to have dental work and has been prescribed an I.M. prophylactic penicillin. Which nursing action is especially important before administering penicillin?
☐ 1. Landmarking the deltoid site correctly
☐ 2. Avoiding aspiration before injection
☐ 3. Checking his platelet count before injection
☐ 4. Checking for allergies to medications

CORRECT ANSWER: 4
Anaphylaxis and death may result if penicillin is given to an allergic individual. Checking for allergies is a safe step in all medication administration. Option 1: The deltoid is too small a muscle for a penicillin injection and wouldn't be used. Option 2: Preventing aspiration is important with any I.M. injection. It isn't specific to penicillin administration. Option 3: Platelets aren't checked routinely before injection. If the history indicates a bleeding tendency, I.M. injections are avoided and an alternate route of medication administration is suggested.
NP: Implementing care
CN: Physiological integrity
CNS: Pharmacological therapies
CL: Application

---

59 The nurse is assessing a febrile child with rheumatic fever and cardiac involvement. Which goal would be the most important?
☐ 1. Preventing joint pain
☐ 2. Promoting rest
☐ 3. Maintaining contact with friends
☐ 4. Treating the maculopapular rash

CORRECT ANSWER: 2
Rest is important to recovery, especially during the febrile period of rheumatic fever and when the child has cardiac involvement (carditis). Rest decreases the oxygen demand of the myocardium, allowing the heart to rest. Option 1: Although preventing joint pain is important, it's less important than limiting the client's activity. Option 3: Allowing the child to maintain contact with friends is important, provided activities aren't too strenuous. However, this isn't the priority. Option 4: The rash is self-limiting and will disappear without treatment.
NP: Planning care
CN: Physiological integrity
CNS: Basic care and comfort
CL: Application

---

60 Planning for prevention of rheumatic fever in noninfected children involves teaching parents about the need to:
☐ 1. have their children properly immunized against strep infections.
☐ 2. have their children's sore throats cultured and treated.
☐ 3. give aspirin as prescribed for joint pain.
☐ 4. ensure that children with carditis maintain bed rest.

CORRECT ANSWER: 2
Group A beta-hemolytic streptococci upper respiratory tract infections can lead to the development of rheumatic fever within weeks of initial infection. Therefore, children should receive prompt medical treatment, which includes culturing and antibiotic therapy. Option 1: No immunization is available for group A streptococci, the causative organisms of rheumatic fever. Option 3: Aspirin is used to treat the joint inflammation that may occur with rheumatic fever; it isn't a preventive measure. Option 4: Bed rest is a treatment, not a preventive measure.
NP: Planning care
CN: Health promotion and maintenance
CNS: Prevention and early detection of disease
CL: Application

61 An adolescent diabetic client is on an American Diabetes Association (ADA) diet. Which nursing action would be best if the client refuses to eat his dinner because he dislikes the food?
☐ 1. Provide him with two snacks at 7 p.m.
☐ 2. Sit with him and force him to eat the entire meal.
☐ 3. Give him less insulin to compensate for his refusal to eat.
☐ 4. Call the dietitian to obtain an acceptable meal substitution.

CORRECT ANSWER: 4
Good diabetic management consists of a balance of adequate nutrition, exercise, and insulin. If a child refuses to follow the prescribed ADA diet, a dietitian can substitute more acceptable foods that provide the correct dietary exchanges. Option 1: Unless the hospital has a protocol that allows nurses to make dietary substitutions, the hospital dietitian should determine the proper exchanges. Also, most snacks can't substitute for dinner. Option 2: Forcing a child to eat is inappropriate; such pressure won't help him to adjust to the lifestyle changes necessary with an illness like diabetes. Option 3: Altering the insulin dosage wouldn't provide the needed nutrition; also, this isn't the nurse's role.
NP: Implementing care
CN: Physiological integrity
CNS: Basic care and comfort
CL: Application

62 In reviewing a diabetic teaching plan, the nurse discusses a mother's concern about having to give candy, juice, or other sweets when her diabetic son feels ill and can't determine his blood sugar level. The mother is upset that this practice may elevate her son's blood sugar level when it's already high. Which response by the nurse would best in this situation?
☐ 1. "Giving candy is correct because brain damage can occur if your son's blood sugar level falls too low."
☐ 2. "This must be a mistake; let me check with your primary nurse."
☐ 3. "You'll need to consult your physician about that question."
☐ 4. "Giving candy is okay because this sheet has been reviewed by the diabetes nurse-educator."

CORRECT ANSWER: 1
The amount of glucose in a piece of candy will elevate the child's blood glucose level only slightly if he already has a high blood sugar level. However, because brain cells die without sugar, this same increase is sufficient to prevent brain damage in someone whose blood sugar level is dangerously low. Options 2 and 3: The nurse should be able to provide the mother with the correct information without consulting the primary nurse or physician; this would only serve to heighten the mother's anxiety unnecessarily. Option 4: Regardless of whether the diabetes nurse-educator has reviewed the sheet, the nurse can provide the mother with the correct information about the effects of glucose to alleviate her anxiety.
NP: Implementing care
CN: Health promotion and maintenance
CNS: Prevention and early detection of disease
CL: Application

63 A 13-year-old girl is being screened for scoliosis. As part of the screening process, the nurse should observe for:
☐ 1. uneven rib hump.
☐ 2. accentuated anteroposterior spinal curvature.
☐ 3. uneven gluteal folds.
☐ 4. inability to hop.

CORRECT ANSWER: 1
Scoliosis is an abnormal lateral curvature of the spine. The rib cage rotation causes a rib hump, which is more noticeable when the child bends at the waist. Option 2: Kyphosis is an accentuated anteroposterior curvature of the spine that causes a hunchback appearance. Option 3: Uneven gluteal folds are assessed to screen for congenital hip dysplasia. Option 4: The ability to hop isn't part of the assessment for scoliosis.
NP: Collecting data
CN: Health promotion and maintenance
CNS: Prevention and early detection of disease
CL: Application

64 A girl with scoliosis is fitted for a Milwaukee brace. Which statement by the client indicates that she has understood the nurse's instructions on proper use of the brace?
- ☐ 1. "I can remove the brace for sleeping."
- ☐ 2. "I can remove the brace four times per day."
- ☐ 3. "I need to wear the brace 23 hours per day."
- ☐ 4. "I have to wear the brace continually."

CORRECT ANSWER: 3
The brace is removed for bathing or showering once per day for 1 hour to achieve maximum effect. Options 1 and 2 would constitute excessive removal and reduce the effectiveness of the brace. Option 4: Continuous use is unnecessary; also, the brace pad would absorb water during bathing and showering.
NP: Evaluating care
CN: Health promotion and maintenance
CNS: Prevention and early detection of disease
CL: Application

---

65 A client is complaining to the nurse about having to wear a Milwaukee brace. Which complaint should be reported immediately?
- ☐ 1. Difficulty sitting comfortably
- ☐ 2. Feeling of being stretched from the neck to the waist
- ☐ 3. Numbness and paresthesia of the legs
- ☐ 4. Clothing not fitting under the brace

CORRECT ANSWER: 3
With any type of brace, pressure against a bone may compress a nerve and cause damage. Numbness or paresthesia is a sign of a compressed nerve. Option 1: Because the brace prevents flexion of the back, sitting normally in a chair is difficult. Sitting on a stool is one alternative. Option 2: The brace's function is to apply traction to stretch and straighten the back. Option 4: The only clothing that should be worn under the brace is cotton underwear, which provides comfort and absorbs perspiration. All other clothing should be worn over the device.
NP: Implementing care
CN: Health promotion and maintenance
CNS: Prevention and early detection of disease
CL: Application

---

66 A toddler is placed in a croupette for treatment of bronchiolitis. Which nursing diagnosis is most important?
- ☐ 1. *Deficient fluid volume*
- ☐ 2. *Hyperthermia*
- ☐ 3. *Hypothermia*
- ☐ 4. *Activity intolerance*

CORRECT ANSWER: 3
The cool mist of the croupette may cause hypothermia, especially if bedding becomes and remains wet. Option 1: The moist environment wouldn't cause deficient fluid volume. Less fluid is lost in a moist environment because the moist air is inhaled. Option 2: Hyperthermia, if present, would be related to the child's infection, not the croupette. Option 4: Activity intolerance would be related to inadequate oxygenation, not the croupette.
NP: Planning care
CN: Physiological integrity
CNS: Reduction of risk potential
CL: Application

67 Which factor is most important to maintain proper croupette functioning?
- ☐ 1. The plastic should be tucked under the mattress on all sides.
- ☐ 2. There should be no condensation on the plastic, and the sheets should remain dry.
- ☐ 3. The child should be in the center of the tent.
- ☐ 4. The liter flow must be maintained, and mist should circulate into the tent.

CORRECT ANSWER: 4
Correct liter flow and circulating mist indicate that the tent is functioning properly and that sufficient air is circulating. Option 1: Although this is important, the primary goal is to contain the mist and oxygen within the tent. The foot area of the tent is placed under the covers, not tucked under the mattress. Option 2: Condensation on the plastic is normal. However, excessive condensation may be controlled by regulating the mist. Dry sheets are important but aren't as important as maintaining liter flow and mist circulation. Option 3: The child's position in the tent isn't important as long as he's breathing the mist.
NP: Implementing care
CN: Safe, effective care environment
CNS: Safety and infection control
CL: Application

68 Which nursing action would be most helpful when preparing a 16-year-old girl for a bone marrow aspiration?
- ☐ 1. Explaining that strong pressure is needed to enter the bone and that the needle entry and aspiration of marrow will hurt
- ☐ 2. Explaining each step of the procedure but avoiding references to pain or discomfort
- ☐ 3. Stressing that a large pressure bandage will be applied after the procedure to prevent bleeding
- ☐ 4. Stressing the importance of not talking during the procedure so that it can be completed quickly

CORRECT ANSWER: 1
This description accurately portrays what the child will feel and adequately prepares her for the procedure. Option 2: Avoiding any references to pain or discomfort doesn't adequately prepare the child. Option 3: The nurse may mention potential complications but shouldn't emphasize them. Also, a small, not large, pressure bandage is typically applied. Option 4: Talking during the procedure may help to distract the client and lessen her anxiety.
NP: Implementing care
CN: Physiological integrity
CNS: Reduction of risk potential
CL: Application

69 Postprocedure care for a child who has had a bone marrow aspiration should include:
- ☐ 1. keeping the child flat in bed for 6 hours.
- ☐ 2. positioning the child on her right side for 2 hours.
- ☐ 3. checking the lumbar spine for leakage.
- ☐ 4. checking the pressure dressing for bleeding.

CORRECT ANSWER: 4
The pressure dressing should be checked because bleeding from the site may occur. If a sedative has been used, the nurse will have to ensure the child's safety until vital signs and level of consciousness return to normal. Options 1 and 2: No special positioning or activity restriction is required. Option 3: The lumbar region isn't punctured for bone marrow aspiration. The iliac crest is the site most often used in children.
NP: Implementing care
CN: Physiological integrity
CNS: Reduction of risk potential
CL: Application

70 A child is being tested for a potentially life-threatening illness. Which statement by the client would indicate that she's having anticipatory grieving?
- ☐ 1. "I think the bone marrow aspiration test was very painful."
- ☐ 2. "I hope I don't get sicker and lose my hair."
- ☐ 3. "I thought I had the flu."
- ☐ 4. "I hope I'm home in time to go to the dance."

CORRECT ANSWER: 2
This response indicates a concern for a future problem that may or may not occur. Option 1: This is a realistic perception of a past event. Option 3: This describes the past, not anticipation of future events. Option 4: This is a common adolescent concern and is unrelated to thought of anticipated illness.
NP: Evaluating care
CN: Psychosocial integrity
CNS: Coping and adaptation
CL: Application

71 A 10-year-old boy with diabetes is being taught self-administration of insulin. Which site chosen by the boy would be acceptable?
☐ 1. Rectus femoris
☐ 2. Deltoid
☐ 3. Lateral thigh
☐ 4. Medial thigh

CORRECT ANSWER: 3
Insulin is administered into an area of subcutaneous tissue, such as the lateral thigh. Options 1 and 2: Both are intramuscular sites, not subcutaneous sites. Option 4: Injections aren't given into medial sites to avoid nerves and large vessels.
NP: Evaluating care
CN: Physiological integrity
CNS: Pharmacological therapies
CL: Application

72 Which statement by a diabetic boy indicates deficient knowledge related to insulin administration?
☐ 1. "I'll clean my skin with alcohol before injecting insulin."
☐ 2. "I may mix my regular and NPH insulins in the same syringe."
☐ 3. "I'll administer my morning injection before breakfast."
☐ 4. "I'll be sure to use a 1¹/₂″ needle."

CORRECT ANSWER: 4
An insulin syringe requires a subcutaneous needle that is ¹/₂″ to 1″ long. The shorter (¹/₂″) needle is preferred for children, who may have little subcutaneous fat. Options 1, 2, and 3 are all correct procedures in insulin administration.
NP: Evaluating care
CN: Physiological integrity
CNS: Pharmacological therapies
CL: Application

73 When administering NPH insulin, which step should be taken?
☐ 1. Use a 3-ml syringe.
☐ 2. Roll the vial to mix the insulin before withdrawal.
☐ 3. Administer the NPH insulin with an I.V. push.
☐ 4. Avoid mixing NPH and regular insulin in the same syringe.

CORRECT ANSWER: 2
NPH insulin is a suspension, and rolling the vial distributes the insulin evenly throughout the suspension. Option 1: Insulin syringes are labeled in units, not milliliters. Both 1- and 0.5-ml syringes are used, depending on the dosage. Option 3: NPH insulin can't be given I.V. Option 4: NPH insulin may be mixed in the same syringe with regular insulin.
NP: Implementing care
CN: Physiological integrity
CNS: Pharmacological therapies
CL: Application

74 What is the nurse's priority when caring for a 10-month-old infant with meningitis?
☐ 1. Maintaining an adequate airway
☐ 2. Maintaining fluid and electrolyte balance
☐ 3. Controlling seizures
☐ 4. Controlling hyperthermia

CORRECT ANSWER: 1
Maintaining an adequate airway is always a top priority. Options 2, 3, and 4 are all important but not as important as an adequate airway.
NP: Implementing care
CN: Physiological integrity
CNS: Reduction of risk potential
CL: Application

75 Which intervention would be appropriate for an infant after cardiac catheterization?
☐ 1. Keep the leg on the operative site flexed to reduce bleeding.
☐ 2. Change the catheterization site dressing immediately to reduce the risk of infection.
☐ 3. Apply pressure if oozing or bleeding is noted.
☐ 4. Keep the infant's temperature below normal to promote vasoconstriction and decrease bleeding.

CORRECT ANSWER: 3
Applying pressure to the site is appropriate if bleeding is noted. Option 1: The leg should be kept straight and immobile to prevent trauma and bleeding. Option 2: The pressure dressing shouldn't be changed, but it may be reinforced if bleeding occurs. Option 4: Hypothermia causes stress in infants and should be avoided.
NP: Implementing care
CN: Physiological integrity
CNS: Reduction of risk potential
CL: Application

76 Which finding would concern the nurse who is caring for an infant after a right femoral cardiac catheterization?
☐ 1. Weak right dorsalis pedis pulse
☐ 2. Elevated temperature
☐ 3. Decreased urine output
☐ 4. Slight bloody drainage around catheterization site dressing

CORRECT ANSWER: 1
The pulse below the catheterization site should be strong and equal to the unaffected extremity. A weakened pulse may indicate vessel obstruction or perfusion problems. Options 2 and 3: These are relatively normal findings after catheterization and may be the result of decreased oral fluids. Option 4: A small amount of bloody drainage is normal; however, the site must be assessed frequently for increased bleeding.
NP: Collecting data
CN: Physiological integrity
CNS: Reduction of risk potential
CL: Application

77 Which guideline should the nurse follow when administering digoxin (Lanoxin) to an infant?
☐ 1. Mix the digoxin with the infant's food.
☐ 2. Double the subsequent dose if a dose is missed.
☐ 3. Give the digoxin with antacids when possible.
☐ 4. Withhold the dose if the apical pulse rate is less than 90 beats/minute.

CORRECT ANSWER: 4
Digoxin is used to decrease heart rate; however, the apical pulse must be carefully monitored to detect a severe reduction. Administering digoxin to an infant with a heart rate of under 90 beats/minute could further reduce the rate and compromise cardiac output. Option 1: Mixing digoxin with other food may interfere with accurate dosage. Option 2: Double-dosing should never be done. Option 3: Antacids may decrease drug absorption.
NP: Implementing care
CN: Physiological integrity
CNS: Pharmacological therapies
CL: Application

78 Which change would the nurse expect after administering oxygen to an infant with uncorrected tetralogy of Fallot?
☐ 1. Disappearance of the murmur
☐ 2. No evidence of cyanosis
☐ 3. Improvement of finger clubbing
☐ 4. Less agitation

CORRECT ANSWER: 4
Supplemental oxygen will help the child to breathe easier and feel less anxious. Options 1, 2, and 3: These findings won't occur as the result of providing supplemental oxygen.
NP: Evaluating care
CN: Physiological integrity
CNS: Basic care and comfort
CL: Analysis

79 A 6-month-old infant with uncorrected tetralogy of Fallot suddenly becomes increasingly cyanotic and diaphoretic, with weak peripheral pulses and an increased respiratory rate. What should the nurse do immediately?
☐ 1. Administer oxygen.
☐ 2. Administer morphine sulfate.
☐ 3. Place the infant in a knee-chest position.
☐ 4. Place the infant in Fowler's position.

CORRECT ANSWER: 3
The knee-chest position reduces the workload of the heart by increasing the blood return to the heart and keeping the blood flow more centralized. Option 1: This should be done quickly but only after placing the infant in the knee-chest position. Option 2: Morphine should be administered after options 3 and 1 are completed. Option 4: Fowler's position wouldn't improve the situation.
NP: Implementing care
CN: Physiological integrity
CNS: Physiological adaptation
CL: Application

80 A 2-year-old child is admitted to the pediatric unit with respiratory distress. Which finding indicates that the problem concerns the child's upper respiratory tract rather than the lower tract?
- ☐ 1. Nasal flaring
- ☐ 2. Pallor
- ☐ 3. Fever
- ☐ 4. Inspiratory stridor

CORRECT ANSWER: 4
Inspiratory stridor is the hallmark assessment finding in cases of upper respiratory distress, such as with croup and foreign body aspiration. Options 1 and 2: These symptoms probably would be present in most children with respiratory distress; they wouldn't help pinpoint the location of the problem. Option 3: Fever may or may not be present in children with respiratory distress.
NP: Evaluating care
CN: Physiological integrity
CNS: Physiological adaptation
CL: Application

---

81 The nurse is caring for a 3-year-old child with laryngotracheobronchitis who is fighting his aerosol treatment. What should the nurse do?
- ☐ 1. Restrain the child's extremities and give the treatment.
- ☐ 2. Document the child's refusal and try again at the next scheduled treatment.
- ☐ 3. Ask for the parents' help.
- ☐ 4. Call the physician.

CORRECT ANSWER: 3
Allowing the parents to participate in the child's care is essential; it decreases the child's anxiety and promotes compliance. Option 1: Restraints only cause the child to work harder to breathe and increase the level of distress. Option 2: Aerosol treatments are an essential part of the child's care and must be administered as prescribed. Option 4: This doesn't help the child get the required medication.
NP: Implementing care
CN: Physiological integrity
CNS: Basic care and comfort
CL: Comprehension

---

82 Which statement about caring for clients with acetaminophen intoxication is true?
- ☐ 1. Acetaminophen is harmless and an overdose isn't serious.
- ☐ 2. Vomiting shouldn't be induced.
- ☐ 3. The recognized antidote is acetylcysteine (Mucomyst).
- ☐ 4. Acetaminophen toxicity causes swollen mucous membranes.

CORRECT ANSWER: 3
Acetylcysteine is the antidote for acetaminophen toxicity and should be administered as a loading dose, followed by a maintenance dose. Option 1: Acetaminophen intoxication is a medical emergency that can cause hepatotoxicity or death. Option 2: Vomiting and lavage are the initial interventions in acetaminophen overdoses. Option 4: Swollen mucous membranes are associated with ingestion of corrosive substances, not acetaminophen.
NP: Implementing care
CN: Physiological integrity
CNS: Physiological adaptation
CL: Application

---

83 Which finding would prompt the nurse to take further action when caring for a 10-year-old boy with nephrotic syndrome?
- ☐ 1. Urine specific gravity of 1.030
- ☐ 2. Sudden loss of appetite
- ☐ 3. Resting blood pressure of 90/60 mm Hg
- ☐ 4. Abdominal girth with 2¹/₃″ (6-cm) increase from previous measurement

CORRECT ANSWER: 4
This is a significant increase and may interfere with the child's respiratory effort. Fluid retention and edema are common in clients with nephrotic syndrome, and abdominal distention must be carefully evaluated for its systemic effects. Option 1: This is expected due to the proteinuria associated with nephrotic syndrome. Option 2: A loss of appetite is common due to protein and fluid losses related to nephrotic syndrome. Option 3: This is a relatively normal blood pressure for a 10-year-old boy.
NP: Evaluating care
CN: Physiological integrity
CNS: Basic care and comfort
CL: Analysis

84 Which regimen would be best for the successful management of type 1 diabetes mellitus?
- [ ] 1. Oral hypoglycemics, diet, and exercise
- [ ] 2. Diet and exercise alone
- [ ] 3. Insulin, diet, and exercise
- [ ] 4. Vigorous workout program

CORRECT ANSWER: 3
Clients with type 1 diabetes mellitus are insulin-dependent; therefore, insulin must be included in the daily regimen. However, diet and exercise are also important aspects of treatment. Option 1: Oral hypoglycemics won't control type 1 diabetes mellitus. Options 2 and 4: Insulin must be part of any regimen for this type of diabetes.
NP: Planning care
CN: Health promotion and maintenance
CNS: Prevention and early detection of disease
CL: Application

---

85 A 10-year-old girl is admitted to the pediatric unit with the following symptoms: weight loss, blurred vision, increased thirst, increased appetite, and increased urination. Which laboratory test would probably provide vital additional information?
- [ ] 1. Platelet count
- [ ] 2. Serum creatinine
- [ ] 3. Serum electrolytes
- [ ] 4. Complete blood count

CORRECT ANSWER: 3
The symptoms presented are classic findings for a child with type 1 diabetes mellitus. Electrolyte studies include a glucose level reading, which will be most important in determining the child's present condition. Options 1, 2, and 4 may be ordered; however, an evaluation of the client's blood glucose level is vital initially.
NP: Implementing care
CN: Physiological integrity
CNS: Reduction of risk potential
CL: Application

---

86 A client with type 1 diabetes mellitus is scheduled for surgery and requires insulin to be added to his I.V. solution. What type of insulin will be used?
- [ ] 1. Semilente
- [ ] 2. NPH
- [ ] 3. Regular
- [ ] 4. Protamine zinc

CORRECT ANSWER: 3
Regular insulin is a short-acting insulin that has an onset of action of 30 minutes to 1 hour. However, if given I.V., regular insulin acts within 10 to 30 minutes. Regular insulin is the only insulin that should be given I.V. Options 1, 2, and 4: These insulins all have a longer onset of action and peak effect, which makes them unsuitable for I.V. use.
NP: Implementing care
CN: Physiological integrity
CNS: Pharmacological therapies
CL: Application

---

87 The nurse is caring for a pediatric client with a chest tube attached to suction. The tube becomes disconnected at the connection site closest to the client, and the suction system is cracked. What should the nurse do?
- [ ] 1. Clamp the chest tube close to the client's chest.
- [ ] 2. Submerge the chest tube attached to the client in saline solution.
- [ ] 3. Obtain and set up a new water-seal system.
- [ ] 4. Connect the wall suction to the chest tube while preparing a new water-seal setup.

CORRECT ANSWER: 2
Submerging the chest tube creates a water-seal and reduces the risk of a tension pneumothorax. Option 1: Clamping the chest tube increases the risk of a tension pneumothorax. Option 3: This compromises the client by allowing atmospheric and intrathoracic pressures to become more equal. Option 4: Wall suction would exert too great a force and should never be used.
NP: Implementing care
CN: Physiological integrity
CNS: Reduction of risk potential
CL: Application

88 Which problem is most frequently encountered by adolescent females with scoliosis?
- [ ] 1. Respiratory distress
- [ ] 2. Poor self-esteem
- [ ] 3. Poor appetite
- [ ] 4. Renal difficulty

CORRECT ANSWER: 2
Poor self-esteem is a major issue with many adolescents. The use of orthopedic appliances such as those used to treat scoliosis make this issue much bigger. Options 1 and 3: Although these problems may surface, they aren't as common as problems with self-esteem. Option 4: Renal problems aren't usually an issue.
NP: Planning care
CN: Health promotion and maintenance
CNS: Growth and development through the life span
CL: Analysis

89 A client who recently suffered a head injury is at risk for developing increased intracranial pressure (ICP). Which measure is appropriate to prevent this?
- [ ] 1. Lower the head of the bed.
- [ ] 2. Hyperflex the neck.
- [ ] 3. Hyperventilate the client.
- [ ] 4. Increase the I.V. rate to twice the usual maintenance rate.

CORRECT ANSWER: 3
Hyperventilation causes the carbon dioxide level to decrease, resulting in vasoconstriction of cerebral blood vessels. This decreased cerebral blood flow temporarily reduces ICP. Options 1, 2, and 4: These measures increase ICP by preventing blood return from the head and by overhydrating with I.V. fluid.
NP: Implementing care
CN: Physiological integrity
CNS: Physiological adaptation
CL: Application

90 Which complication is possible for any pediatric client requiring mechanical ventilation?
- [ ] 1. Pneumothorax
- [ ] 2. High cardiac output
- [ ] 3. Polycythemia
- [ ] 4. Hypovolemia

CORRECT ANSWER: 1
Mechanical ventilation can cause barotrauma, as occurs with pneumothorax; clients receiving mechanical ventilation must be carefully monitored. Option 2: Mechanical ventilation decreases the cardiac output. Option 3: Polycythemia is the result of chronic hypoxia, not mechanical ventilation. Option 4: Mechanical ventilation can cause fluid overload, not dehydration.
NP: Evaluating care
CN: Physiological integrity
CNS: Physiological adaptation
CL: Application

91 The nurse is caring for a child on a mechanical ventilator when the high-pressure alarm sounds. What is the most likely cause?
- [ ] 1. Leaking endotracheal tube cuff
- [ ] 2. Disconnected tubing
- [ ] 3. Increased lung compliance
- [ ] 4. Increased pulmonary secretions

CORRECT ANSWER: 4
Increased pulmonary secretions increase the pressure required to ventilate a client. This creates a high-pressure situation and sounds the alarm. Options 1, 2, and 3: These decrease the pressure required for ventilation.
NP: Evaluating care
CN: Physiological integrity
CNS: Physiological adaptation
CL: Application

92 The nurse observes a 14-year-old boy who suffered a severe head injury and who has been experiencing significant increased intracranial pressure (ICP) over the past 24 hours. Which finding would indicate that the client is improving?
☐ 1. Increasing systolic blood pressure
☐ 2. Widening pulse pressure
☐ 3. Decerebrate posturing to touch
☐ 4. Equal and reactive pupils

CORRECT ANSWER: 4
As ICP rises, pupils become larger, less reactive, and often unequal as the result of interference with the transmission of nerve impulses. Equal and reactive pupils would suggest that the client's condition is improving. Options 1, 2, and 3: These findings indicate that ICP is rising.
NP: Collecting data
CN: Physiological integrity
CNS: Physiological adaptation
CL: Application

---

93 Which of the following definitions best describes Gowers' sign?
☐ 1. A transfer technique
☐ 2. A waddling gait
☐ 3. The position of the pelvis while walking
☐ 4. Muscle twitching that is present after stretching quickly

CORRECT ANSWER: 1
Gower's sign is a transfer technique used during some phases of muscular dystrophy. The child turns on the side or abdomen, extends the knees, and pushes on the torso to achieve an upright position by walking his hands up his legs. Option 2: A waddling gait isn't involved with Gower's sign. Option 3: Gower's sign doesn't involve the position of the pelvis. Option 4: Muscle twitching that is present after a quick stretch is called clonus.
NP: Collecting data
CN: Physiological integrity
CNS: Physiological adaptation
CL: Knowledge

---

94 The nurse is caring for a severely dehydrated child who has received a large volume of I.V. fluid replacement in a relatively short time. What finding would indicate that fluid replacement should be slowed?
☐ 1. Hypertension
☐ 2. Tenting of skin
☐ 3. Capillary refill time of 4 seconds
☐ 4. Weak peripheral pulses

CORRECT ANSWER: 1
Hypertension in a dehydrated child may indicate fluid overload; therefore, the fluid rate should be slowed. Options 2, 3, and 4: These signs are indicative of hypovolemia.
NP: Collecting data
CN: Physiological integrity
CNS: Physiological adaptation
CL: Application

---

95 The physician prescribes albuterol (Proventil) aerosol, as needed, for a 9-year-old boy. Which observation would be an indication for instituting such a treatment?
☐ 1. Wheezing on auscultation
☐ 2. Decreased level of consciousness
☐ 3. Bradypnea
☐ 4. Nasal flaring

CORRECT ANSWER: 1
Albuterol is a bronchodilator used to treat reversible obstructive airway disease. Wheezing is a symptom of lower airway obstruction, and auscultation should be performed before and after all aerosol treatments. Options 2 and 4: These symptoms are often associated with respiratory distress and respiratory failure; however, they aren't as definitive for aerosol treatment as option 1. Option 3: Bradypnea isn't usually seen in clients with respiratory distress, except when such clients approach respiratory failure and require ventilatory assistance.
NP: Collecting data
CN: Physiological integrity
CNS: Pharmacological therapies
CL: Application

96 A 4½-year-old boy is admitted to the pediatric unit for chemotherapy. He's on his last cycle. He turns to his mother and says, "I just want to go home, Mom." His mother looks up at you and says, "We're all so worn out." Which response is best initially?
- [ ] 1. "You've come this far; just hang in there."
- [ ] 2. "Only a couple more months, and he'll be done."
- [ ] 3. "I understand this must be very hard on both of you."
- [ ] 4. "All of your effort will be rewarded in the future."

CORRECT ANSWER: 3
The nurse's initial response should be to acknowledge the difficulty the mother and child are having with the psychological impact of the illness and its treatment. Options 1 and 2: They already know that the treatments are coming to an end but feel as though this will never occur. The nurse should acknowledge their feelings, not focus on their awareness of the length of treatment. Option 4: This offers a false sense of security and is inappropriate.
NP: Implementing care
CN: Psychosocial integrity
CNS: Coping and adaptation
CL: Analysis

---

97 Which instruction should the nurse include when discharging a client receiving chemotherapy?
- [ ] 1. "Decrease spicy food intake to prevent stomach upset."
- [ ] 2. "Decrease fluid intake to prevent overworking the kidneys."
- [ ] 3. "Be sure to include such foods as liver to help prevent anemia."
- [ ] 4. "Eat foods low in purines to prevent increased urate deposits."

CORRECT ANSWER: 4
The child is at risk for hyperuricemia from rapid lysis of neoplastic cells. The breakdown of purines produces uric acid, which can add to the already high levels of uric acid and urate deposits in the kidneys, leading to renal failure. Option 1: There is no chemotherapeutic or physiologic reason to address intake of spicy foods. Option 2: Increased fluid intake is essential to prevent urate deposits and calculi formation. Option 3: Liver contains purines and should be avoided.
NP: Implementing care
CN: Health promotion and maintenance
CNS: Prevention and early detection of disease
CL: Comprehension

---

98 A 1-year-old girl has been admitted to the pediatric unit with a left-sided neck mass that has been identified as swollen lymphatic glands. She's provisionally diagnosed as having bubonic plague. What precautions should be used when caring for this client?
- [ ] 1. Full isolation, including a gown, mask, and gloves
- [ ] 2. Reverse isolation precautions
- [ ] 3. Standard precautions
- [ ] 4. Use of a mask

CORRECT ANSWER: 3
Bubonic plague organisms infect the lymphatic system and can eventually invade the vascular system. The client may have fever and lymphadenitis. The bacilli are transferred by client body fluids; therefore, standard precautions are essential. Options 1 and 4: Pulmonic, not bubonic, plague requires full isolation precautions and use of a mask due to airborne droplets from the client's coughing. Option 2: Reverse isolation is primarily used for clients with immunosuppressive diseases.
NP: Planning care
CN: Safe, effective care environment
CNS: Safety and infection control
CL: Application

99 A 2-year-old girl who is receiving chloramphenicol (Chloromycetin) has been sitting in a high chair eating her dinner. The nurse observes a large amount of vomitus 10 minutes after the child finishes her meal. After first determining that there is no medical emergency, the nurse should take which action?
☐ 1. Notify the physician of a relapse in the client's condition.
☐ 2. Give the child nothing by mouth for the next several hours.
☐ 3. Rock and cuddle the child and give her clear fluids as she demands.
☐ 4. Give the child another dinner.

CORRECT ANSWER: 3
After cleaning the client, the nurse should try to soothe the child and let her know that she's safe. Nausea and vomiting are possible adverse effects of chloramphenicol use. Options 2 and 4: Because the child hasn't vomited before this incident, the nurse can offer her clear liquids and, after these are tolerated, begin food again at the child's request. Option 1: The physician may be notified, but vomiting isn't necessarily a relapse of the child's condition.
NP: Implementing care
CN: Physiological integrity
CNS: Pharmacological therapies
CL: Application

---

100 Which statement is best to say to a child when preparing him for removal of a nasogastric (NG) tube?
☐ 1. "This may be a bit uncomfortable, but it will be over pretty quickly."
☐ 2. "Hold your breath while the tube is being removed."
☐ 3. "Would you like to do this yourself?"
☐ 4. "I'll give you pain medication before removing the tube."

CORRECT ANSWER: 1
Removal of an NG tube isn't necessarily painful, but it can be quite uncomfortable. It usually proceeds quickly and without complications. Option 2: Holding the breath isn't necessary. Option 3: Although it's important to allow children to do things for themselves to master a sense of control, this procedure must be done by the nurse or a trained caregiver. Option 4: Pain medication is unnecessary.
NP: Planning care
CN: Psychosocial integrity
CNS: Coping and adaptation
CL: Application

---

101 A 10-year-old girl has femur fractures in both legs and is in bilateral skeletal traction. Five days after being admitted, she begins ringing for the nurse every 30 minutes and requesting the bedpan. She voids only 20 to 40 ml each time, but there is no evidence of a urinary tract infection. The nurse teaches the child to perform Kegel exercises. The purpose of these exercises is to help:
☐ 1. strengthen the child's arms so that she can better use the trapeze to lift up for bedpan placement and removal.
☐ 2. strengthen the child's calf muscles so that she's less likely to get leg cramps.
☐ 3. distract the child.
☐ 4. maintain good perineal muscle tone by tightening the pubococcygeus muscle.

CORRECT ANSWER: 4
Kegel exercises involve tightening the perineal muscles to help strengthen the pubococcygeus muscle and increase its elasticity. This helps to keep the child from becoming incontinent. Options 1, 2, and 3 are incorrect.
NP: Implementing care
CN: Physiological integrity
CNS: Basic care and comfort
CL: Application

---

102 A client with bilateral fractured femurs is scheduled for a double-hip spica cast. She says to the nurse, "Only 3 more months, and I can go home." Further investigation reveals that the client and her family believe she'll be hospitalized until the cast comes off. The nurse should explain to the client and her family that she:
☐ 1. may be hospitalized 2 to 4 months.
☐ 2. will go home 2 to 4 days after casting.
☐ 3. will go home a week after casting.
☐ 4. will go home as soon as she can move around.

CORRECT ANSWER: 2
The cast will dry fairly rapidly with the use of fiberglass casting material. The time spent in the hospital after casting, typically 2 to 4 days, will be for teaching the client and family how to care for her at home and for evaluating the client's skin integrity and neurovascular status before discharge. Options 1, 3, and 4: The time frames given are inaccurate.
NP: Implementing care
CN: Health promotion and maintenance
CNS: Prevention and early detection of disease
CL: Application

103 A boy with diabetes is on a 1,500-calorie American Diabetes Association diet while in the hospital. He had lunch 1 hour ago but complains that he's very hungry. Which action should the nurse take?
☐ 1. Tell him that he just ate and he'll have to wait for dinner.
☐ 2. Encourage him to drink a glass of water and play a game to distract him.
☐ 3. Offer him dietetic gelatin, carrot sticks, and a diet soft drink.
☐ 4. Offer him graham crackers and an apple.

CORRECT ANSWER: 3
Many clients with diabetes feel satisfied with three meals and two snacks per day, with the snacks taken between mealtimes. However, sometimes clients don't feel satisfied at mealtime and are hungry before snack time. Sugar-free snacks can be given to hold the client until the next meal or snack. Option 1 is inappropriate. Option 2: Diversional activities are helpful if the problem is boredom rather than hunger. Option 4 includes sugar-containing foods that may be incorporated into the planned meals or snacks.
NP: Implementing care
CN: Physiological integrity
CNS: Basic care and comfort
CL: Comprehension

104 A 3-month-old boy has been admitted to the hospital with pneumonia and possible pertussis. He has spasmodic coughing episodes in which he becomes cyanotic. During a coughing episode, the nurse realizes that mucus is clogging the infant's nasal passages. He appears agitated and dusky as his mother holds him up to her shoulder. A blow-by oxygen mask is running. What should the nurse do next?
☐ 1. Remove the infant from the mother and lay him in the crib.
☐ 2. Using a bulb syringe, suction the infant's mouth and nares while the mother is holding him.
☐ 3. Take the infant from the mother and place the oxygen mask firmly to his face.
☐ 4. Do nothing until the infant has calmed down.

CORRECT ANSWER: 2
Suctioning the infant's airway with a bulb syringe to remove the mucus helps to open the airway. Bronchial spasms and the effort to cough up mucous plugs are causing the infant's agitation and dusky appearance. Option 1: The mother's presence and attempt to soothe her son are helping to reduce some of infant's fear and anxiety. Option 3: It may be necessary to remove the infant and use more aggressive treatments if he becomes limp or remains dusky. Option 4: Doing nothing is inappropriate and compromises the infant's condition.
NP: Implementing care
CN: Physiological integrity
CNS: Physiological adaptation
CL: Application

105 Which terms are used to describe the three stages of pertussis?
☐ 1. Catarrhal, paroxysmal, and convalescent
☐ 2. First, second, and third
☐ 3. Paroxysmal, contagious, and convalescent
☐ 4. Infectious, paroxysmal, and convalescent

CORRECT ANSWER: 1
Pertussis is commonly described in terms of three stages: catarrhal, paroxysmal, and convalescent. The catarrhal stage, which lasts 1 to 2 weeks, is the most contagious. During the paroxysmal stage, which lasts 2 to 4 weeks, symptoms are most pronounced. The convalescent stage marks the time of recovery and typically lasts 1 to 2 weeks. However, the client may have coughing episodes for up to 1 year. Options 2, 3, and 4 are incorrect.
NP: Collecting data
CN: Health promotion and maintenance
CNS: Prevention and early detection of disease
CL: Knowledge

106 An 8-month-old boy is admitted to the pediatric unit with a diagnosis of pneumonia. Laboratory analysis of a nasal swab indicates that he's positive for RSV, which stands for:
- ☐ 1. respiratory syncytial virus.
- ☐ 2. rhinosalpingitis.
- ☐ 3. respiratory sinus virus.
- ☐ 4. rhinosporidiosis.

CORRECT ANSWER: 1

Respiratory syncytial virus (RSV) is a form of pneumonia most prevalent in infants and children. Option 2: Rhinosalpingitis is the inflammation of the nasal mucosa and eustachian tubes. Option 3 doesn't exist. Option 4: Rhinosporidiosis is a fungal disease—not a virus—that is characterized by the development of polyps on the mucosa of the nose, eyes, ears and, sometimes, the penis or vagina.

NP: Collecting data
CN: Health promotion and maintenance
CNS: Prevention and early detection of disease
CL: Knowledge

---

107 A client is receiving oxygen via a nasal cannula at 2 L/minute. What percentage of oxygen concentration is coming through the cannula?
- ☐ 1. 23% to 30%
- ☐ 2. 30% to 40%
- ☐ 3. 40% to 60%
- ☐ 4. 50% to 75%

CORRECT ANSWER: 1

The percent of oxygen concentration as it passes out of the nasal cannula at 2 L/minute is 23% to 30%. Option 1: The oxygen concentration via cannula at 3 to 5 L/minute is 30% to 40%. Option 3: A simple mask at 6 to 8 L/minute delivers 40% to 60% of oxygen. Option 4: A partial rebreather mask at 8 to 11 L/minute delivers 50% to 75% of oxygen.

NP: Collecting data
CN: Physiological integrity
CNS: Reduction of risk potential
CL: Comprehension

---

108 A child with respiratory syncytial virus (RSV) has been in the hospital for 36 hours and now requires oxygen. His mother doesn't understand why his condition is worsening. Which response by the nurse is best?
- ☐ 1. "Your son isn't responding to antibiotics and is getting worse."
- ☐ 2. "Your son is very sick and will be getting different antibiotics soon."
- ☐ 3. "With this virus, he'll get a little worse before he starts to get better."
- ☐ 4. "Don't worry, we're doing all we can for him."

CORRECT ANSWER: 3

RSV begins with coldlike symptoms and becomes more severe over several days. A child brought to the hospital within the first couple of days of illness may need oxygen as his respiratory system becomes compromised. Options 1 and 2: Antibiotics aren't generally used because RSV is caused by a virus; however, if the client also manifests evidence of a bacterial infection, antibiotics may be ordered. Within 3 to 5 days after onset, the client typically wheezes audibly and becomes sicker. This may last another 2 to 5 days, after which he begins to improve. Option 4: Platitudes aren't good therapeutic communications and don't provide comfort or reduce parental anxiety.

NP: Implementing care
CN: Psychosocial integrity
CNS: Coping and adaptation
CL: Application

109 The nurse determines that a client's oxygen saturation is 89% by using a pulse oximeter. What action should the nurse take?
- ☐ 1. Increase the oxygen flow until the saturation level is above 90%.
- ☐ 2. Assess the client's color, breathing status, and skin temperature.
- ☐ 3. Notify the physician about the oximeter finding.
- ☐ 4. Retest the client in 30 minutes.

CORRECT ANSWER: 2
The nurse should never rely solely on mechanical devices to determine a client's condition; client assessment is integral to the nursing process. Pallor or duskiness and signs of respiratory distress are more accurate measures of the client's condition than what a mechanical reading can provide. Option 1: In this case, the client may require more oxygen; however, this can be determined only after performing a nursing assessment and confirming the accuracy of the oximeter test result. Option 3: If the nurse determines that the oxygen flow may need to be increased, the physician should be notified because this may be a sign that the client's condition is worsening. Option 4: Cold fingers and toes can give a low reading on an oximeter. If this is the case, the nurse should warm the extremity and try again.
NP: Implementing care
CN: Physiological integrity
CNS: Reduction of risk potential
CL: Application

---

110 An 11-year-old boy with a head injury has been in the hospital for 16 days. He's receiving physical, occupational, and speech therapies. He can swallow and has adequate oral intake; however, his speech is slow and sometimes he makes inappropriate statements. He's usually cooperative but occasionally has combative and violent outbursts. His parents are upset and want to know what is wrong with him. What is the best response by the nurse?
- ☐ 1. "He probably didn't receive enough discipline growing up and is throwing tantrums."
- ☐ 2. "He needs to be restrained during these episodes."
- ☐ 3. "This is a stage of healing for him."
- ☐ 4. "He'll need to be on lifetime medication to control his temper."

CORRECT ANSWER: 3
Clients with head injuries may pass through eight stages during their recovery. Stage 1, marked by unresponsiveness, is the worst stage. Stage 8, characterized by purposeful, appropriate behavior, is the final stage of healing. This client is somewhere between stage 4 (confused, agitated behavior) and stage 6 (confused, appropriate behavior) because sometimes he can answer appropriately but at other times becomes confused and angry, resorting to violent behavior. Options 1, 2, and 4 are incorrect.
NP: Implementing care
CN: Health promotion and maintenance
CNS: Prevention and early detection of disease
CL: Analysis

---

111 Which statement about nutrition is most appropriate for a client with diabetes?
- ☐ 1. "You're prohibited from eating cakes, pies, potato chips, and fast-food hamburgers and from drinking cola."
- ☐ 2. "It's important that you eat regular nutritious meals that are low in fat and high in complex carbohydrates."
- ☐ 3. "You must follow a specific American Diabetes Association (ADA) diet that will be ordered by your physician."
- ☐ 4. "Nutrition isn't important in controlling your diabetes because you'll be taking insulin."

CORRECT ANSWER: 2
The goal for a client with diabetes is to follow a regular nutritious diet that includes 10% to 20% protein, a low amount of fat, and a relatively constant amount of complex carbohydrates. Options 1 and 3: A client with diabetes isn't prohibited from eating certain foods. The diet recommended by the ADA isn't specific or individualized. Option 4: Diet is integral to controlling diabetes along with insulin and exercise.
NP: Implementing care
CN: Health promotion and maintenance
CNS: Prevention and early detection of disease
CL: Application

112 The nurse is teaching a 23-year-old first-time mother about her 7-month-old infant's nutritional needs. What recommendations should the nurse provide about beginning to introduce foods?
- ☐ 1. Begin feeding food, usually rice cereal.
- ☐ 2. Begin feeding foods, such as bananas or sweet potatoes.
- ☐ 3. Begin feeding soft finger foods.
- ☐ 4. Begin feeding moist, soft table foods that are served at family meals.

CORRECT ANSWER: 2
By 6 to 8 months of age, most infants can start to eat foods, such as rice cereal, fruits, and vegetables. Option 1: Infants begin to eat baby food, usually rice cereal, at 4 to 6 months. Option 3: By 8 to 10 months, most infants enjoy soft finger foods. Option 4: At 12 months, infants eat most soft table foods that are served at family meals.
NP: Implementing care
CN: Health promotion and maintenance
CNS: Growth and development through the life span
CL: Application

---

113 The nurse at a family health clinic is teaching a group of parents about normal infant development. At what age can most children sit alone without support?
- ☐ 1. 2 to 4 months
- ☐ 2. 4 to 6 months
- ☐ 3. 6 to 8 months
- ☐ 4. 8 to 10 months

CORRECT ANSWER: 3
By the age of 6 to 8 months, most infants can sit alone without support. Option 1: Infants age 2 to 4 months can turn from side to back. Option 2: At 4 to 6 months, babies can usually support most of their weight when held standing. Option 4: By 8 to 10 months, babies can crawl or pull the body with the arms.
NP: Collecting data
CN: Health promotion and maintenance
CNS: Growth and development through the life span
CL: Knowledge

---

114 A 4-month-old is admitted to the pediatric unit to be hospitalized for 1 day or more. What toys should the nurse encourage the parents to provide?
- ☐ 1. Large blocks
- ☐ 2. Teething toys
- ☐ 3. Mobiles
- ☐ 4. Soft toys with contrasting colors

CORRECT ANSWER: 4
At age 3 to 6 months, most babies enjoy rattles, stuffed animals, and soft toys with contrasting colors. Options 1 and 2: Large blocks and teething toys are appropriate for a 6- to 12-month-old baby. Option 3: Mobiles are used for infants from birth to 2 months.
NP: Implementing care
CN: Health promotion and maintenance
CNS: Growth and development through the life span
CL: Application

---

115 The nurse is assessing a 6-year-old child who shows some signs of urinary tract infection (UTI). The signs and symptoms of UTI in children over age 2 include:
- ☐ 1. nausea and vomiting.
- ☐ 2. lethargy and failure to gain weight.
- ☐ 3. frequency and strong smelling urine.
- ☐ 4. renal tenderness and crying.

CORRECT ANSWER: 3
Fever, dysuria, frequency, and strong smelling urine are signs and symptoms of UTI in children. Options 1, 2, and 4: Nausea, vomiting, lethargy, and renal tenderness are signs and symptoms of UTI in infants, not children.
NP: Collecting data
CN: Physiological integrity
CNS: Physiological adaptation
CL: Comprehension

116 The nurse at a family health clinic is teaching a group of parents about normal infant development. What patterns of communication should the nurse tell parents to expect from a baby at age 1?
- ☐ 1. Squeals and makes pleasure sound
- ☐ 2. Understands "no" and other simple commands
- ☐ 3. Uses speechlike rhythm when talking with an adult
- ☐ 4. Uses multisyllabic babbling

CORRECT ANSWER: 2

At age 1, most babies understand the word "no" and other simple commands. Children at this age also learn one or two other words. Options 1 and 4: Babies squeal, make pleasure sounds, and use multisyllabic babbling at age 3 to 6 months. Option 3: Using speechlike rhythm when talking with an adult usually occurs between ages 6 and 9 months.
NP: Collecting data
CN: Health promotion and maintenance
CNS: Growth and development through the life span
CL: Knowledge

---

117 The nurse is caring for neonates in the hospital nursery. What is the normal respiratory rate for a neonate?
- ☐ 1. 12 to 20 breaths/minute
- ☐ 2. 16 to 20 breaths/minute
- ☐ 3. 20 to 40 breaths/minute
- ☐ 4. 30 to 80 breaths/minute

CORRECT ANSWER: 4

The normal respiratory range for a newborn is 30 to 80 breaths/minute. Option 1: Adult respirations range from 12 to 20 breaths/minute. Option 2: At age 10, respiratory rates range from 16 to 22 breaths/minute. Option 3: Children at age 1 usually have respiratory rates ranging from 20 to 40 breaths/minute.
NP: Collecting data
CN: Health promotion and maintenance
CNS: Growth and development through the life span
CL: Knowledge

---

118 A 2-week old neonate in acute respiratory distress is brought to the emergency department by his parents. What findings does the nurse expect to see in a neonate in respiratory distress?
- ☐ 1. Flaring, grunting, and retracting
- ☐ 2. Bradycardia
- ☐ 3. Bradypnea
- ☐ 4. Weak cough

CORRECT ANSWER: 1

In a neonate, the classic signs of respiratory distress are flaring, grunting, and retracting. Options 2 and 3: Bradycardia and bradypnea are seen in adult respiratory distress. Option 4: Coughing isn't seen in a neonate.
NP: Collecting data
CN: Physiological integrity
CNS: Physiological adaptation
CL: Application

---

119 The nurse is assessing a 3-year-old female at a family health center. The normal heart rate range for a 3-year-old is:
- ☐ 1. 100 to 170 beats/minute.
- ☐ 2. 80 to 130 beats/minute.
- ☐ 3. 70 to 120 beats/minute.
- ☐ 4. 60 to 100 beats/minute.

CORRECT ANSWER: 3

The normal heart rate for a 3-year-old is 70 to 120 beats/minute. Option 1: Newborns have a heart rate range from 100 to 170 beats/minute. Option 2: Children up to age 2 have heart rates ranging from 80 to 130 beats/minute. Option 4: Heart rates of 60 to 100 beats/minute are observed in children ages 10 to 16.
NP: Collecting data
CN: Health promotion and maintenance
CNS: Growth and development through the life span
CL: Knowledge

120 The nurse is assessing a 3-year-old child brought to a family health center for a routine examination. The median systolic and diastolic blood pressure values for a 3-year-old child are:
☐ 1. 70/50 mm Hg.
☐ 2. 90/50 mm Hg.
☐ 3. 114/65 mm Hg.
☐ 4. 120/70 mm Hg.

CORRECT ANSWER: 2
The median systolic and diastolic blood pressure values for a 3-year-old child is 90/50 mm Hg. Option 1: Newborns have a median systolic and diastolic blood pressure value of 70/50 mm Hg. Option 3: A median systolic and diastolic blood pressure value of 114/65 mm Hg can be observed in 15-year-old adolescents. Option 4: A systolic and diastolic value of 120/70 mm Hg is observed in clients age 18 and older.
NP: Collecting data
CN: Health promotion and maintenance
CNS: Growth and development through the life span
CL: Knowledge

121 The nurse is teaching a developmental health class for parents at a community health clinic. Which instruction should the nurse provide when teaching parents about caring for their toddler?
☐ 1. Learn to accept the child's need for self-mastery.
☐ 2. Learn to allow the child to explore the surrounding environment.
☐ 3. Learn to accept rejection without deserting.
☐ 4. Learn to support the emergence of the child as an individual.

CORRECT ANSWER: 1
According to Erikson's development tasks, toddlers ages 1 to 3 are at the development stage of *autonomy versus doubt and shame*. Parents need to accept the child's growing need for freedom while setting consistent and realistic limits and offering support and understanding when separation anxiety occurs. Option 2: Exploring surrounding environments is a developmental task that should be accomplished during preschool years (ages 3 to 6). Option 3: Learning to accept rejection without deserting is usually accomplished by the time a child is at school age (ages 6 to 12). Option 4: Learning to support the emergence of the child's success and defeat is accomplished as an adolescent (ages 12 to 19).
NP: Collecting data
CN: Health promotion and maintenance
CNS: Growth and development through the life span
CL: Application

122 A 6-month-old infant is waiting for assessment by the nurse in a family health center. Which activity best describes the social development of a 6-month-old infant?
☐ 1. He clings to his parent in unfamiliar situations.
☐ 2. He attends to an adult's face and voice with eye contact.
☐ 3. He complies with simple verbal commands.
☐ 4. He starts to imitate sounds.

CORRECT ANSWER: 4
A 6-month-old infant starts to imitate sounds and vocalize one-syllable sounds such as "ma." Option 1: At age 12 months, the infant clings to the parent in unfamiliar situations. Option 2: A newborn attends to the adult's face and voice with eye contact. Option 3: By age 9 months, the infant complies with simple verbal commands.
NP: Collecting data
CN: Health promotion and maintenance
CNS: Growth and development through the life span
CL: Comprehension

123 A nurse on the pediatric unit is caring for a 2-year-old toddler who is about to be discharged. Which activity of daily living should the nurse expect the toddler to be able to perform?
☐ 1. Dressing himself
☐ 2. Demonstrating concern for personal cleanliness and appearance
☐ 3. Performing simple hygiene measures
☐ 4. Demonstrating toilet training

CORRECT ANSWER: 1
By age 2 or 3, the child can begin to dress himself. Option 2: A child usually demonstrates concern for personal cleanliness and appearance between ages 6 and 12. Options 3 and 4: A 2-year-old toddler begins to develop bowel and bladder control but isn't able to demonstrate toilet training or perform simple hygiene measures until age 4 or 5.
NP: Collecting data
CN: Health promotion and maintenance
CNS: Growth and development through the life span
CL: Comprehension

124 The nurse is observing a group of school-age children in an after-school art program. Which activities should the nurse expect to observe in a school-age child?
☐ 1. Associative play
☐ 2. Parallel play
☐ 3. Cooperative play
☐ 4. Dramatic play

CORRECT ANSWER: 3
One characteristic of school-age children is cooperative play — the ability to cooperate with others and play a part in contributing to a unified whole. Option 1: Playing side by side while each child engages in his own activities is called associative play and is usually observed in preschoolers. Option 2: Parallel play, or playing side by side and occasionally trading toys and words, is usually observed in toddlers. Option 4: Dramatic play, or living out the dramas of life, is observed in preschoolers.
NP: Collecting data
CN: Health promotion and maintenance
CNS: Growth and development through the life span
CL: Comprehension

125 The school nurse is assessing a 13-year-old male student after his involvement in a fight on the soccer field. Which developmental tasks must be accomplished in adolescence?
☐ 1. Self-control without the loss of self-esteem
☐ 2. Creativity, productivity, and concern for others
☐ 3. Coherent sense of self
☐ 4. Acceptance of worth and uniqueness of one's own life

CORRECT ANSWER: 3
According to Erikson's development tasks, the central task of adolescence is *identity versus role confusion*. During this stage, the adolescent learns to actualize his abilities and develop a coherent sense of self. Option 1: Self-control without the loss of self-esteem should be developed in early childhood. Option 2: Creativity, productivity, and concern for others are observed in adulthood. Option 4: Acceptance of worth and the uniqueness of one's own life is usually accomplished at maturity (age 65 and older).
NP: Collecting data
CN: Health promotion and maintenance
CNS: Growth and development through the life span
CL: Comprehension

126 The nurse is instructing a first-time mother in proper breast-feeding technique. She explains that the infant demonstrates the rooting reflex by:
☐ 1. extension and adduction of the extremities in response to sudden jarring.
☐ 2. leaving the hands open with the fingers remaining curved in response to jarring.
☐ 3. prancing movements of the legs when a neonate is held upright.
☐ 4. turning the head in the direction of anything that touches the cheek.

CORRECT ANSWER: 4
The infant turns the head in the direction of anything that touches the cheek, in anticipation of food. Options 1 and 2: Extension and adduction of the extremities and leaving the hands open with the fingers curved are part of the Moro reflex. Option 3: Prancing movements of the legs when a neonate is held upright is called the dancing reflex.
NP: Collecting data
CN: Health promotion and maintenance
CNS: Growth and development through the life span
CL: Knowledge

127 The nurse is assessing a 3-month-old male infant during a routine examination in a family health center. The nurse notes the presence of bluish discolorations of the skin. Such markings, which are common in babies of Black, Native American, and Mediterranean descent, are called:
☐ 1. milia.
☐ 2. Mongolian spots.
☐ 3. lanugo.
☐ 4. vernix caseosa.

CORRECT ANSWER: 2
Bluish discolorations of the skin, which are common in babies of Black, Native American, and Mediterranean races, are called Mongolian spots. Option 1: Pinpoint pimples caused by obstruction of sebaceous glands are called milia. Option 3: The fine hair covering the body of a neonate is called lanugo. Option 4: Vernix caseosa is a cheeselike substance that covers the skin of a neonate.
NP: Collecting data
CN: Health promotion and maintenance
CNS: Growth and development through the life span
CL: Knowledge

128 The nurse is collecting a health history of a 5-year-old. The mother notes that the child enjoys dressing in her parents' clothes and jewelry. This behavior is characteristic of which adaptive mechanism?
☐ 1. Imagination
☐ 2. Identification
☐ 3. Introjection
☐ 4. Intellectualization

CORRECT ANSWER: 2
Identification occurs when a child perceives himself like another person and behaves like that person. Option 1: Imagination occurs when the child fantasizes in play such as pretending that a chair is a throne. Option 3: Introjection occurs when the child assimilates the attributes of others such as a younger sister telling her older brother not to talk to strangers. Option 4: Intellectualization occurs when an uncomfortable or painful incident is avoided or evaded by the use of rational explanations.
NP: Collecting data
CN: Health promotion and maintenance
CNS: Growth and development through the life span
CL: Comprehension

129 The nurse is reviewing the theory of Erikson's development tasks in preparation for an upcoming examination. In which of Erikson's development tasks do lack of self-confidence, pessimism, and fear of wrongdoing indicate a negative resolution?
☐ 1. Trust versus mistrust
☐ 2. Autonomy versus shame and doubt
☐ 3. Initiative versus guilt
☐ 4. Industry versus inferiority

CORRECT ANSWER: 3
According to Erikson's development tasks, lack of self-confidence, pessimism, and fear of wrongdoing all indicate failure to resolve the development task of *initiative versus guilt* at ages 3 to 5. Option 1: Mistrust and withdrawn behavior are indicators of negative resolution of *trust versus mistrust* from birth to 18 months. Option 2: Compulsive self-restraint or compliance indicates negative resolution of *autonomy versus shame and doubt* at ages 18 months to 3 years. Option 4: Loss of hope and sense of being mediocre is indicative of failure to resolve *industry versus inferiority* at ages 6 to 12.
NP: Collecting data
CN: Health promotion and maintenance
CNS: Growth and development through the life span
CL: Comprehension

130 A child is admitted to the medical-surgical unit with complaints of weight loss and lack of energy. The child's ears and cheeks are flushed and the nurse observes an acetone odor to the client's breath. The blood glucose level is 325. The blood pressure is 104/60 mm Hg, pulse is 88, and respirations are 16 breaths/minute. Which of the following does the nurse expect the physician to order first?
☐ 1. Subcutaneous administration of glucagon
☐ 2. Administration of regular insulin by continuous infusion pump
☐ 3 Subcutaneous administration of regular insulin every 4 hours as needed by sliding scale insulin
☐ 4. Administration of I.V. fluids in boluses of 20 ml/kg

CORRECT ANSWER: 2
Weight loss, lack of energy, acetone odor to the breath, and a blood glucose level of 325 indicate diabetic ketoacidosis. Insulin is given by continuous infusion pump at a rate not to exceed 100 mg/dl/hour. Faster reduction of hypoglycemia could be related to the development of cerebral edema. Option 1: Glucagon is administered for mild hypoglycemia. Option 3: Sliding scale insulin isn't as effective as the administration of insulin by continuous infusion pump in the treatment of diabetic ketoacidosis. Option 4: Administration of I.V. fluids in boluses of 20 ml/kg is recommended for the treatment of shock.
NP: Implementing care
CN: Physiological integrity
CNS: Physiological adaptation
CL: Application

131 The nurse is planning teaching about insulin administration for a 5-year-old child diagnosed with diabetes mellitus. Which developmental guideline should the nurse use?
☐ 1. The parents should take responsibility for the child's care.
☐ 2. The child can give his own injections with supervision.
☐ 3. The child can learn to measure and mix insulin.
☐ 4. The child can tell where the injection should be given.

CORRECT ANSWER: 4
Children under age 6 should be able to tell where an injection should be given. Option 1: Parents shouldn't take total responsibility for children over age 4; preschool-age children should be able to participate in some aspects of care. Options 2 and 3: Usually, a child is age 7 or over before he can administer, measure, or mix insulin, and then only with supervision.
NP: Implementing care
CN: Physiological integrity
CNS: Physiological adaptation
CL: Application

132 A child diagnosed with diabetes mellitus is being evaluated for complaints of headache, fatigue, and hunger. The nurse notes that the child is alert and oriented to person and place. The parent states that the child was behaving aggressively toward his friends just prior to his admission at the ambulatory center. Which intervention should the nurse expect to be performed first?
☐ 1. Administration of glucagon subcutaneously
☐ 2. Administration of 10 units of regular insulin subcutaneously
☐ 3. Administration of orange juice orally
☐ 4. Administration of glucose I.V.

CORRECT ANSWER: 3
Fatigue, headache, and aggressive or antisocial behavior are symptoms of hypoglycemia reaction in children. The child is alert and oriented and should be able to drink orange juice without aspiration. Options 1 and 4: Glucagon and glucose are administered I.V. only if the child is unable to take a sugar source orally. Option 2: Insulin is administered for hyperglycemia, not hypoglycemia.
NP: Implementing care
CN: Physiological integrity
CNS: Physiological adaptation
CL: Application

133 The nurse is assessing a child diagnosed with type 1 diabetes mellitus. The physician ordered Lispro-Humalog insulin. The nurse knows that the onset of action for Lispro-Humalog insulin is:
☐ 1. 5 to 15 minutes.
☐ 2. $^1/_2$ to 1 hour.
☐ 3. 1 to 2 hours.
☐ 4. 4 to 6 hours.

CORRECT ANSWER: 1
The onset of Lispro-Humalog insulin is 5 to 15 minutes. Option 2: The onset of regular insulin is $^1/_2$ to 1 hour. Option 3: Intermediate-acting insulin or NPH has an onset of 1 to 2 hours. Option 4: Long-acting insulin or ultralente has an onset of 4 to 6 hours.
NP: Collecting data
CN: Physiological integrity
CNS: Pharmacological therapies
CL: Application

134 The physician orders a mixed dose of regular and NPH insulin for a child at 8:00 a.m. The child ate 100% of the breakfast tray and 25% of the lunch tray. At what time is the child most at risk for experiencing a hypoglycemia reaction?
☐ 1. 0800 to 1000
☐ 2. 1000 to 1200
☐ 3. 1200 to 1400
☐ 4. 1400 to 1600

CORRECT ANSWER: 4
The peak action of intermediate insulin is 6 to 12 hours; therefore, the NPH insulin administered at 0800 begins to peak between the hours of 1400 to 1600. The client ate only 25% of the lunch tray; therefore, the risk of experiencing a hypoglycemic reaction is greatest in midafternoon. The peak action of regular insulin is 2 to 4 hours. The client ate 100% of the breakfast tray, which decreases the risk of experiencing a hypoglycemic reaction during the morning hours. Options 1, 2, and 3: The other times are incorrect.
NP: Collecting data
CN: Physiological integrity
CNS: Physiological adaptation
CL: Application

135 An infant who appears to be younger than age 1 is admitted to the emergency room. On assessment, the nurse observes that the baby is lethargic and drowsy and is having respiratory difficulty. The parent describes seizure activity, which occurred at home just before their arrival. There are no external signs of injury. Which condition should the nurse suspect?
☐ 1. Epilepsy
☐ 2. Shaken baby syndrome
☐ 3. Failure to thrive
☐ 4. Infantile spasms

CORRECT ANSWER: 2
Signs and symptoms of shaken baby syndrome include apnea, seizures, lethargy, drowsiness, bradycardia, respiratory difficulty, and coma. Subdural and retinal hemorrhages in the absence of external signs of injury are strong indicators of the syndrome. Option 1: Epilepsy is a recurrent and chronic seizure disorder with onset usually between ages 4 and 8. Option 3: Infants with failure to thrive show delayed development without physical cause. Option 4: Infantile spasms are sudden brief, symmetric muscle contractions accompanied by rolling of the eyes.
NP: Collecting data
CN: Physiological integrity
CNS: Physiological adaptation
CL: Comprehension

---

136 The nurse is assessing a 14-year-old who received numerous insect and, possibly, tick bites on a recent camping trip. Which of the following signs and symptoms does the nurse expect to observe in a child with Lyme disease?
☐ 1. Jaundice, fever, and malaise
☐ 2. Bluish white spots on a red background
☐ 3. A slowly expanding red rash at the site of a bite
☐ 4. A red rash that begins on the cheeks

CORRECT ANSWER: 3
The most typical early symptom of Lyme disease is a slowly progressing red rash at the site of the bite. Option 1: Jaundice, fever, and malaise occur in hepatitis. Option 2: Bluish white spots on a red background are called Koplik's spots and occur with measles. Option 4: A red rash that begins on the cheeks is characteristic of erythema infectiosum.
NP: Collecting data
CN: Physiological integrity
CNS: Physiological adaptation
CL: Comprehension

---

137 The nurse is caring for a 9-year-old child diagnosed with Lyme disease. Nursing management for a child with Lyme disease includes which intervention?
☐ 1. Observing closely for prolonged or unusual bleeding
☐ 2. Administering aspirin to provide relief for fever
☐ 3. Administering antibiotics as ordered
☐ 4. Observing closely for seizure activity

CORRECT ANSWER: 3
There is a high risk for infection in clients with Lyme disease. The nurse should administer antibiotics as ordered. Option 1: Prolonged or unusual bleeding isn't a characteristic of Lyme disease. Option 2: Nonaspirin products are used to provide relief of pain and fever in children. Option 4: Seizures don't usually occur with Lyme disease.
NP: Implementing care
CN: Physiological integrity
CNS: Physiological adaptation
CL: Application

---

138 A 5-year-old male child is admitted to the medical-surgical unit with a diagnosis of nephrotic syndrome. Which symptom is the characteristic symptom of nephrosis?
☐ 1. Hyperproteinemia
☐ 2. Edema
☐ 3. Hypolipidemia
☐ 4. Osmotic diuresis

CORRECT ANSWER: 2
The characteristic symptom of nephrosis is edema. Edema may occur slowly, appearing first about the eyes and ankles and later becoming generalized. Options 1 and 3: The client may also develop hypoproteinemia and hyperlipidemia, but these symptoms aren't considered the characteristic symptom of nephrosis. Option 4: In osmotic diuresis, urine output is clear and increased. In nephrotic syndrome, urine output may be dark and decreased.
NP: Collecting data
CN: Physiological integrity
CNS: Physiological adaptation
CL: Knowledge

139 A 7-year-old child is brought to the emergency department in respiratory distress. His parents tell the nurse that he has asthma. Which signs indicate respiratory distress in a child with a diagnosis of asthma?
- ☐ 1. Fever, cough, and increased breathing
- ☐ 2. Nasal flaring and chest retractions
- ☐ 3. Restlessness, flushed skin, and decreased respirations
- ☐ 4. Flushed skin, decreased pulse, and decreased respirations

CORRECT ANSWER: 2
In children, nasal flaring and chest retractions indicate respiratory distress. Option 1: Fever may or may not be present, but it's usually more indicative of infection than respiratory difficulty. Options 3 and 4: Asthma clients are usually pale, with tachypnea (increased respirations).
NP: Collecting data
CN: Physiological integrity
CNS: Physiological adaptation
CL: Comprehension

---

140 A 16-year-old adolescent is brought to the emergency department exhibiting signs of respiratory distress after ingesting an unknown substance. Which signs indicate imminent respiratory arrest?
- ☐ 1. Dyspnea, bradycardia, and cyanosis
- ☐ 2. Tachycardia, tachypnea, and diaphoresis
- ☐ 3. Nasal flaring, retractions, and wheezing
- ☐ 4. Confusion, grunting, and diaphoresis

CORRECT ANSWER: 1
Dyspnea, bradycardia, cyanosis, stupor, and coma are signs of imminent respiratory arrest and occur because the client's oxygen deficit is overwhelming and beyond spontaneous recovery. Option 2: Tachycardia, tachypnea, and diaphoresis are initial signs of respiratory failure. The client's behavior and vital signs reflect that the oxygen supply is inadequate and that compensation and early hypoxia are occurring. Option 3: Nasal flaring, retractions, wheezing, and confusion are signs of early decompensation. The child is attempting to use accessory muscles to take in more oxygen. Hypoxia persists and decompensation occurs. Option 4: Diaphoresis and grunting may be early signs of respiratory failure and decompensation, but confusion is a sign of imminent respiratory arrest.
NP: Collecting data
CN: Physiological integrity
CNS: Physiological adaptation
CL: Comprehension

---

141 The nurse is caring for a 1-week-old infant who was abandoned and rescued from a nearby alley. Signs of severe dehydration in an infant include:
- ☐ 1. thirst and slight oliguria.
- ☐ 2. increased heart rate, restlessness, and irritable behavior.
- ☐ 3. marked thirst, sunken anterior fontanel, and restlessness.
- ☐ 4. increased heart and respiratory rates and lethargic behavior.

CORRECT ANSWER: 4
An infant with severe dehydration demonstrates lethargic or comatose behavior and has cold and clammy skin and increased heart and respiratory rates. Option 1: Slight oliguria and thirst indicate mild dehydration. Options 2 and 3: Increased heart rate, restlessness, irritable behavior, and marked thirst with a sunken anterior fontanel indicate moderate dehydration.
NP: Collecting data
CN: Physiological integrity
CNS: Physiological adaptation
CL: Comprehension

142 A 1-year old child diagnosed with dehydration is admitted to the pediatric unit. The physician orders 500 ml of dextrose 5% in normal saline solution to run over 10 hours. At what rate should the nurse infuse the fluids using a microdrip that delivers 60 gtt/ml?
☐ 1. 40 gtt/minute
☐ 2. 50 gtt/minute
☐ 3. 60 gtt/minute
☐ 4. 70 gtt/minute

CORRECT ANSWER: 2
The nurse should administer 50 gtt/minute using a microdrip that delivers 60 gtt/ml in order to infuse 500 ml of fluid I.V. over 10 hours. The correct formula is:
amount of fluid × mini or macro drip factor ÷ hours × minutes

$$\frac{500\ ml \times 60}{50 \times 10} = \frac{30000.00}{600} = 50\ gtt/minute.$$

Options 1, 3, and 4 are incorrect.
NP: Implementing care
CN: Physiological integrity
CNS: Pharmacological therapies
CL: Application

143 The nurse is caring for a 9-month-old infant diagnosed with acquired immunodeficiency syndrome (AIDS). The most common signs and symptoms in infants with this diagnosis are:
☐ 1. failure to thrive and enlargement of the liver and spleen.
☐ 2. development of Kaposi's sarcoma.
☐ 3. fever, anorexia, and night sweats.
☐ 4. lethargy, poor sucking reflex, and a high-pitched, shrill cry.

CORRECT ANSWER: 1
Infants with AIDS often fail to thrive and have chronic diarrhea, liver and spleen enlargement, and repeated respiratory infections. Option 2: Development of Kaposi's sarcoma isn't usually seen in children. Option 3: Fever, anorexia, and night sweats are usually observed with tuberculosis. Option 4: Lethargy, poor sucking reflex, and a high-pitched, shrill cry are observed with increased intracranial pressure.
NP: Collecting data
CN: Physiological integrity
CNS: Physiological adaptation
CL: Comprehension

144 A child has been diagnosed with acute glomerulonephritis. Which food should be eliminated from his diet?
☐ 1. Turkey sandwich with mayonnaise
☐ 2. Hot dog with ketchup
☐ 3. Chocolate cake with vanilla icing
☐ 4. Apple with peanut butter

CORRECT ANSWER: 2
Foods that are high in sodium content should be eliminated from the child's diet. Because hot dogs contain a great deal of sodium, they should be eliminated from the diet. Snacks such as pretzels and potato chips shouldn't be encouraged. Options 1, 3, and 4: Any other food that the child likes should be encouraged.
NP: Evaluating care
CN: Physiological integrity
CNS: Basic care and comfort
CL: Application

145 A 16-month-old male baby is brought to the emergency department for evaluation. The nurse observes that the baby is kicking, drawing his legs toward his abdomen, and crying loudly. The child is vomiting a stomach content that is greenish yellow. The parent states that the child's bowel movements have diminished. Which condition should the nurse suspect?
☐ 1. Inguinal hernia
☐ 2. Pyloric stenosis
☐ 3. Intussusception
☐ 4. Umbilical hernia

CORRECT ANSWER: 3
Intussusception, when a portion of the bowel telescopes into a distal portion, usually occurs in males before age 5, with the highest incidence between ages 6 and 18 months. The nurse usually observes the child kicking and drawing his legs, crying loudly, and vomiting bilious or greenish yellow stomach contents. Options 1 and 4: The child with an inguinal or umbilical hernia may be asymptomatic. Option 2: Pyloric stenosis is usually characterized by vomiting.
NP: Collecting data
CN: Physiological integrity
CNS: Physiological adaptation
CL: Application

146 The nurse is working overnight in the emergency department when a child is admitted in sickle cell crisis. Which intervention should the nurse expect to perform?
☐ 1. Giving blood transfusions
☐ 2. Giving antibiotics
☐ 3. Increasing fluid intake and giving analgesics
☐ 4. Preparing the child for a splenectomy

CORRECT ANSWER: 3
The primary therapy for sickle cell crisis is to increase fluid intake according to age and to give analgesics. Option 1: Blood transfusions are only given conservatively to avoid iron overload. Option 2: Antibiotics are given to children with fever. Option 4: Routine splenectomy isn't recommended. Splenectomy in children with sickle cell is controversial.
NP: Implementing care
CN: Physiological integrity
CNS: Physiological adaptation
CL: Application

147 The nurse is caring for a 2-year-old male toddler diagnosed with Kawasaki disease. The nurse knows that this disease is:
☐ 1. an inflammation that usually follows group A beta-hemolytic streptococci.
☐ 2. an inflammatory illness with an unknown etiology that is characterized by fever.
☐ 3. an inflammation of the lining, valves, and arterial vessels of the heart.
☐ 4. a chronic, inflammatory process limited to the mucosa that can involve the entire length of the bowel.

CORRECT ANSWER: 2
Kawasaki disease (also known as mucocutaneous lymph node syndrome) is characterized by a fever, generally over 104.5° F (40.3° C), of 5 days' duration or longer. The disease's etiology is unknown. Option 1: Rheumatic fever is an inflammatory illness that usually follows group A beta-hemolytic streptococci. Option 3: Endocarditis involves an inflammation of the lining, valves, and arterial vessels of the heart. Option 4: Ulcerative colitis is a chronic, inflammatory process that is limited to the mucosa and can involve the entire length of the bowel.
NP: Collecting data
CN: Physiological integrity
CNS: Physiological adaptation
CL: Comprehension

148 The nurse is caring for a 2-year-old toddler diagnosed with Kawasaki disease. The nurse must assess for which signs and symptoms in a child with Kawasaki disease?
☐ 1. Chest pain, dyspnea, fever, and headache
☐ 2. Fever, headache, and erythema marginatum, a rash characterized by pink macules and blanching in the middle of the lesions
☐ 3. Bilateral conjunctivitis
☐ 4. Weight loss, abdominal pain, and cramping

CORRECT ANSWER: 3
Bilateral conjunctivitis is typically observed early in the illness. Option 1: Chest pain and dyspnea are sometimes observed in endocarditis. Option 2: Erythema marginatum is a rash observed in rheumatic fever. Option 4: Weight loss, abdominal pain, and cramping are characteristic of ulcerative colitis.
NP: Collecting data
CN: Physiological integrity
CNS: Physiological adaptation
CL: Comprehension

149 The nurse is assessing a 5-year-old male child who exhibits signs of possible lead poisoning. Signs and symptoms of lead poisoning include:
☐ 1. nausea, vomiting, seizures, and coma.
☐ 2. jaundice, confusion, and coagulation abnormalities.
☐ 3. insomnia, weight loss, diarrhea, and gingivitis.
☐ 4. general fatigue, difficulty concentrating, tremors, and headache.

CORRECT ANSWER: 4
Signs and symptoms of lead poisoning depend on the degree of toxicity. General fatigue, difficulty concentrating, tremors, and headache indicate moderate toxicity. Option 1: Nausea, vomiting, seizures, and coma are observed in salicylate and iron poisoning. Option 2: Jaundice, confusion, and coagulation abnormalities are observed in acetaminophen poisoning. Option 3: Insomnia, weight loss, diarrhea, and gingivitis are observed in mercury poisoning.
NP: Collecting data
CN: Physiological integrity
CNS: Physiological adaptation
CL: Comprehension

150 The nurse is caring for a 7-year-old child admitted with possible acetaminophen poisoning. Which laboratory data should the nurse monitor closely?
- [ ] 1. Glucose and potassium levels
- [ ] 2. Blood urea nitrogen (BUN) level
- [ ] 3. Liver function studies
- [ ] 4. Complete blood count (CBC)

CORRECT ANSWER: 3
Acetaminophen is metabolized by the liver, so liver damage is a major concern. Elevated liver function studies should be reported to the physician. Options 1, 2, and 4: Glucose, potassium, and BUN levels and a CBC aren't major concerns when caring for a client with acetaminophen poisoning.
NP: Implementing care
CN: Physiological integrity
CNS: Physiological adaptation
CL: Application

151 The nurse is assessing a 6-year-old female client with recurrent tonsillitis. Which signs and symptoms are associated with tonsillitis?
- [ ] 1. Facial pain, headache, and fever
- [ ] 2. Sore throat with breathing and swallowing difficulties, persistent redness of the anterior pillars, and enlargement of the cervical lymph nodes
- [ ] 3. Sore throat, minimal throat redness, pain, and mild lymphadenopathy
- [ ] 4. Sore throat, dysphonia, and dysphagia

CORRECT ANSWER: 2
Frequent sore throat with difficulty swallowing and breathing, accompanied by persistent redness of the anterior pillars and enlargement of the cervical lymph nodes, is characteristic of tonsillitis. Option 1: Fever, headache, and facial pain indicate sinusitis. Option 3: Sore throat, minimal throat redness, pain, and mild lymphadenopathy are observed in strep throat. Option 4: Sore throat, dysphonia, and dysphagia are seen in children with epiglottiditis.
NP: Collecting data
CN: Physiological integrity
CNS: Physiological adaptation
CL: Comprehension

152 The nurse is assessing a 9-year-old male client brought to the emergency department with signs of possible metabolic acidosis. Signs and symptoms of metabolic acidosis include:
- [ ] 1. nausea and vomiting.
- [ ] 2. decreased rate and depth of respirations accompanied by neuromuscular irritability.
- [ ] 3. increased respiratory rate, confusion, and headache.
- [ ] 4. muscle cramping and carpal or pedal spasms.

CORRECT ANSWER: 3
Metabolic acidosis is characterized by increased rate and depth of respirations (Kussmaul respirations). Confusion, headache, and drowsiness may also occur. Options 1 and 2: Nausea, vomiting, and increased rate and depth of respirations accompanied by neuromuscular irritability may be observed in metabolic alkalosis. Option 4: Muscle cramping and carpal or pedal spasms are signs and symptoms of respiratory alkalosis.
NP: Collecting data
CN: Physiological integrity
CNS: Physiological adaptation
CL: Comprehension

153 The nurse is assessing a 14-year-old female client brought to the emergency department with signs of possible metabolic alkalosis. Which electrolyte imbalance often occurs with metabolic alkalosis?
- [ ] 1. Hypokalemia
- [ ] 2. Hyperkalemia
- [ ] 3. Hypernatremia
- [ ] 4. Hyponatremia

CORRECT ANSWER: 1
Hypokalemia (decreased serum potassium levels) often occurs simultaneously with metabolic alkalosis. Option 2: Hyperkalemia (increased serum potassium levels) often occurs with metabolic acidosis. Option 3: Hypernatremia (increased serum sodium levels) occurs with water loss, inadequate water intake, or increased sodium intake. Option 4: Hyponatremia (decreased serum sodium levels) occurs with inadequate sodium intake, excessive sodium loss, or increased water intake.
NP: Collecting data
CN: Physiological integrity
CNS: Physiological adaptation
CL: Comprehension

154 The nurse is assessing the laboratory results for a 9-year-old child hospitalized with severe vomiting and diarrhea. What is the normal serum potassium range in a child?
☐ 1. 4.5 to 7.2 mmol/L
☐ 2. 3.7 to 5.2 mmol/L
☐ 3. 3.5 to 5.8 mmol/L
☐ 4. 3.5 to 5.5 mmol/L

CORRECT ANSWER: 3
The normal potassium level in children ranges from 3.5 to 5.8 mmol/L. Option 1: Levels of 4.5 to 7.2 mmol/L are observed in premature infants. Option 2: Potassium levels of 3.7 to 5.2 mmol/L are observed in full-term infants. Option 4: Potassium levels of 3.5 to 5.5 mmol/L are usually seen in adults.
NP: Collecting data
CN: Physiological integrity
CNS: Reduction of risk potential
CL: Knowledge

155 The nurse is instructing the parents of a child at risk for hyperkalemia. What response from the father indicates understanding of the nurse's instructions about foods to avoid?
☐ 1. "Chicken should be avoided."
☐ 2. "Dates, figs, and orange juice should be avoided."
☐ 3. "Dark green vegetables should be avoided."
☐ 4. "Whole grain cereals should be restricted."

CORRECT ANSWER: 2
Clients with hyperkalemia (excessive serum potassium) are placed on a potassium-restricted diet. Dates, figs, and oranges should be avoided for clients on a potassium-restricted diet. Option 1: Chicken is high in calcium, not potassium. Options 3 and 4: Dark green vegetables and whole grains are high in magnesium, not potassium.
NP: Evaluation
CN: Physiological integrity
CNS: Reduction of risk potential
CL: Application

156 Which of the following conditions can result from an overdose of acetaminophen?
☐ 1. Brain damage
☐ 2. Heart failure
☐ 3. Hepatic damage
☐ 4. Kidney damage

CORRECT ANSWER: 3
Damage to the hepatic system resulting from an overdose of acetaminophen isn't caused by the drug but by one of the metabolites of the drug. This metabolite binds to liver cells in large quantities. Options 1, 2, and 4: Brain damage, heart failure, and kidney damage may develop but not initially.
NP: Collecting data
CN: Physiological integrity
CNS: Physiological adaptation
CL: Knowledge

157 The nurse is assessing a 7-year-old child with possible hyperaldosteronism. Which factor is the nurse's top priority in assessing a child with hyperaldosteronism?
☐ 1. Blood glucose level
☐ 2. Breath sounds
☐ 3. Arterial blood gas levels
☐ 4. Weekly weights

CORRECT ANSWER: 2
Aldosterone is secreted by the adrenal cortex. One of its major functions is causing the kidneys to retain saline in the body. A child with hyperaldosteronism should be observed for signs of respiratory distress, crackles, and the use of accessory muscles. Options 1 and 3: Blood glucose level and arterial blood gas levels aren't immediate priorities when assessing a child with hyperaldosteronism. Option 4: Rapid weight gains can indicate fluid volume excess, but the child should be weighed daily, not weekly.
NP: Collecting data
CN: Physiological integrity
CNS: Physiological adaptation
CL: Comprehension

158 The nurse in a family health clinic is assessing an 11-year-old male client who shows signs of possible pheochromocytoma. Which signs are the classic triad observed in pheochromocytoma?

☐ 1. New onset hypertension, new or worsening diabetes mellitus, and hypertension crisis

☐ 2. Salt craving, poor weight gain, and hyperpigmentation

☐ 3. Excessive weight gain, moon face appearance, and buffalo hump

☐ 4. Enlarged, nontender thyroid gland; bulging eyes; and emotional lability

CORRECT ANSWER: 1
New onset hypertension, new or worsening diabetes mellitus, and hypertension crisis are the triad of signs usually observed in pheochromocytoma, a chromaffin cell tumor of the adrenal medulla. Option 2: Salt craving, poor weight gain, and hyperpigmentation are signs and symptoms of Addison's disease. Option 3: Excessive weight gain, moon face appearance, and a buffalo hump are observed in clients with Cushing's syndrome. Option 4: An enlarged, nontender thyroid gland, bulging eyes, and emotional lability are signs and symptoms in clients with hyperthyroidism.
NP: Collecting data
CN: Physiological integrity
CNS: Physiological adaptation
CL: Comprehension

---

159 The nurse is caring for a 17-year old female client who had a subtotal thyroidectomy to treat hyperthyroidism. Which sign or symptom could indicate bleeding at the incision site?

☐ 1. Hoarseness

☐ 2. Severe stridor

☐ 3. Complaints of feelings of pressure at the incision site

☐ 4. Difficulty swallowing

CORRECT ANSWER: 3
Complaints of pressure at the incision site indicate postoperative bleeding. Options 1 and 2: Hoarseness or severe stridor indicates damage to the laryngeal nerve. Option 4: Difficulty swallowing doesn't indicate postoperative hemorrhage.
NP: Collecting data
CN: Physiological integrity
CNS: Physiological adaptation
CL: Application

---

160 The nurse is assessing a 15-year-old adolescent to determine if her fitness level is sufficient to join the high-school basketball team. Which signs and symptoms would the nurse expect to find in a child with suspected aplastic anemia?

☐ 1. Purpura, petechiae, and fatigue

☐ 2. Frequent epistaxis and darkening of the skin

☐ 3. Pain, fever, and tissue engorgement

☐ 4. Nail bed deformities, tachycardia, and systolic heart murmur

CORRECT ANSWER: 1
Aplastic anemia — a deficiency of the red blood cells — is characterized by purpura, petechiae, and fatigue. Option 2: Frequent epistaxis and darkening of the skin is observed in children with B-thalassemia. Option 3: Pain, fever, and tissue engorgement are observed in clients in sickle cell crisis. Option 4: Nail bed deformities, tachycardia, and systolic heart murmurs are manifested in clients with delayed iron deficiency anemia.
NP: Collecting data
CN: Physiological integrity
CNS: Physiological adaptation
CL: Comprehension

---

161 The nurse is caring for a 12-year-old client on the pediatric oncology unit. Common signs of childhood cancer include:

☐ 1. fever, vomiting, diarrhea, and persistent pain.

☐ 2. projectile vomiting, failure to gain weight, dehydration, and hyperbilirubinemia.

☐ 3. weight loss, delayed growth, nutritional deficiencies, and arthralgia.

☐ 4. pain, cachexia, infection, anemia, and bruising.

CORRECT ANSWER: 4
Many of the signs and symptoms of cancer in adults are also commonly observed in childhood illness. Some typical signs of childhood cancer include pain, cachexia, anemia, infection, and bruising. Option 1: Fever, vomiting, diarrhea, and persistent pain are observed in children receiving chemotherapy. Option 2: Failure to gain weight, dehydration and hyperbilirubinemia, and projectile vomiting are signs and symptoms of pyloric stenosis. Option 3: Weight loss, delayed growth, and nutritional deficiencies can be observed in children with ulcerative colitis.
NP: Collecting data
CN: Physiological integrity
CNS: Physiological adaptation
CL: Comprehension

162 A 1-year-old infant is hospitalized with a diagnosis of eczema. Which signs and symptoms does the nurse expect to observe?
☐ 1. Exudative, crusty, papulovesicular and erythematous lesions on the cheeks, scalp, forehead, and arms
☐ 2. Erythematous, dry, scaly, well-circumscribed, papular, thickened, and lichenified pruritic lesions on wrists, hands, and neck
☐ 3. Large thickened and lichenified plaques on face, neck, and back
☐ 4. Erythematous papules with oozing, crusting, and edema

CORRECT ANSWER: 1
Exudative, crusty, papulovesicular, and erythematous lesions on the cheeks, scalp, forehead, and arms are observed in children ages 2 months to 2 years with a diagnosis of eczema. Option 2: Erythematous, dry, scaly, well-circumscribed, papular, thickened, and lichenified pruritic lesions on the wrists, hands, and neck are observed in children ages 2 years to puberty. Option 3: In adolescents, lesions on the face, neck, and back consist of large plaques that are thickened and lichenified. Option 4: Erythematous papules with oozing, crusting, and edema are characteristic of contact dermatitis.
NP: Collecting data
CN: Physiological integrity
CNS: Physiological adaptation
CL: Comprehension

163 The nurse is caring for a 12-year-old child with a diagnosis of eczema. Which nursing interventions are appropriate for a child with eczema?
☐ 1. Administer antibiotics as prescribed.
☐ 2. Administer antifungals as ordered.
☐ 3. Administer tepid baths and pat dry or air-dry the affected areas.
☐ 4. Administer hot baths and use moisturizers immediately after the bath.

CORRECT ANSWER: 3
Tepid baths and moisturizers are indicated to keep the infected areas clean and minimize itching. Option 1: Antibiotics are given only when there is superimposed infection. Option 2: Antifungals aren't usually administered in the treatment of eczema. Option 4: Hot baths can exacerbate the condition and increase itching.
NP: Implementing care
CN: Physiological integrity
CNS: Physiological adaptation
CL: Application

164 A 9-year-old child is brought to the emergency department with extensive burns received in a restaurant fire. What is the most important aspect of caring for the burned child?
☐ 1. Administering antibiotics to prevent superimposed infections
☐ 2. Conducting wound management
☐ 3. Administering liquids orally to replace fluid
☐ 4. Administering frequent small meals to support nutritional requirements

CORRECT ANSWER: 2
The most important aspect of caring for a burned child is wound management. The goals of wound care are to speed debridement, protect granulation tissue and new grafts, and conserve body heat and fluids. Option 1: Antibiotics aren't always administered prophylactically. Option 3: Fluids are administered I.V. according to the child's body weight to replace volume. Option 4: Enteral feedings, rather than meals, are initiated within the first 24 hours after the burn to support the child's increased nutritional requirements.
NP: Implementing care
CN: Physiological integrity
CNS: Physiological adaptation
CL: Application

165 The nurse is assessing a child involved in a motor vehicle accident. As the child is admitted to the emergency department, the parent tells the nurse that the child was thrown into the dashboard. The nurse watches closely for which early sign of increased intracranial pressure (ICP)?
☐ 1. Bradycardia
☐ 2. Irregular respirations
☐ 3. Increased systolic blood pressure
☐ 4. Seizures

CORRECT ANSWER: 4
Headache, visual disturbances, and seizures are some of the early signs of increased ICP. Options 1, 2, and 3: Irregular respirations, increased systolic blood pressure, and bradycardia are late signs of increased ICP.
NP: Collecting data
CN: Physiological integrity
CNS: Physiological adaptation
CL: Comprehension

Pediatric Nursing

166 The nurse is assessing an infant with infantile spasms. Which signs and symptoms would the nurse observe?
- ☐ 1. Head, extremity, or body contractions with no loss of consciousness
- ☐ 2. Dropping of the head, flexion of neck, extension of arms, and flexion of legs accompanied by possible loss of consciousness
- ☐ 3. Loss of muscle tone with momentary loss of consciousness
- ☐ 4. Recovery in seconds with no postictal period

CORRECT ANSWER: 2
Dropping of the head, flexion of neck, extension of arms, and flexion of legs accompanied by possible loss of consciousness are characteristic signs of infantile spasms. Options 1 and 4: Head, extremity, or body contractions with no loss of consciousness and recovery without a postictal period are observed in children with myoclonic seizures. Option 3: Loss of muscle tone with momentary loss of consciousness can be observed in children with akinetic or atonic seizures.
NP: Collecting data
CN: Physiological integrity
CNS: Physiological adaptation
CL: Comprehension

---

167 A 1-month-old male infant is admitted to the pediatric unit and diagnosed with bacterial meningitis. Which signs or symptoms does the nurse observe in this client?
- ☐ 1. Hemorrhagic rash, first appearing as petechiae
- ☐ 2. Photophobia
- ☐ 3. Fever, change in feeding pattern, vomiting, or diarrhea
- ☐ 4. Fever, lethargy, and purpura or large necrotic patches

CORRECT ANSWER: 3
Fever, change in feeding patterns, vomiting, and diarrhea are often observed in children with bacterial meningitis. Options 1, 2, and 4: Hemorrhagic rashes, petechiae, photophobia, fever, lethargy, and purpura are observed in older children with meningitis.
NP: Collecting data
CN: Physiological integrity
CNS: Physiological adaptation
CL: Comprehension

---

168 The nurse is assessing a 1-month-old male infant during a routine examination at a family health center. Which method does the nurse use to test for Babinski's sign?
- ☐ 1. Raise the child's leg with the knee flexed and then extend the child's leg at the knee to determine if resistance is noted.
- ☐ 2. With the knee flexed, dorsiflex the foot to determine if there is pain in the calf of the leg.
- ☐ 3. Flex the child's head while he's in a supine position to determine if the knees or hips flex involuntarily.
- ☐ 4. Stroke the bottom of the foot to determine if there is fanning and dorsiflexion of the big toe.

CORRECT ANSWER: 4
To test for Babinski's sign, stroke the bottom of the foot to determine if there is fanning and dorsiflexion of the big toe. Option 1: Raising the child's leg with the knee flexed and then extending the leg at the knee to determine if resistance is noted tests for Kernig's sign. Option 2: Dorsiflexion of the foot with the knee flexed to determine if there is pain in the calf of the leg tests for Homans' sign. Option 3: Flexing the child's head while he's in a supine position to determine if the knees or hips flex involuntarily tests for Brudzinski's sign.
NP: Implementing care
CN: Physiological integrity
CNS: Physiological adaptation
CL: Knowledge

---

169 What behavioral responses to pain would a nurse observe from an infant under age 1?
- ☐ 1. Localized withdrawal and resistance of the entire body
- ☐ 2. Passive resistance, clenching fists, and holding body rigid
- ☐ 3. Reflex withdrawal to stimulus and facial grimacing
- ☐ 4. Low frustration level and striking out physically

CORRECT ANSWER: 3
Infants under age 1 become irritable and exhibit reflex withdrawal to the painful stimulus. Facial grimacing also occurs. Option 1: Localized withdrawal is experienced by toddlers ages 1 to 3 in response to pain. Option 2: The nurse would observe passive resistance in school-age children. Option 4: Preschoolers show a low frustration level and strike out physically.
NP: Collecting data
CN: Physiological integrity
CNS: Physiological adaptation
CL: Comprehension

170 A nurse on the pediatric unit is reviewing the signs and symptoms of fluid volume deficit and excess. What are the signs and symptoms of extracellular fluid volume deficit?
☐ 1. Full, bounding pulse
☐ 2. Distended neck veins
☐ 3. Thready, rapid pulse
☐ 4. Decreased hemoglobin level and hematocrit

CORRECT ANSWER: 3
Cardiac reflex responses to decreased vascular volume result in a thready, rapid pulse. Options 1, 2, and 4: A full, bounding pulse, distended neck veins, and decreased hemoglobin level and hematocrit are observed in fluid volume excess.
NP: Collecting data
CN: Physiological integrity
CNS: Physiological adaptation
CL: Comprehension

171 The nurse is assessing a 4-year-old child who exhibits signs of possible rubeola (measles). What signs and symptoms is the nurse most likely to observe in a child with rubeola?
☐ 1. Lymphadenopathy and sore throat
☐ 2. Anorexia, abdominal pain, fatigue, and headache
☐ 3. Fever, conjunctivitis, and cough
☐ 4. Red rash that begins on the cheeks, accompanied by circumoral rash

CORRECT ANSWER: 3
Signs and symptoms of rubeola include fever, conjunctivitis, and cough. Option 1: Lymphadenopathy and a sore throat are usually signs of chronic fatigue syndrome. Option 2: A maculopapular rash, anorexia, abdominal pain, fatigue, and headache may occur in children with mononucleosis. Option 4: A red rash that begins on the cheeks, accompanied by a circumoral rash, is characteristic of erythema infectiosum.
NP: Collecting data
CN: Physiological integrity
CNS: Physiological adaptation
CL: Comprehension

172 The nurse is assessing an 11-month-old infant who recently emigrated with his parents from a densely populated area of a developing country. The infant exhibits signs that could indicate tuberculosis. Signs and symptoms of tuberculosis in infants include:
☐ 1. night sweats and fatigue.
☐ 2. absence of symptoms.
☐ 3. weight loss or failure to gain weight, fever, and persistent cough.
☐ 4. low-grade fever, weight loss, and night sweats.

CORRECT ANSWER: 3
Signs and symptoms of tuberculosis in infants include a persistent cough, weight loss or failure to gain weight, and fever. Wheezing and tachypnea may also be observed. Options 1 and 4: Night sweats, fatigue, and low-grade fever are signs and symptoms of tuberculosis in adults. Option 2: Older children with tuberculosis may be asymptomatic.
NP: Collecting data
CN: Physiological integrity
CNS: Physiological adaptation
CL: Comprehension

173 The nurse is caring for a child who was exposed to an adult with tuberculosis. Nursing care includes administering:
☐ 1. rifampin (Rifadin).
☐ 2. isoniazid (INH).
☐ 3. pyrazinamide.
☐ 4. ethambutol (Magambutol).

CORRECT ANSWER: 2
Isoniazid is given to a child who was exposed to an adult with infectious tuberculosis even if the child has a negative skin test. If the skin test is negative after 3 months, the medication is discontinued. If the skin test is positive, the child needs a complete regimen of therapy. Options 1, 3, and 4: Rifampin, pyrazinamide, and ethambutol are part of the medication therapy for clients diagnosed with tuberculosis.
NP: Implementing care
CN: Physiological integrity
CNS: Pharmacological therapies
CL: Application

174 The nurse is observing a child admitted to the pediatric unit with a diagnosis of cystic fibrosis. Which clinical feature would be found in a child with cystic fibrosis?
☐ 1. Inflammation of the pulmonary parenchyma
☐ 2. A chromosomal abnormality inherited as an autosomal-dominant trait
☐ 3. A multisystem disorder affecting the exocrine or mucus-producing glands
☐ 4. A chronic lung disease related to high concentrations of oxygen and ventilation

CORRECT ANSWER: 3
Cystic fibrosis affects many organs as well as the exocrine or mucus-producing glands. Option 1: Inflammation of the pulmonary parenchyma describes pneumonia, not cystic fibrosis. Option 2: In cystic fibrosis, an autosomal-recessive abnormality, the child receives defective genes from both parents. Option 4: Bronchopulmonary dysplasia is related to high concentrations of oxygen and ventilation.
NP: Collecting data
CN: Physiological integrity
CNS: Physiological adaptation
CL: Knowledge

175 The nurse is caring for a 5-year-old male child admitted to the pediatric unit with cystic fibrosis. Stools of a child with cystic fibrosis are characteristically:
☐ 1. black and tarry.
☐ 2. frothy, foul-smelling, and steatorrheaic.
☐ 3. clay-colored.
☐ 4 orange or green.

CORRECT ANSWER: 2
The stools of a child with cystic fibrosis are frothy, foul-smelling, and steatorrheaic. Option 1: Black and tarry stools are observed in clients who have upper GI bleeding, are on iron medications, or who consume diets high in red meat and dark-green vegetables. Option 3: Clay-colored stools indicate possible bile obstruction. Option 4: Orange or green stools may indicate intestinal infection.
NP: Collecting data
CN: Physiological integrity
CNS: Physiological adaptation
CL: Comprehension

176 The nurse is planning care for a 9-year-old male child with heart failure. Which nursing diagnosis should receive priority?
☐ 1. *Ineffective tissue perfusion (cardiopulmonary, renal) related to sympathetic response to heart failure*
☐ 2. *Imbalanced nutrition: Less than body requirements related to rapid tiring while feeding*
☐ 3. *Anxiety (parent) related to unknown nature of child's illness*
☐ 4. *Decreased cardiac output related to cardiac defect*

CORRECT ANSWER: 4
The primary nursing diagnosis for a child with heart failure is *Decreased cardiac output related to cardiac defect*. The most common cause of heart failure in children is congenital heart defects. Some defects result in the blood being pumped from the left side of the heart to the right side of the heart. The heart is unable to manage the extra volume, resulting in the pulmonary system becoming overloaded. Options 1, 2, and 3: Ineffective tissue perfusion, imbalanced nutrition, and anxiety don't take priority over decreased cardiac output. The child's heart must produce cardiac output sufficient to meet the body's metabolic demands.
NP: Planning care
CN: Physiological integrity
CNS: Physiological adaptation
CL: Application

177 The nurse is caring for a child immediately after a cardiac catheterization to test for a congenital heart defect. An essential nursing procedure for the client at this time is to:
☐ 1. maintain the child on strict bed rest for the first 24 hours.
☐ 2. restrict oral fluid and food intake for the first 24 hours.
☐ 3. apply a pressure dressing over the site for 6 hours.
☐ 4. assess neurovascular status of the lower extremity once every hour for 4 hours.

CORRECT ANSWER: 3
To prevent postprocedure bleeding and hematoma formation, the nurse applies a pressure dressing over the site for the first 6 hours. Option 1: The child should be placed on strict bed rest for the first 6 hours and limited activity for the next 24 hours. Option 2: Oral fluid and food intake isn't generally restricted for the first 24 hours but may be gradually resumed as soon as the child is alert. Option 4: The client's neurovascular status should be assessed every 15 minutes for the first hour after the procedure, and then once every 30 minutes for the next hour.
NP: Implementing care
CN: Physiological integrity
CNS: Physiological adaptation
CL: Application

178 A 3-day-old infant is admitted to the hospital with a diagnosis of tetralogy of Fallot. Which signs and symptoms should the nurse expect to observe?
☐ 1. No symptoms and normal growth
☐ 2. Diaphoresis and facial edema
☐ 3. Hepatomegaly and frequent respiratory infections
☐ 4. Hypoxia and cyanosis

CORRECT ANSWER: 4
As the ductus arteriosus closes, an infant with tetralogy of Fallot becomes cyanotic and hypoxic and a systolic murmur may be heard in the pulmonic area. Metabolic acidosis, poor growth, clubbing, and exercise intolerance may develop. Option 1: Children with acyanotic heart defects may have no symptoms and grow normally. Option 2: Diaphoresis and facial edema are some of the signs and symptoms of heart failure in infants and toddlers. Option 3: Hepatomegaly and frequent respiratory infections are observed in some children with acyanotic heart conditions.
NP: Collecting data
CN: Physiological integrity
CNS: Physiological adaptation
CL: Comprehension

179 The nurse is assessing an 8-year-old child admitted to the emergency unit following a school bus accident. Which early signs of shock may be observed?
☐ 1. Confusion and lethargy
☐ 2. Increased systolic blood pressure and absent distal pulses
☐ 3. Mottled skin appearance and decreased urine output
☐ 4. Bradycardia and profound hypotension

CORRECT ANSWER: 3
Early signs of shock include skin that appears mottled and decreased urine output. The child experiencing early signs of shock becomes irritable or combative. Options 1 and 2: Confusion, lethargy, tachycardia, and absent distal pulses can be assessed in a child who progresses to uncompensated shock. Option 4: Bradycardia and hypotension are observed in a child in profound shock.
NP: Collecting data
CN: Physiological integrity
CNS: Physiological adaptation
CL: Comprehension

180 The nurse is assessing a 1-year-old child diagnosed with gastroesophageal reflux. Which clinical manifestation is the nurse likely to observe?
- [ ] 1. Frequent hunger and weight loss regardless of eating
- [ ] 2. Projectile vomiting and poor skin turgor
- [ ] 3. Nausea and vomiting
- [ ] 4. Constipation alternating with diarrhea and vomiting

CORRECT ANSWER: 1
Frequent hunger, weight loss regardless of eating, and irritability are some of the signs and symptoms assessed in a client with gastroesophageal reflux. Option 2: Children with pyloric stenosis experience frequent vomiting. Option 3: Children with small-bowel obstruction experience nausea and vomiting. Option 4: Constipation alternating with diarrhea and vomiting and dehydration are signs and symptoms of Hirschsprung's disease.
NP: Collecting data
CN: Physiological integrity
CNS: Physiological adaptation
CL: Comprehension

181 The nurse is assessing a 6-month-old infant in the pediatric clinic. The parent states that the child has been experiencing diarrhea, vomiting, and anorexia and has stopped gaining weight. The parent works full-time and the infant goes to a local day-care center. The nurse suspects that these signs and symptoms are most likely the result of:
- [ ] 1. toxocariasis.
- [ ] 2. giardiasis.
- [ ] 3. enterobiasis (pinworm).
- [ ] 4. ascariasis (roundworm).

CORRECT ANSWER: 2
Signs and symptoms of giardiasis include diarrhea, vomiting, anorexia, and failure to thrive. Older children may experience abdominal cramps with loose, foul-smelling, pale, and greasy stools. Option 1: Most cases of toxocariasis are asymptomatic. Severe symptoms may include hepatomegaly and neurologic disturbances. Option 3: Symptoms of enterobiasis include intense perianal itching, irritability, and restlessness. Option 4: Mild ascariasis may be asymptomatic. Severe infestation may result in intestinal obstruction.
NP: Collecting data
CN: Physiological integrity
CNS: Physiological adaptation
CL: Comprehension

182 The nurse is instructing the parents of a full-term male neonate before discharge. Which instruction should the nurse provide when teaching the parents how to alleviate colic?
- [ ] 1. Use a bottle with a disposable and collapsible bag.
- [ ] 2. The breast-feeding mother should increase the amount of milk in her diet.
- [ ] 3. Place the infant in a prone position on his abdomen immediately after eating.
- [ ] 4. Feed the infant less frequently, giving larger quantities.

CORRECT ANSWER: 1
The parents should use a bottle with a collapsible bag to prevent the infant from sucking air. Option 2: The breast-feeding mother should eliminate milk products and spicy or gas-producing foods from her diet. Option 3: The infant should be held upright for $1/2$ hour after feeding. Option 4: The parents should feed smaller amounts and burp the infant frequently.
NP: Implementing care
CN: Physiological integrity
CNS: Physiological adaptation
CL: Comprehension

183 A 3-year-old female child is diagnosed with biliary atresia complicated by cirrhosis. In caring for this client, the nurse should monitor for:
☐ 1. steatorrhea, failure to gain weight, and anemia.
☐ 2. fever, anorexia, nausea, and vomiting.
☐ 3. crampy abdominal pain followed by diarrhea.
☐ 4. projectile vomiting, failure to gain weight, dehydration, and hyperbilirubinemia.

CORRECT ANSWER: 1
Steatorrhea, failure to gain weight, and anemia can be observed in children diagnosed with cirrhosis. Clubbing of the fingers and cyanosis are other common findings. Option 2: Fever, anorexia, nausea, and vomiting may be experienced by children with hepatitis. Option 3: Crampy abdominal pain followed by diarrhea is experienced by children with Crohn's disease. Option 4: Projectile vomiting, failure to gain weight, dehydration, and hyperbilirubinemia are observed in children with pyloric stenosis.
NP: Collecting data
CN: Physiological integrity
CNS: Physiological adaptation
CL: Comprehension

184 A 5-year-old child is hospitalized with ascites due to nephritic syndrome. Nursing care for the child includes which of the following?
☐ 1. Administering lactulose
☐ 2. Restricting protein, fluids, and sodium
☐ 3. Administering neomycin (Neo-Tabs) or other nonabsorbable antibiotics as ordered
☐ 4. Administering B complex and K vitamins as ordered

CORRECT ANSWER: 2
The nurse should restrict fluids, sodium, and protein to prevent ascites (the accumulation of fluids in the abdominal cavity). Option 1: Lactulose controls ammonia levels and is administered in clients with hepatic encephalopathy. Option 3: Neomycin or other nonabsorbable antibiotics are administered to clients with hepatic encephalopathy to suppress the activity of bacterial flora in the intestinal tract. Option 4: Vitamin K is administered to children with hemorrhage, which may be caused by esophageal varices.
NP: Implementing care
CN: Physiological integrity
CNS: Physiological adaptation
CL: Application

185 A 13-year-old with structural scoliosis has Harrington rods inserted. Which of the following positions would be best during the postoperative period?
☐ 1. Supine in bed
☐ 2. Side-lying
☐ 3. Semi-Fowler's
☐ 4. High Fowler's

CORRECT ANSWER: 1
After placement of Harrington rods, the client must remain flat in bed. The gatch on a manual bed should be taped and electric beds should be unplugged to prevent the client from raising the head or foot of the bed. Options 2, 3, and 4: Other positions, such as the side-lying, semi-Fowler, and high Fowler positions, could prove damaging because the rods couldn't maintain the spine in a straight position.
NP: Implementing care
CN: Physiological integrity
CNS: Reduction of risk potential
CL: Application

186 A Mantoux test is ordered for a 6-year-old child. Which direction about this test is accurate?
☐ 1. Read results within 24 hours.
☐ 2. Read results within 48 to 72 hours.
☐ 3. Use the large muscle of the upper leg.
☐ 4. Massage the site to increase absorption.

CORRECT ANSWER: 2
The test should be read within 48 to 72 hours after placement by measuring the diameter of the induration that develops at the site. Option 1: Reading results in 24 hours wouldn't give an accurate test reading. Option 3: The purified protein derivative is injected intradermally on the volar surface of the forearm. Option 4: Massaging the site could cause leakage from the injection site.
NP: Analysis
CN: Physiological integrity
CNS: Reduction of risk potential
CL: Knowledge

Psychiatric Nursing

1 The nurse asks the parents of a 12-year-old boy for more information about their son's recent behavioral changes. Which information would be most useful to obtain initially?
☐ 1. Academic interests
☐ 2. Relationships with girls
☐ 3. Relationships with extended family
☐ 4. Any changes in daily activities

CORRECT ANSWER: 4
Changes in daily activities often signal changes in mental health and should be explored first. Option 1: The child's academic interests probably are unrelated to his mental health. Options 2 and 3: Relationships with girls and extended family may or may not be significant and wouldn't be the primary concern.
NP: Collecting data
CN: Psychosocial integrity
CNS: Coping and adaptation
CL: Application

2 A mother asks the nurse what she should do about her son's behavior, which has been erratic for 6 months. Which response is best?
☐ 1. Tell her how to set daily goals for her son.
☐ 2. Reassure her that her child is going through a phase that will pass.
☐ 3. Discuss the child's specific behaviors and suggest possible actions to take.
☐ 4. Explain that the child seems fragile and that she needs to be patient with him.

CORRECT ANSWER: 3
This parent requires guidance and direction to consider possible alternatives. Option 1: The child needs to set his own goals. Option 2: Erratic behavior isn't typical of a passing phase. Option 4: More than patience is needed to deal with erratic behavior that persists for 6 months.
NP: Implementing care
CN: Psychosocial integrity
CNS: Coping and adaptation
CL: Application

3 Which outcome criteria is most appropriate for a teenager who hasn't slept well in 6 months, is irritable, and has dropped out of social activities?
☐ 1. The client will sleep well at night.
☐ 2. The parents will stop worrying about the client.
☐ 3. The client will obtain appropriate mental health services.
☐ 4. The parents will impose strict behavior guidelines for the client to follow.

CORRECT ANSWER: 3
Mental health services can protect the client and offer the best means of regaining mental health. Option 1: The client could reestablish a healthy sleeping pattern without addressing underlying issues. Option 2: The parents' worrying is unrelated to the child's immediate need for help. Option 4: The child's behavior suggests the need for professional service, not disciplinary measures.
NP: Planning care
CN: Psychosocial integrity
CNS: Coping and adaptation
CL: Application

4 A client's husband tells the community nurse that his wife has just begun taking isocarboxazid (Marplan) for depression. He states that the instructions on the bottle say to "follow food and medication restrictions" and asks what that means. The nurse explains that the last dose of this medication needs to be taken before 4 p.m. and that, while taking this medication, the client must avoid ingesting:
☐ 1. apples and green bananas.
☐ 2. cottage cheese and whole milk.
☐ 3. processed meats and aged cheeses.
☐ 4. over-the-counter cold remedies, such as NyQuil and aspirin.

CORRECT ANSWER: 3
Foods and drugs containing tyramine, the active ingredient in isocarboxazid, must be avoided to prevent hypertensive crisis. Tyramine-containing substances include overripe fruits, processed meats, beer, wine, aged cheeses, flava beans, chocolate (should be limited to no more than 1 oz per day), avocados, monosodium glutamate, yogurt (limited to no more than 8 oz per day), and sympathomimetic drugs. The items in options 1, 2, and 4 don't contain tyramine.
NP: Implementing care
CN: Psychosocial integrity
CNS: Psychosocial adaptation
CL: Knowledge

5 A depressed female client doesn't use the dining room, doesn't participate in any unit activities and instead, remains in bed all day. Which nursing action would be best?
☐ 1. Assist the client with getting up and dressed each day and accompany her to unit activities.
☐ 2. Require the client to do only as much activity as her current energy level allows.
☐ 3. Avoid paying attention to the client's inappropriate behavior.
☐ 4. Tell the client that she'll lose privileges if she refuses to get up.

CORRECT ANSWER: 1
The client's lack of energy is preventing her from independently taking action. She'll require assistance to perform activities of daily living. Option 2: To externalize her energy, the client must be made to move around. Options 3 and 4: The client won't become physically or psychologically motivated on her own; she'll need much prodding and assistance.
NP: Implementing care
CN: Psychosocial integrity
CNS: Psychosocial adaptation
CL: Application

6 Clients experiencing grief and those experiencing depression often manifest similar behaviors. Which behavior isn't typical of someone experiencing grief?
☐ 1. Loss of self-esteem
☐ 2. Disturbed sleep patterns
☐ 3. Lack of interest in most daily activities
☐ 4. Spiritual distress

CORRECT ANSWER: 1
Grieving clients usually don't have a loss of self-esteem. Options 2, 3, and 4: These behaviors are characteristic of both grief and depression.
NP: Collecting data
CN: Psychosocial integrity
CNS: Psychosocial adaptation
CL: Knowledge

7 A client who began receiving fluoxetine (Prozac) 2 weeks ago tells the nurse that the medicine isn't working because he still feels the same. Which response is best?
☐ 1. Explain how this medication works.
☐ 2. Consult the physician about a possible medication change.
☐ 3. Explain that some clients don't respond to this drug.
☐ 4. Reassure the client that he'll feel better in 2 to 4 weeks.

CORRECT ANSWER: 1
Explain that up to 4 weeks may be necessary for this medication to alter the client's depression. Option 2: Initiating a medication change so soon would be premature. Option 3: Although true, this information isn't helpful at this time. Option 4: Although most clients begin to feel better in 2 to 4 weeks, this isn't always the case.
NP: Implementing care
CN: Psychosocial integrity
CNS: Psychosocial adaptation
CL: Application

8 Which of the following indicates the highest risk of suicide?
☐ 1. Suicide plan, handy means of carrying out plan, and history of previous attempt
☐ 2. Preoccupation with morbid thoughts and limited support system
☐ 3. Suicidal ideation, active suicide planning, and family history of suicide
☐ 4. Threats of suicide, recent job loss, and intact support system

CORRECT ANSWER: 1
A lethal plan with a handy means of carrying out the plan poses the highest risk and requires immediate intervention. Options 2, 3, and 4: Although all the remaining risk factors can lead to suicide, they aren't considered as high a risk as a formulated lethal plan and the means at hand. However, a client exhibiting any of these risk factors should be taken seriously and considered at risk for suicide.
NP: Collecting data
CN: Psychosocial integrity
CNS: Psychosocial adaptation
CL: Application

---

9 A client with bulimia and a history of purging by vomiting is hospitalized for further observation because she's at risk for:
☐ 1. diabetes mellitus.
☐ 2. cardiac arrhythmias and electrolyte imbalances.
☐ 3. GI obstruction or paralytic ileus.
☐ 4. septicemia from a low white blood cell count.

CORRECT ANSWER: 2
People who purge by vomiting are at great risk for electrolyte imbalance and resulting cardiac arrhythmias. Options 1, 3, and 4: Purging doesn't lead to any of these conditions.
NP: Collecting data
CN: Physiological integrity
CNS: Reduction of risk potential
CL: Application

---

10 Which nursing diagnosis should the nurse expect to find in the nursing plan of care of a client with bulimia?
☐ 1. *Decreased cardiac output related to muscle spasms in the hands and feet*
☐ 2. *Risk for infection related to enlargement of salivary and parotid glands*
☐ 3. *Disturbed thought processes related to personal identity disturbance*
☐ 4. *Ineffective denial related to underlying need for acceptance*

CORRECT ANSWER: 4
An unmet need for acceptance can cause denial about self-destructive behaviors and is congruent with the underlying dynamics of eating disorders. Option 1: Decreased cardiac output isn't caused by muscle spasms in the hands and feet. Option 2: Enlarged parotid and salivary glands don't cause infection. Option 3: Disturbed thought processes aren't caused by personal identity disturbance.
NP: Planning care
CN: Psychosocial integrity
CNS: Psychosocial adaptation
CL: Application

---

11 A 45-year-old male client has entered the hospital for renal dialysis. A few hours before he's to receive the treatment, the nurse notices that he's irritable, easily distracted, hypersensitive to light and noise, and disoriented. Which of the following most accurately describes what the client is experiencing?
☐ 1. Delirium
☐ 2. Reye's syndrome
☐ 3. Normal pressure hydrocephalus
☐ 4. Early Wernicke-Korsakoff syndrome

CORRECT ANSWER: 1
The symptoms described in this scenario are typical of delirium. Option 2: This disease of children is characterized by increasing fever, agitation, and lethargy. Option 3: Symptoms include dementia, erratic gait, and incontinence. Option 4: Appropriate symptoms would include confusion and amnesia.
NP: Collecting data
CN: Psychosocial integrity
CNS: Psychosocial adaptation
CL: Application

12 The best way to help a client with mild Alzheimer's disease to remain functional is to:
- ☐ 1. obtain a physician's order for a mild anxiolytic to control behavior.
- ☐ 2. call attention to all mistakes so they can be quickly corrected.
- ☐ 3. advise the client to move into a retirement center.
- ☐ 4. maintain a stable, predictable environment and daily routine.

CORRECT ANSWER: 4
Clients in the early stages of Alzheimer's disease remain fairly functional with familiar surroundings and a predictable routine. They become easily disoriented with surprises and social overstimulation. Option 1: Anxiolytics can impair memory and worsen the problem. Option 2: This is nonproductive and serves to lower the client's self-esteem. Option 3: Moving to an unfamiliar environment will heighten the client's agitation and confusion.
NP: Planning care
CN: Psychosocial integrity
CNS: Psychosocial adaptation
CL: Application

---

13 Which activity is most appropriate for a client in the middle (moderate) stage of Alzheimer's disease?
- ☐ 1. Putting together a 300-piece puzzle
- ☐ 2. Playing charades
- ☐ 3. Playing a simple board game such as checkers
- ☐ 4. Tossing a soft-foam ball

CORRECT ANSWER: 4
Tossing a soft-foam ball requires little concentration and provides large-muscle activity. Option 1: This requires too much concentration. Option 2: This activity requires abstract thought. Option 3: This activity requires the ability to concentrate and follow rules.
NP: Planning care
CN: Psychosocial integrity
CNS: Psychosocial adaptation
CL: Application

---

14 An 80-year-old female client with Alzheimer's disease often climbs out of bed at night and wanders the halls. At a team meeting, one staff member strongly advocates the use of nighttime restraints for this client. Which response would be best in this situation?
- ☐ 1. "The use of restraints will only increase the client's agitation."
- ☐ 2. "Maybe we should consider placing her mattress on the floor."
- ☐ 3. "The physician should prescribe a stronger sedative."
- ☐ 4. "That probably would be the best way to keep her safe."

CORRECT ANSWER: 2
Suggesting that the client's mattress be placed on the floor is an easy solution and it ensures the client's safety. Option 1: Using restraints will increase the client's agitation. Option 3: Use of a stronger sedative in an 80-year-old client increases the risk of adverse effects and other possible problems. Option 4: Such a statement blocks the lines of communication and stops the problem-solving process.
NP: Planning care
CN: Psychosocial integrity
CNS: Psychosocial adaptation
CL: Analysis

---

15 A 22-year-old woman was brought to the hospital by her parents because of her bizarre behavior at home. The parents reported that she stayed in her room, refused to eat meals with the family, and talked to herself almost constantly. She lost interest in her job and had been fired because of her inability to perform. During the intake process, the nurse notes that the client is unkempt, has body odor, exhibits illogical thought patterns, and appears to be listening to someone no one else can see or hear. Which nursing goal is the priority for this client?
- ☐ 1. Maintain safety.
- ☐ 2. Ensure adequate nutrition.
- ☐ 3. Orient the client.
- ☐ 4. Provide hygiene measures.

CORRECT ANSWER: 1
Whenever a client is hallucinating or otherwise out of touch with reality, safety is always the primary concern. Options 2, 3, and 4: Although these are valid concerns, they're all secondary to ensuring a safe environment.
NP: Planning care
CN: Safe, effective care environment
CNS: Safety and infection control
CL: Application

16 A client who appears to be listening to someone no one else can see or hear is experiencing:
☐ 1. altered thought processes.
☐ 2. sensory-perceptual alteration.
☐ 3. potential cognitive impairment.
☐ 4. impaired adjustment.

CORRECT ANSWER: 2
Such a client is experiencing an auditory hallucination. Option 1: Altered thought processes refer to delusions, illogical thoughts, and looseness of association. Option 3: Cognitive impairment refers to memory deficits related to organic processes. Option 4: Impaired adjustment refers to an inability to adjust behavior to accommodate changes in health.
NP: Collecting data
CN: Psychosocial integrity
CNS: Psychosocial adaptation
CL: Analysis

17 Which nursing intervention is most important for a client with schizophrenia?
☐ 1. Teach the client about the illness.
☐ 2. Initiate a behavioral contract with the client.
☐ 3. Require the client to attend all unit functions.
☐ 4. Provide a consistent, predictable environment.

CORRECT ANSWER: 4
A consistent, predictable environment helps the client remain as functional as possible and prevents sensory overload. Option 1 is important but not a priority. Options 2 and 3 aren't particularly effective with schizophrenia.
NP: Implementing care
CN: Psychosocial integrity
CNS: Psychosocial adaptation
CL: Application

18 When the parents of a schizophrenic client arrive to visit her, the client tells them she's too busy to see them but then clears off a space on her bed for them to sit. Her behavior is indicative of:
☐ 1. anhedonia.
☐ 2. automatism.
☐ 3. ambivalence.
☐ 4. avoidance.

CORRECT ANSWER: 3
The client is experiencing ambivalence, or two opposing needs: To drive her parents away and to draw them closer. Option 1: Anhedonia is the inability to experience pleasure. Option 2: Automatism is slow, repetitive movement. Option 4: Avoidance is a form of withdrawal.
NP: Collecting data
CN: Psychosocial integrity
CNS: Psychosocial adaptation
CL: Comprehension

19 The mother of a schizophrenic client approaches the nurse's station in tears. She says that she's upset about her daughter's behavior. Which response is best?
☐ 1. "What is it that upsets you the most?"
☐ 2. "Are you afraid your daughter will never get well?"
☐ 3. "Her behavior is typical of someone with schizophrenia."
☐ 4. "Let me give you some information about her illness."

CORRECT ANSWER: 1
Option 1 permits the nurse to collect data reported in the mother's own words. Option 2 narrows the data collection process prematurely. Also, it's important to hear what the mother has to say without planting suggestions about her daughter's condition. Options 3 and 4 close off the data collection process too soon.
NP: Collecting data
CN: Psychosocial integrity
CNS: Coping and adaptation
CL: Application

20 A client who has been taking thiothixene (Navane) for the past 10 days approaches the nurse's station. The nurse notices that the client is exhibiting stooped posture, shuffling gait, drooling, and tremulous arms. Which condition is this client probably experiencing?
- [ ] 1. Akathisia
- [ ] 2. Dyskinesia
- [ ] 3. Parkinsonism
- [ ] 4. Akinesia

CORRECT ANSWER: 3
These symptoms are characteristic of parkinsonism. Option 1: Akathisia describes a restless behavior. Option 2: Dyskinesia involves muscle rigidity. Option 4: Akinesia is typified by slow movements.
NP: Collecting data
CN: Physiological integrity
CNS: Pharmacological therapies
CL: Comprehension

---

21 The reason for administering the abnormal involuntary movement scale (AIMS) is to assess for:
- [ ] 1. extrapyramidal adverse effects.
- [ ] 2. client's ability to perform manual tasks.
- [ ] 3. need for an anticholinergic medication.
- [ ] 4. effectiveness of the client's neuroleptic medication.

CORRECT ANSWER: 1
AIMS assesses the ability to move body parts in a coordinated manner. Extrapyramidal adverse effects are uncoordinated body movements. Options 2 and 3: AIMS isn't used to assess the client's ability to perform manual tasks or need for an anticholinergic. Option 4 is determined by the relief of the client's symptoms for which a neuroleptic is prescribed.
NP: Collecting data
CN: Physiological integrity
CNS: Pharmacological therapies
CL: Comprehension

---

22 A client is to begin electroconvulsive therapy (ECT) in 3 days. Which physician's order is likely to be included in this client's chart?
- [ ] 1. Give liquid breakfast after ECT treatments.
- [ ] 2. Begin phenelzine (Nardil) 15 mg three times per day.
- [ ] 3. Administer succinylcholine (Anectine) 50 mg 30 minutes before ECT.
- [ ] 4. Discontinue lithium carbonate (Lithobid) STAT.

CORRECT ANSWER: 4
Psychotropic medications aren't generally given simultaneously with ECT. Option 1: No dietary restrictions are necessary after ECT. Option 2: Phenelzine is typically discontinued because it alters the seizure threshold. Option 3: Succinylcholine is administered only seconds before the treatment is given and after the client is anesthetized.
NP: Planning care
CN: Physiological integrity
CNS: Reduction of risk potential
CL: Knowledge

---

23 A male client who is actively manic has disrupted his roommate's sleep for the past 2 nights. Which intervention would be best for this client?
- [ ] 1. Obtain a physician's order for a nighttime sedative.
- [ ] 2. Allow the client to sleep in an open seclusion room.
- [ ] 3. Take the client to the gymnasium for a vigorous workout before bedtime.
- [ ] 4. Institute a behavioral contract to help the client stay quiet at night.

CORRECT ANSWER: 2
The client's nocturnal behaviors won't disrupt the sleep of others if the client is placed in an unoccupied room. Option 1: A bedtime sedative usually is ineffective with acutely manic clients. With option 3, the client would become even more energized and unable to settle down. Option 4 is also ineffective because acutely manic people can't follow behavior contracts.
NP: Implementing care
CN: Psychosocial integrity
CNS: Psychosocial adaptation
CL: Application

24 When established patterns of coping no longer work, a person generally experiences:
☐ 1. "as if" behavior.
☐ 2. suicidal ideation.
☐ 3. mental illness.
☐ 4. a crisis.

CORRECT ANSWER: 4
A crisis is generally defined as the loss of ability to cope. Option 1: "As if" behavior is exhibited by those with self-identity problems and those who are covering unacceptable feelings. Options 2 and 3: People in crisis aren't necessarily mentally ill or suicidal.
NP: Collecting data
CN: Psychosocial integrity
CNS: Coping and adaptation
CL: Knowledge

---

25 A woman enters a crisis center and implores the nurse on duty to help her. Which of the following is most important for the nurse to assess first?
☐ 1. The woman's family history
☐ 2. The woman's perception of her situation
☐ 3. What she wants the nurse to do for her
☐ 4. What she's willing to do to resolve her problem

CORRECT ANSWER: 2
The nurse must attempt to understand the client's perception of the situation. Option 1: A family history isn't paramount to crisis intervention. Although options 3 and 4 provide useful information, they aren't priorities.
NP: Collecting data
CN: Psychosocial integrity
CNS: Coping and adaptation
CL: Application

---

26 One of the goals of crisis intervention with a suicidal adolescent is to:
☐ 1. prevent the adolescent from embarrassing himself.
☐ 2. show the adolescent how to cope with his life situation.
☐ 3. assist the adolescent to consider other options for coping with the situation.
☐ 4. change the adolescent's situation, thereby eliminating the need for suicide.

CORRECT ANSWER: 3
An adolescent who can identify coping alternatives is less likely to view suicide as a solution. Option 1: The goal of crisis intervention is to restore equilibrium through problem solving, not to prevent embarrassment. Option 2 is wrong; people are responsible for finding their own viable solutions. Option 4 is also incorrect because the nurse can't change anyone's life situation.
NP: Planning care
CN: Psychosocial integrity
CNS: Coping and adaptation
CL: Comprehension

---

27 A 14-year-old boy tells the nurse that he wishes to talk about a friend who is contemplating killing himself. Which response is best in this situation, initially?
☐ 1. "Who is this friend?"
☐ 2. "Tell me about this friend."
☐ 3. "Has your friend ever told anyone else?"
☐ 4. "Sounds like your friend needs to talk to someone."

CORRECT ANSWER: 2
Option 2 conveys interest and allows the client to proceed at his own rate. He's probably talking about himself and is testing the nurse's reaction. Options 1, 3, and 4 block communication or ask for information that is irrelevant.
NP: Implementing care
CN: Psychosocial integrity
CNS: Coping and adaptation
CL: Application

28 While performing a suicide assessment, the nurse discovers that the client is moderately depressed and somewhat withdrawn and that he can name only one person to call in times of need. The client seems to have a relatively stable lifestyle but reports that he attempted suicide 1 year ago by taking fifty 25-mg tablets of Benadryl. He claims to have increased thoughts about attempting suicide again and is still formulating a plan. The most accurate assessment of this client's suicide risk is:
- ☐ 1. low.
- ☐ 2. high.
- ☐ 3. moderate.
- ☐ 4. unpredictable.

CORRECT ANSWER: 3
The client's previous suicide attempt makes the risk moderate. Option 1: The risk isn't low because of the previous suicide attempt. Option 2: The fact that the client is still formulating a plan and has a stable lifestyle keeps him from being at high risk. Option 4: A client's risk for suicide usually can be predicted using various criteria.
NP: Collecting data
CN: Psychosocial integrity
CNS: Coping and adaptation
CL: Analysis

29 The nurse is caring for a female client who had been extremely suicidal but now appears very serene. She says she has finally gotten things worked out. What would be the best way to respond to this client?
- ☐ 1. "I'm glad things are working out for you."
- ☐ 2. "How have you managed to work things out so quickly?"
- ☐ 3. "I'm not clear about what has changed for you; tell me more."
- ☐ 4. "You look so much better; you must be feeling relieved."

CORRECT ANSWER: 3
Option 3 allows the nurse to seek further clarification without placing words in the client's mouth. Options 1 and 4 block further exploration and indicate the nurse's lack of insight. Option 2 allows the client to give an answer that hides underlying intent (for example, the client may respond, "I prayed about it and believe that God is now in charge of my life").
NP: Implementing care
CN: Psychosocial integrity
CNS: Coping and adaptation
CL: Application

30 Which activity is best for a client with bipolar disorder who is in the manic phase?
- ☐ 1. Swimming laps in a pool
- ☐ 2. Reading quietly in her room
- ☐ 3. Attending the unit bingo party
- ☐ 4. Playing volleyball

CORRECT ANSWER: 1
Option 1 provides large-muscle activity without overstimulating the client. Option 2 is inappropriate because manic clients can't sit quietly at this phase of their disorder. Options 3 and 4 provide too much stimulation for a manic client who is already overstimulated.
NP: Planning care
CN: Psychosocial integrity
CNS: Psychosocial adaptation
CL: Application

31 Which nursing diagnosis is the priority for a client with bipolar disorder during the manic phase?
- ☐ 1. *Impaired adjustment*
- ☐ 2. *Disturbed sensory perception*
- ☐ 3. *Disturbed sleep pattern*
- ☐ 4. *Ineffective role performance*

CORRECT ANSWER: 3
A manic client who doesn't receive adequate rest is at high risk for physiologic collapse. Options 1 and 4 aren't priority diagnoses at this time. Option 2 is incorrect because the client isn't hallucinating.
NP: Planning care
CN: Psychosocial integrity
CNS: Psychosocial adaptation
CL: Analysis

32 A client on the sixth floor of a psychiatric unit has a morbid fear of elevators. She's scheduled to attend occupational therapy, which is located on the ground floor of the hospital. The client refuses to take the elevator, insisting that the stairs are safer. Which nursing action would be best given the client's refusal to use the elevator?
- ☐ 1. Insist that she take the elevator.
- ☐ 2. Offer a special reward if she rides the elevator.
- ☐ 3. Withhold her occupational therapy privileges until she's able to ride the elevator.
- ☐ 4. Allow her to use the stairs.

CORRECT ANSWER: 4
This client has a phobia and must not be forced to ride the elevator because of the risk of panic-level anxiety, which can occur if she's forced to contact the phobic object. Option 4 is the only reasonable answer. Options 1 and 2: This client can't control her fear; therefore, stating that she must take the elevator or promising a reward won't work. Option 3: Occupational therapy is a treatment the client needs, not a reward.
NP: Implementing care
CN: Psychosocial integrity
CNS: Psychosocial adaptation
CL: Application

33 Which nursing diagnosis would the nurse expect to find on the plan of care of a client with a phobia about elevators?
- ☐ 1. *Social isolation related to a lack of social skills*
- ☐ 2. *Disturbed thought processes related to a fear of elevators*
- ☐ 3. *Ineffective individual coping related to poor coping skills*
- ☐ 4. *Anxiety related to fear of elevators*

CORRECT ANSWER: 3
Poor coping skills can cause ineffective coping. Option 1: Such a client isn't relegated to social isolation and lack of social skills has nothing to do with phobia. Options 2 and 4: Fear of elevators is a manifestation, not the cause, of altered thoughts and anxiety.
NP: Planning care
CN: Psychosocial integrity
CNS: Psychosocial adaptation
CL: Analysis

34 Which statement most accurately characterizes clients with generalized anxiety disorder?
- ☐ 1. They believe their situation is hopeless.
- ☐ 2. They tend to worry about most aspects of their lives.
- ☐ 3. They experience anxiety mostly when exposed to trigger events.
- ☐ 4. They can't control their anxiety without medication.

CORRECT ANSWER: 2
Clients with generalized anxiety disorder worry about everything. Option 1: Those with this disorder believe that they can be helped. Option 3: Such clients have no particular triggers that stimulate their anxiety. Option 4: Behavioral techniques have proven effective for many clients with generalized anxiety disorder. If needed, medication is only used short-term.
NP: Collecting data
CN: Psychosocial integrity
CNS: Psychosocial adaptation
CL: Knowledge

35 A client enters the crisis center and tells the nurse that she needs help. She relays that she was nearly killed 4 months ago after being kidnapped from a convenience store, assaulted, then left for dead along the interstate highway. She says that she can't sleep at night because of recurring nightmares, can't use the freeway because of acute anxiety, can't function at work because of preoccupation with her experience, and is very tense and irritable most of the time. Which disorder is this client most likely experiencing?
- ☐ 1. Panic disorder
- ☐ 2. Briquet's syndrome
- ☐ 3. Posttraumatic stress disorder
- ☐ 4. Generalized anxiety disorder

CORRECT ANSWER: 3
This client's description of events and symptoms is characteristic of posttraumatic stress disorder. Option 1 is characterized by unpredictable attacks of panic-level anxiety. Option 2 is characterized by numerous somatic complaints. Option 4 is characterized by excessive worry and fear of doing things poorly.
NP: Collecting data
CN: Psychosocial integrity
CNS: Psychosocial adaptation
CL: Knowledge

36 While working with a kidnap victim with post-traumatic stress disorder, the focus of nursing sessions should be to help the client:

☐ 1. confront her assailant by taking legal action against him.

☐ 2. understand why she has let this experience dominate her life.

☐ 3. suppress this experience and get on with her life.

☐ 4. gain cognitive mastery over this experience.

CORRECT ANSWER: 4

Before this client can move on with her life, she must gain cognitive mastery over the experience and thereby put it into perspective. Options 1 and 2 may be addressed but they aren't the primary focus. Option 3: Suppressing the experience is contrary to gaining cognitive mastery over it.

NP: Planning care
CN: Psychosocial integrity
CNS: Psychosocial adaptation
CL: Application

---

37 The primary goal initially when working with a kidnap victim with posttraumatic stress disorder is to:

☐ 1. have the client describe, in detail, the kidnapping and assault.

☐ 2. help the client to understand that her life is no longer in danger.

☐ 3. help the client to feel less irritable when feeling stressed.

☐ 4. ensure that the client sleeps restfully for 6 consecutive hours each night.

CORRECT ANSWER: 1

Before accomplishing anything else, the client must develop cognitive mastery of the kidnapping and assault. Options 2 and 4 will follow when cognitive mastery has been achieved. Option 3 is unmeasurable and not of immediate concern.

NP: Planning care
CN: Psychosocial integrity
CNS: Psychosocial adaptation
CL: Analysis

---

38 The etiology for posttraumatic stress disorder is typically:

☐ 1. ineffective coping.

☐ 2. a life-threatening or catastrophic event.

☐ 3. posttraumatic phobia and uncontrolled anxiety.

☐ 4. altered role performance.

CORRECT ANSWER: 2

Posttraumatic stress disorder is usually caused by some life-threatening or catastrophic event, such as a war, rape, or natural disaster. Options 1, 3 and 4 are all manifestations, not causes, of this disorder.

NP: Collecting data
CN: Psychosocial integrity
CNS: Psychosocial adaptation
CL: Knowledge

---

39 A female client describes her unpredictable episodes of acute anxiety as "just awful." She says that she feels like she's about to die and can hardly breathe. These symptoms are most characteristic of:

☐ 1. agoraphobia.

☐ 2. dissociative disorder.

☐ 3. posttraumatic stress disorder.

☐ 4. panic disorder.

CORRECT ANSWER: 4

This client is describing the characteristics of someone with panic disorder. Option 1 is characterized by fear of public places; option 2, by lost periods of time; and option 3, by hypervigilance and sleep disturbance.

NP: Collecting data
CN: Psychosocial integrity
CNS: Psychosocial adaptation
CL: Knowledge

---

40 A 14-year-old girl exercises vigorously and believes that she's grossly obese (she's actually 20 lb underweight). She's a self-described perfectionist with a straight-A average and a state-level track and field contender. Although she's well liked by her teachers and the track coach, she has few friends. Which inference about the client can the nurse make based on this profile?

☐ 1. She has somatoform disorder.

☐ 2. She's just overanxious.

☐ 3. She has obsessive-compulsive disorder.

☐ 4. She has an eating disorder.

CORRECT ANSWER: 4

Such a profile is typical of someone with an eating disorder. Option 1: A client with somatoform disorder would have many physical complaints unsupported by medical findings. Option 2: Someone who is merely overanxious would worry excessively about life events. Option 3: Obsessive-compulsive disorder is characterized by unwanted thoughts and ritualistic behavior.

NP: Collecting data
CN: Psychosocial integrity
CNS: Psychosocial adaptation
CL: Application

41 Which of the following is the treatment team's priority in planning the care of a client with an eating disorder?

☐ 1. Preventing the client from performing any muscle-building exercises
☐ 2. Keeping the client on bed rest until she attains a specified weight
☐ 3. Meeting daily to discuss countertransferences and splitting behaviors
☐ 4. Monitoring the client's weight and vital signs daily

CORRECT ANSWER: 3
Clients with eating disorders commonly use manipulative ploys to resist weight gain if they restrict food intake or to maintain purging practices if they are bulimic. They frequently play staff members against one other and hone in on their caretakers' vulnerabilities. Option 1: Muscle building is acceptable because, compared with aerobic exercise, it burns relatively few calories. Option 2 can result in unnecessary power struggles and prevents staff from focusing on more pertinent issues and problems. Option 4 is important but not vital on a daily basis unless the client's physiologic condition warrants such close scrutiny.
NP: Planning care
CN: Psychosocial integrity
CNS: Psychosocial adaptation
CL: Application

42 A nurse's friend has bulimia nervosa and is receiving therapy for her disorder. The nurse is aware that the friend continues to purge when feeling stressed. Which action concerning the purging is appropriate for the nurse to take in this situation?

☐ 1. Do nothing because the friend is responsible for her own well-being.
☐ 2. Call the friend's therapist and report what is going on.
☐ 3. Take over some of the friend's responsibilities to decrease her stress level.
☐ 4. Monitor the friend's behavior to prevent her from purging.

CORRECT ANSWER: 1
The nurse isn't a therapist and can't control her friend's behavior. However, she can express her concern. Option 2 is invasive and probably oversteps the boundaries of friendship. Option 3 would place undue burden on the nurse and does nothing to solve the friend's underlying problems. Option 4: Monitoring the friend's behavior would be fruitless because the nurse has no control over the friend's choices.
NP: Implementing care
CN: Psychosocial integrity
CNS: Coping and adaptation
CL: Application

43 A 15-year-old girl with an eating disorder says to the nurse, "You're the only one who understands me." Which reply is best?

☐ 1. "I'm glad you think that I understand you."
☐ 2. "What is it you want nurses to understand about you?"
☐ 3. "What do I do that is more helpful than others do?"
☐ 4. "I think the other staff understand more than you think."

CORRECT ANSWER: 2
This attempts to clarify the client's statement without engaging in splitting (options 1 and 3). Option 4 is defensive and sets the nurse up for taking sides. The client needs to communicate her desires directly to the other nurses.
NP: Implementing care
CN: Psychosocial integrity
CNS: Psychosocial adaptation
CL: Application

44 A 26-year-old woman is admitted to the psychiatric unit after a suicide attempt that was precipitated by her husband's overseas assignment with his army reserve unit. During the admission assessment, the nurse learns that this is her 10th suicide attempt in 9 years, that she can't tolerate being alone, and that she places people and events into mutually exclusive dichotomous categories (such as good versus bad and positive versus negative). Which is the most reasonable inference about the client the nurse can make based on this profile?
☐ 1. She has borderline personality disorder.
☐ 2. She has narcissistic personality disorder.
☐ 3. She has passive-aggressive personality disorder.
☐ 4. She has histrionic personality disorder.

CORRECT ANSWER: 1
Based on this profile, the client probably has a borderline personality disorder. Option 2: A client with a narcissistic personality disorder displays characteristics of entitlement. Option 3: Someone who has passive-aggressive personality disorder is typically unable to directly express anger. Option 4: A client with histrionic personality disorder displays flamboyance and seductiveness.
NP: Collecting data
CN: Psychosocial integrity
CNS: Psychosocial adaptation
CL: Knowledge

---

45 In planning care for a client with borderline personality disorder, the nurse must realize that the client will probably:
☐ 1. be unable to make decisions independently.
☐ 2. act out when feeling afraid, alone, or devalued.
☐ 3. believe she deserves special privileges not accorded to others.
☐ 4. display inappropriately seductive appearance and behavior.

CORRECT ANSWER: 2
Those with borderline personality disorder have an intense fear of abandonment. Option 1 isn't true. Option 3 is characteristic of a person with narcissistic personality disorder; Option 4 is characteristic of someone with histrionic personality disorder.
NP: Planning care
CN: Psychosocial integrity
CNS: Psychosocial adaptation
CL: Application

---

46 A client with borderline personality disorder confides in one nurse that she's disappointed in the other nurses because of their lack of sensitivity to her. What is the best action for the nurse to take now?
☐ 1. Explain the other nurses' behaviors to the client.
☐ 2. Ask for more information about the client's disappointment.
☐ 3. Call a team meeting to help others understand the client better.
☐ 4. Advise the client to seek out the nurses and tell them directly.

CORRECT ANSWER: 4
One communication strategy when working with a client with borderline personality disorder is to never engage in third-party conversations. Options 1, 2, and 3 all encourage splitting behaviors and are nonproductive.
NP: Implementing care
CN: Psychosocial integrity
CNS: Psychosocial adaptation
CL: Application

---

47 A client's confiding in one nurse about other staff is an example of:
☐ 1. splitting.
☐ 2. projection.
☐ 3. entitlement.
☐ 4. displacement.

CORRECT ANSWER: 1
Splitting is a defense mechanism that prevents the unification of one's good and bad aspects or image of another person. Option 2: Projection is crediting another person with an undesired personal quality. Option 3: Entitlement is feeling deserving of unmerited recognition. Option 4: Displacement is venting feelings (usually anger) to a safe object or person rather than directly to the source.
NP: Collecting data
CN: Psychosocial integrity
CNS: Psychosocial adaptation
CL: Application

48 Which psychotropic medication is considered a controlled substance and should therefore kept in a locked cupboard?
☐ 1. fluoxetine (Prozac)
☐ 2. doxepin (Sinequan)
☐ 3. clonazepam (Klonopin)
☐ 4. thiothixene (Navane)

CORRECT ANSWER: 3
Clonazepam falls within schedule IV of controlled substances and should be kept locked. The medications in options 1, 2, and 4 aren't habit-forming and produce no tolerance adverse effects.
NP: Planning care
CN: Physiological integrity
CNS: Pharmacological therapies
CL: Comprehension

49 Of the following psychotropic medications, which one has an adverse effect of tolerance?
☐ 1. thioridazine (Mellaril)
☐ 2. fluphenazine (Prolixin)
☐ 3. carbamazepine (Tegretol)
☐ 4. alprazolam (Xanax)

CORRECT ANSWER: 4
Alprazolam is the only drug listed for which a client can sustain tolerance. Therefore, options 1, 2, and 3 are incorrect.
NP: Planning care
CN: Physiological integrity
CNS: Pharmacological therapies
CL: Knowledge

50 A client calls the clinic at 4 p.m. to say that he forgot to take his 8 a.m. dose of imipramine (Tofranil). The nurse should instruct him to take:
☐ 1. the medication as directed for the next scheduled dose.
☐ 2. the missed dose now and cut the next scheduled dose in half.
☐ 3. a little more of the medication at the next scheduled time.
☐ 4. half of the missed dose now and the full amount at the next scheduled time.

CORRECT ANSWER: 1
Nurses aren't authorized to change medication dosages without a physician's order. With most medications, a single missed dose causes little harm.
NP: Implementing care
CN: Physiological integrity
CNS: Pharmacological therapies
CL: Application

51 Which medication is found in all body fluids and excreted through the kidneys?
☐ 1. triazolam (Halcion)
☐ 2. benztropine (Cogentin)
☐ 3. lithium carbonate (Lithobid)
☐ 4. phenelzine (Nardil)

CORRECT ANSWER: 3
Lithium is the only drug excreted by the kidneys. Therefore, options 1, 2, and 4 are incorrect.
NP: Planning care
CN: Physiological integrity
CNS: Pharmacological therapies
CL: Comprehension

52 Which symptoms suggest abuse of anxiolytic medication?
☐ 1. Hypotension, dry mouth, and syncope
☐ 2. Slurred speech, ataxia, and faintness
☐ 3. Fine tremors, metallic taste in the mouth, and confusion
☐ 4. Muscle rigidity, hyperpyrexia, and fluctuating vital signs

CORRECT ANSWER: 2
These symptoms are classic indicators of anxiolytic overdose. Option 1: Dry mouth isn't an adverse effect of anxiolytic agents. Options 3 and 4: These are symptoms of lithium toxicity and neuroleptic syndrome, respectively.
NP: Evaluating care
CN: Physiological integrity
CNS: Pharmacological therapies
CL: Comprehension

53 A young woman arrives at the emergency department with mild euphoria, dilated pupils, restlessness, hand tremors, and a pulse rate of 116 beats/minute. She states that she has been taking street drugs. Which drug would the nurse suspect the client has taken?
☐ 1. lysergic acid diethylamide (LSD)
☐ 2. Amphetamines
☐ 3. Crack cocaine
☐ 4. phencyclidine (PCP)

CORRECT ANSWER: 2
The client's symptoms are consistent with amphetamine use. Options 1 and 4: Looseness of association and bizarre behavior would be characteristic for LSD or PCP. Option 3: Grandiosity is characteristic of crack cocaine use.
NP: Collecting data
CN: Psychosocial integrity
CNS: Psychosocial adaptation
CL: Comprehension

---

54 Acute intoxication with lysergic acid diethylamide (LSD) may mimic which mental illness?
☐ 1. Schizophrenia
☐ 2. Multiple personality disorder
☐ 3. Generalized anxiety disorder
☐ 4. Acute mania

CORRECT ANSWER: 1
Visual distortions and gross distortions of reality are found in both LSD intoxication and schizophrenia. Options 2, 3, and 4: LSD intoxication doesn't manifest in switching personalities; total anxiety and tenseness; or hyperactivity, euphoria, or emotional liability.
NP: Collecting data
CN: Psychosocial integrity
CNS: Psychosocial adaptation
CL: Knowledge

---

55 A male client returns to the psychiatric unit after being on a 6-hour pass. The nurse observes that the client is somewhat agitated and ataxic and that he exhibits nystagmus and general muscle hypertonicity. The nurse suspects that the client was using drugs while away from the unit. His symptoms are most indicative of intoxication with which drug?
☐ 1. phencyclidine (PCP)
☐ 2. Crack cocaine
☐ 3. Heroin
☐ 4. Cannabis

CORRECT ANSWER: 1
The client's behavior suggests the use of PCP. Option 2: Crack intoxication is characterized by euphoria, grandiosity, aggressiveness, paranoia, and depression. Option 3: Heroin intoxication is characterized by euphoria followed by sleepiness. Option 4: Cannabis intoxication is characterized by panic state and visual hallucinations.
NP: Collecting data
CN: Psychosocial integrity
CNS: Psychosocial adaptation
CL: Knowledge

---

56 The nurse is caring for a client who typically consumes 15 to 20 beers per week and is extremely defensive about his alcohol intake. He admits to experiencing blackouts and has had three alcohol-related accidents. The best action this client can take is to:
☐ 1. monitor his alcohol intake.
☐ 2. switch to low-alcohol beer or wine coolers.
☐ 3. limit his intake to no more than three beers per drinking occasion.
☐ 4. abstain from alcohol altogether.

CORRECT ANSWER: 4
This client demonstrates behaviors consistent with middle-stage addiction. Once addicted, the only way to control intake is to abstain altogether. Therefore, options 1, 2, and 3 are incorrect.
NP: Planning care
CN: Psychosocial integrity
CNS: Psychosocial adaptation
CL: Comprehension

57 A 30-year-old woman signed herself into an alcohol treatment program. During this first visit with the nurse, she vehemently maintains that she has no problem with alcohol. She states that she's in this program only because her husband issued an ultimatum. Which response is best?
- ☐ 1. "I wonder why your husband would issue such an ultimatum?"
- ☐ 2. "Because you came voluntarily, you're free to leave anytime you wish."
- ☐ 3. "From your point of view, what is most important for me to know about you?"
- ☐ 4. "You sound pretty definite about not having a problem with alcohol."

CORRECT ANSWER: 3
Option 3 allows the nurse to collect more information. Option 1 focuses on the husband, who isn't the client. Option 2 is abrasive and blocks communication. Option 4 doesn't allow for further exploration.
NP: Implementing care
CN: Psychosocial integrity
CNS: Psychosocial adaptation
CL: Application

58 Within 8 hours of her last drink, an alcoholic client experiences tremors, loss of appetite, disordered thinking, and insomnia. The nurse believes that this client is in second-stage withdrawal. The best action for the nurse to take now is to:
- ☐ 1. give disulfiram (Antabuse) as prescribed.
- ☐ 2. obtain a physician's order for lorazepam (Ativan).
- ☐ 3. help the client to engage in progressive muscle-relaxation exercises.
- ☐ 4. provide the client with constant one-on-one monitoring.

CORRECT ANSWER: 2
A client in second-stage withdrawal should be medicated with a benzodiazepine, such as lorazepam, to prevent progression of symptoms to delirium tremens, a life-threatening withdrawal syndrome. Option 1: Disulfiram is used during early recovery, not during detoxification. Option 3: Progressive muscle relaxation isn't particularly effective during withdrawal. Option 4: Close monitoring during withdrawal is appropriate after the client has been medicated for withdrawal symptoms.
NP: Implementing care
CN: Psychosocial integrity
CNS: Psychosocial adaptation
CL: Application

59 A client with alcoholism who has completed a residential treatment program can reasonably expect that:
- ☐ 1. her family will no longer be dysfunctional.
- ☐ 2. she'll need ongoing support to remain abstinent.
- ☐ 3. she doesn't need to be concerned about abusing alcohol in the future.
- ☐ 4. she can learn to consume alcohol without problems.

CORRECT ANSWER: 2
Addiction is a relapsing illness. Support is helpful to most people in maintaining an abstinent lifestyle. Option 1: The family dynamics probably will change as a result of the client's abstinence; however, there is no way to predict whether these changes will be healthy. Option 3: An alcoholic client always remains at risk for abusing alcohol. Option 4: Most addicted people can't consume alcohol in moderation.
NP: Planning care
CN: Psychosocial integrity
CNS: Coping and adaptation
CL: Application

60 When providing discharge instructions to a schizophrenic client who is taking haloperidol, the nurse should advise him to:
☐ 1. monitor his sodium and fluid intake.
☐ 2. avoid strenuous activities.
☐ 3. discontinue the medication if dry mouth becomes a problem.
☐ 4. consult a physician before taking any over-the-counter medications.

CORRECT ANSWER: 4
Haloperidol shouldn't be taken with other medications, including over-the-counter drugs, without a physician's approval because many medications contain substances that interact with haloperidol. Option 1 is irrelevant. Option 2: Caution should be exercised when performing activities that require psychomotor coordination skills; however, these activities need not be avoided. Option 3: This drug shouldn't be discontinued without a physician's approval. Dry mouth can be relieved with candy or by using mouthwash.
NP: Planning care
CN: Physiological integrity
CNS: Pharmacological therapies
CL: Application

61 A client with a diagnosis of paranoid type schizophrenia is receiving an antipsychotic medication. His physician has just prescribed benztropine mesylate (Cogentin). The nurse realizes that this medication was most likely prescribed because of the client's:
☐ 1. tardive dyskinesia.
☐ 2. hypertensive crisis.
☐ 3. acute dystonia.
☐ 4. orthostatic hypotension.

CORRECT ANSWER: 3
Benztropine mesylate is used as adjunctive therapy in parkinsonism and for all conditions and medications that produce extrapyramidal symptoms, except tardive dyskinesia (option 1). Its anticholinergic effect reduces the extrapyramidal effects associated with antipsychotic drugs. Options 2 and 4 aren't associated with extrapyramidal symptoms.
NP: Evaluating care
CN: Physiological integrity
CNS: Pharmacological therapies
CL: Analysis

62 The nurse assesses a schizophrenic client for auditory hallucinations. Which of the following is most suggestive of this symptom?
☐ 1. Speaking loudly when engaged in conversation
☐ 2. Ignoring comments by the nurse
☐ 3. Responding only to the same person
☐ 4. Tilting the head to one side

CORRECT ANSWER: 4
A client who is having auditory hallucinations may tilt his head to one side, as if listening to someone or something. Options 1, 2, and 3 are indicative of hearing deficit, anxiety, and paranoid behavior, respectively.
NP: Collecting data
CN: Psychosocial integrity
CNS: Psychosocial adaptation
CL: Analysis

63 A client with a medical diagnosis of major depression has been taking 20 mg of fluoxetine (Prozac) orally twice daily since her admission to the psychiatric unit 2 weeks ago. On admission, the client verbalized serious thoughts of suicide; however, her mood has improved in the past 2 weeks. Which nursing intervention is most appropriate for this client now?
☐ 1. Compliment the client on her progress.
☐ 2. Continue close supervision for suicide attempts.
☐ 3. Keep the client on locked unit.
☐ 4. Notify the physician of the client's progress.

CORRECT ANSWER: 2
A client who was too depressed to carry out a suicidal plan at the time of admission but shows signs of improvement later should be watched closely. Her medication may have lifted her depression enough to enable her to carry out a suicidal plan. Options 1 and 3 may be appropriate but don't provide the close supervision required by this client. Option 4: Suicide precautions are a nursing function, not a medical order.
NP: Implementing care
CN: Psychosocial integrity
CNS: Psychosocial adaptation
CL: Analysis

64 Which question would be most appropriate for the nurse to ask to determine the extent of cognitive changes in a client with depression?
- [ ] 1. "How would you describe your usual mood?"
- [ ] 2. "Have you had any thoughts of harming yourself?"
- [ ] 3. "How is your ability to concentrate?"
- [ ] 4. "How do you feel about yourself?"

CORRECT ANSWER: 3
Cognitive changes deal with thinking and thought processes. A depressed client may have a diminished ability to concentrate, suggesting a decrease in overall cognitive functioning. Options 1, 2, and 4 don't elicit data about cognitive ability.
NP: Collecting data
CN: Psychosocial integrity
CNS: Psychosocial adaptation
CL: Application

---

65 A depressed client states that she prefers to remain in her room and not socialize with other clients on the unit. Which response by the nurse is most appropriate?
- [ ] 1. Allow the client to remain in her room.
- [ ] 2. Insist that the client interact with others throughout the day.
- [ ] 3. Sit with the client in her room for brief intervals to establish a trusting relationship.
- [ ] 4. Have other clients go to the client's room to keep her company.

CORRECT ANSWER: 3
Depressed people shouldn't be allowed to isolate themselves, as isolation only further lowers their self-esteem. Brief periods of interaction would accomplish two goals: To prevent the client's withdrawal, and to begin establishing trust and demonstrating genuine interest in the client. Option 1 wouldn't be therapeutic. Options 2 and 4 would be too threatening to the client at this time.
NP: Implementing care
CN: Psychosocial integrity
CNS: Psychosocial adaptation
CL: Application

---

66 Which nursing intervention would be most appropriate for a depressed client with a nursing diagnosis of *Sleep disturbance related to disrupted sleep pattern?*
- [ ] 1. Consult the physician about prescribing a bedtime sleep medication.
- [ ] 2. Allow the client to sit at the nurse's station for comfort.
- [ ] 3. Allow the client to watch television until sleepy.
- [ ] 4. Encourage the client to take a warm bath before retiring.

CORRECT ANSWER: 4
Sleep-inducing activities, such as a warm bath, help promote relaxation and sleep. Although option 1 is possible, it wouldn't be the best nursing intervention for this client. Options 2 and 3 wouldn't necessarily promote sleep. In fact, they may provide too much stimulation, further preventing sleep.
NP: Implementing care
CN: Physiological integrity
CNS: Basic care and comfort
CL: Application

---

67 A client with a diagnosis of bipolar disorder, manic phase, is at risk for exhaustion and inadequate food intake. How can the nurse best meet this client's nutritional needs?
- [ ] 1. Establish a set time to eat meals.
- [ ] 2. Order high-protein milk shakes between meals.
- [ ] 3. Allow family members to bring the client's favorite foods to the hospital.
- [ ] 4. Provide finger foods that can be eaten on the go.

CORRECT ANSWER: 4
Finger food that can be eaten quickly while the client is in a highly energetic state are best. This client can't sit still long enough to eat (option 1). Options 2 and 3 help with caloric intake but don't necessarily provide balanced nutrition.
NP: Implementing care
CN: Physiological integrity
CNS: Basic care and comfort
CL: Application

68 Which activity is appropriate for a client with a diagnosis of bipolar disorder, manic phase?
☐ 1. Playing a card game
☐ 2. Playing a vigorous basketball game
☐ 3. Playing a board game
☐ 4. Painting

CORRECT ANSWER: 4
An activity, such as painting, that promotes minimal stimulation is the best choice. Options 1, 2, and 3: Activities that may escalate hyperactivity should be avoided.
NP: Implementing care
CN: Psychosocial integrity
CNS: Psychosocial adaptation
CL: Application

---

69 Seclusion may be appropriate during a manic episode when the client:
☐ 1. engages in frantic, aimless physical activity.
☐ 2. shouts loudly and continuously.
☐ 3. shows extreme excitement when discussing something.
☐ 4. plays the radio loudly.

CORRECT ANSWER: 1
A manic client who is engaged in frantic, aimless physical activity is at risk for self-injury. Such clients have poor judgment and are impulsive; they can exhaust themselves physically if not controlled. Options 2, 3, and 4: These activities wouldn't lead to physical exhaustion and pose no risk to the client.
NP: Implementing care
CN: Safe, effective care environment
CNS: Safety and infection control
CL: Application

---

70 Setting limits would be most appropriate when the manic client:
☐ 1. engages in frantic, aimless physical activity.
☐ 2. repeatedly changes the television station in the community room without asking others.
☐ 3. frequently questions staff about mealtimes.
☐ 4. asks for help with using the telephone.

CORRECT ANSWER: 2
Clients in manic phase of bipolar disorder may have trouble distinguishing boundaries and frequently intrude on the space of others. Such a situation may become volatile if the other clients understand boundary limits. Option 1 requires structure for safety and option 3 is anxious behavior; neither requires limits. Option 4 is a processing issue, not a limit setting one.
NP: Implementing care
CN: Psychosocial integrity
CNS: Psychosocial adaptation
CL: Application

---

71 When providing discharge instructions for a client with bipolar disorder who is receiving lithium carbonate, the nurse should stress the need to:
☐ 1. take medication with food.
☐ 2. have blood serum levels checked regularly.
☐ 3. take medication on an empty stomach.
☐ 4. avoid operating heavy machinery.

CORRECT ANSWER: 2
Regularly checking serum lithium levels is a critical part of medication management. The client is at high risk for toxicity with this drug, so regular monitoring is key to the success of treatment. Options 1, 3, and 4 aren't necessary for this medication.
NP: Implementing care
CN: Physiological integrity
CNS: Reduction of risk potential
CL: Application

---

72 Which nursing intervention best meets the behavioral needs of a manic client?
☐ 1. Discourage the client from making expensive purchases.
☐ 2. Focus on building the client's self-esteem.
☐ 3. Help the client become aware of his underlying anger.
☐ 4. Define acceptable behaviors, then set limits.

CORRECT ANSWER: 4
The hyperactivity characteristic of the manic phase of bipolar disorder is likely to cause the client to engage in unacceptable behaviors and test staff limits. Therefore, limit setting is important. Options 1, 2, and 3 wouldn't meet the client's behavioral needs.
NP: Implementing care
CN: Psychosocial integrity
CNS: Psychosocial adaptation
CL: Application

73 When planning the care of a client with general anxiety disorder, which intervention is most important to include?
- [ ] 1. Encourage the client to engage in activities that increase feelings of power and self-esteem.
- [ ] 2. Promote the client's interaction and socialization with others.
- [ ] 3. Assist the client to make plans for regular periods of leisure time.
- [ ] 4. Encourage the client to use a diary to record when anxiety occurred, its cause, and which interventions may have helped.

CORRECT ANSWER: 4
One of the nurse's goals is to help the client associate symptoms with an event, thereby beginning to learn appropriate ways to eliminate or reduce distress. A diary can be a beneficial tool for this purpose. Although options 1, 2, and 3 may be appropriate for this client, they aren't the priority.
NP: Planning care
CN: Psychosocial integrity
CNS: Psychosocial adaptation
CL: Application

---

74 A client states that she's experiencing flashbacks about a rape that occurred 6 months ago. After the flashbacks, she becomes immobilized with extreme distress. Which nursing diagnosis is most applicable to this client's current state?
- [ ] 1. *Disturbed sensory perception*
- [ ] 2. *Ineffective individual coping*
- [ ] 3. *Risk for posttrauma syndrome*
- [ ] 4. *Disturbed sleep pattern*

CORRECT ANSWER: 3
This client is suffering from posttraumatic stress disorder. In such cases, flashbacks can precipitate extreme distress, resulting in the client's immobility. The diagnostic categories listed in options 1, 2, and 4 may be established for this client at a later time.
NP: Planning care
CN: Psychosocial integrity
CNS: Psychosocial adaptation
CL: Application

---

75 Which of the following should the nurse be most concerned about when caring for a client taking an antianxiety medication?
- [ ] 1. Physical and psychological dependence
- [ ] 2. Transient hypertension
- [ ] 3. Abrupt withdrawal
- [ ] 4. Constipation

CORRECT ANSWER: 3
Abrupt discontinuation of an antianxiety drug can lead to withdrawal symptoms. Option 1: Antianxiety medications usually are prescribed for short periods. However, if used over a prolonged period, such drugs may produce psychological or physical dependence. Options 2 and 4 aren't associated with antianxiety drugs.
NP: Planning care
CN: Physiological integrity
CNS: Pharmacological therapies
CL: Application

---

76 A 40-year-old client is admitted to the hospital for diagnostic tests after complaining of shortness of breath and indigestion. His wife tells the nurse that he's been under a lot of stress lately. The client states that he feels fine. What type of defense mechanism is he using?
- [ ] 1. Regression
- [ ] 2 Displacement
- [ ] 3. Denial
- [ ] 4. Projection

CORRECT ANSWER: 3
Denial is an attempt to screen or ignore reality by refusing to acknowledge what is happening. Option 1: Regression is reverting to an earlier level of functioning that is more comfortable. Option 2: Displacement is transferring emotions, ideas, or impulses from their original object to a substitute. Option 4: Projection is blaming others for things that are happening to the client.
NP: Collecting data
CN: Psychosocial integrity
CNS: Coping and adaptation
CL: Knowledge

77 A 51-year-old male client is scheduled for cardiac catheterization. The nurse is explaining the procedure when the client develops slight increases in heart and respiratory rates. The client maintains composure and asks many relevant questions. Which level of anxiety is indicated by these behaviors?
☐ 1. Mild
☐ 2. Moderate
☐ 3. Severe
☐ 4. Panic

CORRECT ANSWER: 2
Behaviors that indicate moderate anxiety include voice changes, increased muscle tension, narrow focus of attention, slight increase in heart and respiratory rates, and mild gastric symptoms. Option 1: A person with mild anxiety exhibits mild restlessness but no changes in heart and respiratory rates. Option 3: A severely anxious person exhibits communication difficulties, inability to focus or concentrate, tachycardia, hyperventilation, headache, nausea, and dizziness. Option 4: A person in a panic state exhibits all the symptoms of severe anxiety plus an inability to communicate, distorted perception, and many other physical symptoms.
NP: Collecting data
CN: Psychosocial integrity
CNS: Psychosocial adaptation
CL: Knowledge

78 The nurse is teaching a 53-year-old male client with the nursing diagnosis *Anxiety related to lack of knowledge about an impending surgical procedure.* Which is an appropriate nursing intervention?
☐ 1. Reassure the client that there are many treatments for the problem.
☐ 2. Calmly ask the client to describe the procedure that is to be done.
☐ 3. Instruct the client that the nursing staff will help in any way they can.
☐ 4. Tell the client that he shouldn't keep his feelings to himself.

CORRECT ANSWER: 2
An appropriate short-term goal in this case is, "The client will repeat to the nurse the major points of the procedure." By asking the client to describe the procedure, the nurse can assess his level of understanding and address his anxiety by providing necessary teaching. Options 1, 3, and 4: These options don't address the client's anxiety or lack of knowledge about the procedure.
NP: Evaluating care
CN: Psychosocial integrity
CNS: Coping and adaptation
CL: Comprehension

79 The nurse is caring for a 39-year-old male client who recently underwent surgery and is having difficulty accepting changes in his body image. Which nursing intervention is appropriate?
☐ 1. Allow the client to express both positive and negative feelings about his body and body image.
☐ 2. Restrict the client's opportunity to view the incision and dressing because it's upsetting.
☐ 3. Assist the client to focus on future plans for recovery.
☐ 4. Assist the client to repress anger while discussing the body image alteration.

CORRECT ANSWER: 1
The nurse needs to observe for any indication that the client is ready to address his body image change. Option 2: The client should be allowed to look at the incision and dressing if he wants to do so. Option 3: It's too soon to focus on the future with this client. Option 4: The nurse should allow the client to express his feelings and not repress them, because repression prolongs recovery.
NP: Planning care
CN: Psychosocial integrity
CNS: Coping and adaptation
CL: Application

80 The nurse is caring for a 41-year-old male client with obsessive-compulsive disorder. Which behavior indicates that the client's stress level is increasing?
☐ 1. The client withdraws from people close to him.
☐ 2. The client exhibits increased reliance on his ritualistic behavior.
☐ 3. The client uses meaningless phrases when communicating.
☐ 4. The client becomes increasingly aggressive.

CORRECT ANSWER: 2
As the client's level of stress increases, his reliance on obsessive-compulsive behaviors also increases. Option 1: Withdrawn behavior isn't associated with obsessive-compulsive disorder. Options 3 and 4: Obsessive-compulsive clients have no difficulty with verbal communication skills and aren't aggressive.
NP: Evaluating care
CN: Psychosocial integrity
CNS: Psychosocial adaptation
CL: Comprehension

81 A 31-year-old female is admitted to the nursing unit complaining of feeling depressed, nervous, and lifeless. The client explains that she wants help and wants to feel like herself again. What is the nurse's most appropriate response?
☐ 1. "Don't worry; everything will be all right."
☐ 2. "How do you think this hospital can help you?"
☐ 3. "I can see that you are upset and feeling bad. What brought this on?"
☐ 4. "We're all here to make you feel better."

CORRECT ANSWER: 3
The nurse should acknowledge the client's feelings and seek more information about what lead to the hospitalization. Option 1: Telling the client not to worry provides false reassurance to make her feel better. Option 2: Asking the client how she thinks the hospital can help focuses on the hospital and not the client. Option 4: Telling the client "We're all here to make you feel better" doesn't acknowledge the client's feelings or allow the nurse to obtain further information.
NP: Collecting data
CN: Psychosocial integrity
CNS: Coping and adaptation
CL: Comprehension

82 A 50-year-old male client was admitted to the nursing unit 1 week ago with the diagnosis of major depression. The physician prescribed amitriptyline (Elavil) 50 mg by mouth, twice per day. The client is now complaining of difficulty urinating. What should the nurse do first?
☐ 1. Encourage fluids to increase urine output.
☐ 2. Ask the client when his last dose of amitriptyline was and readjust the next dose.
☐ 3. Palpate the client's abdomen for any signs of urine retention.
☐ 4. Redirect the client's activity in case he's seeking attention.

CORRECT ANSWER: 3
Amitriptyline (Elavil) is a tricyclic antidepressant. Common adverse effects of the anticholinergic effect are blurred vision, dry mouth, constipation, tachycardia, urine retention, and cognitive dysfunction. Option 1: Encouraging the client to increase his fluid intake might worsen the problem because the client has urine retention. Option 2: The nurse never readjusts a medication dose without first checking with the physician. Option 4: The nurse should always listen to a complaint and assess for evidence to support the complaint. Complaints should never be ignored.
NP: Implementing care
CN: Physiological integrity
CNS: Pharmacological therapies
CL: Application

83 A client who is being treated at home with imipramine (Tofranil) phones the nurse to say that his medication doesn't work. The nurse notes that he has been on the medication for 6 days. In her response to the client, which of the following statements should the nurse include?
☐ 1. The dose needs to be increased.
☐ 2. The medication needs to be changed.
☐ 3. The client isn't following the appropriate diet.
☐ 4. The therapeutic effect may not be achieved for 2 to 4 weeks.

CORRECT ANSWER: 4
Tricyclic antidepressants, such as imipramine, take 2 to 4 weeks to begin working effectively. Options 1 and 2: The client hasn't been on the medication long enough to know if the dose needs to be increased or if the medication needs to be changed. Option 3: There is no appropriate diet to follow.
NP: Planning care
CN: Physiological integrity
CNS: Pharmacological therapies
CL: Application

84 A client undergoing treatment for severe depression is being started on phenelzine (Nardil) 45 mg by mouth daily. Which of the following foods should the client avoid?
- [ ] 1. Aged cheese
- [ ] 2. Tomatoes
- [ ] 3. Chicken
- [ ] 4. Grapes

CORRECT ANSWER: 1
Phenelzine is a monoamine oxidase (MAO) inhibitor and specific dietary restrictions should be followed before, during, and after MAO inhibitor therapy. Options 2, 3, and 4: Tomatoes, chicken, and grapes are allowed with MAO inhibitors.
NP: Implementing care
CN: Physiological integrity
CNS: Pharmacological therapies
CL: Knowledge

---

85 The nurse is caring for a 27-year-old male client who is in the panic level of anxiety. Which of the following is the nurse's highest priority?
- [ ] 1. Encourage the client to discuss his feelings.
- [ ] 2. Provide for the client's safety needs.
- [ ] 3. Decrease the environmental stimuli.
- [ ] 4. Respect the client's personal space.

CORRECT ANSWER: 2
A client in a panic level of anxiety doesn't comprehend and can't follow instructions or care for his own basic needs. Option 1: The client is unable to express feelings due to the level of anxiety. Option 3: Decreased environmental stimulus is needed but only after the client's safety needs and other basic needs are met. Option 4: The nurse needs to enter the client's personal space to provide personal care because a client in panic is unable to do this for himself.
NP: Planning care
CN: Psychosocial integrity
CNS: Coping and adaptation
CL: Knowledge

---

86 The nurse is working with a 20-year-old female client diagnosed with severe obsessive-compulsive hand washing disorder. Which of the following is important for the nurse to remember?
- [ ] 1. Psychotherapy isn't usually beneficial.
- [ ] 2. Keeping the client to the schedule on the unit has first priority.
- [ ] 3. The client needs to be taught how to interrupt the ritualistic behavior.
- [ ] 4. The nurse needs to observe for skin breakdown from the ritualistic behavior.

CORRECT ANSWER: 4
Obsessive-compulsive clients wash their hands many times daily and experience red, chapped, irritated hands if the nursing staff doesn't intervene. Option 1: Psychotherapy is usually beneficial. Option 2: Keeping to the unit's schedule is low priority until the ritualistic behavior is under control. Option 3: Attempting to teach the client how to interrupt the ritualistic behavior would increase the client's anxiety and ritualistic behavior.
NP: Implementing care
CN: Psychosocial integrity
CNS: Coping and adaptation
CL: Knowledge

---

87 The nurse is completing a nursing plan of care for a 45-year-old male client with a psychophysiological disorder. Which intervention should be included?
- [ ] 1. Don't include any physical symptoms that aren't life-threatening.
- [ ] 2. Consider only the physical symptoms that are distressing to the client.
- [ ] 3. Include physical, psychosocial, and spiritual problems.
- [ ] 4. Consider only psychosocial symptoms.

CORRECT ANSWER: 3
Physical, psychosocial, and spiritual problems are thoroughly and continuously assessed with each client. Option 1: The nurse needs to include all symptoms, even those that aren't life threatening. Option 2: Consider all physical symptoms, even those the client doesn't find distressing. Option 4: Psychosocial symptoms should be considered but all three areas must be assessed to provide a thorough plan of care.
NP: Planning care
CN: Psychosocial integrity
CNS: Psychosocial adaptation
CL: Comprehension

88 Two 16-year-old clients are being treated in an adolescent unit. During a recreational activity they begin a physical fight. How should the nurse intervene?
- [ ] 1. Remove the teenagers to separate areas and set limits.
- [ ] 2. Remind the teenagers of the unit rules.
- [ ] 3. Obtain an order to place the teenagers in seclusion.
- [ ] 4. Obtain an order to place the teenagers in restraints.

CORRECT ANSWER: 1
Setting limits and removing the clients from the situation is the best way to handle aggression. Option 2: Reminders of appropriate behaviors aren't likely to be effective at this time. Options 3 and 4: Seclusion and restraints are reserved for more serious situations.
NP: Implementing care
CN: Psychosocial integrity
CNS: Psychosocial adaptation
CL: Application

89 A 35-year-old female client is diagnosed with conversion disorder with paralysis of the legs. What is the best nursing intervention for the nurse to use?
- [ ] 1. Discuss with the client ways to live with the paralysis.
- [ ] 2. Focus interactions on the results of medical tests.
- [ ] 3. Encourage the client to move the legs as much as possible.
- [ ] 4. Avoid focusing on the client's physical limitations.

CORRECT ANSWER: 4
The paralysis is used as an unhealthy way of expressing unmet psychological needs. The nurse should avoid speaking about the paralysis to shift the client's attention and focus on the mental aspect of the disorder. Options 1, 2, and 3: The other options focus too much on the paralysis, which doesn't allow recognition of the underlying psychological motivations.
NP: Implementing care
CN: Psychosocial integrity
CNS: Psychosocial adaptation
CL: Application

90 The nurse is instructing a 38-year-old male client undergoing treatment for anxiety and insomnia. The physician has prescribed lorazepam (Ativan) 1 mg by mouth three times per day. The nurse should instruct the client to:
- [ ] 1. avoid caffeine.
- [ ] 2. avoid aged cheeses.
- [ ] 3. avoid sunlight.
- [ ] 4. maintain an adequate salt intake.

CORRECT ANSWER: 1
Lorazepam is a benzodiazepine used to treat various forms of anxiety and insomnia. Caffeine is contraindicated because it's a stimulant and increases anxiety. Option 2: A client on a monoamine oxidase inhibitor should avoid aged cheeses. Option 3: Clients taking certain antipsychotic medications should avoid sunlight. Option 4: Salt intake has no effect on lorazepam.
NP: Implementing care
CN: Physiological integrity
CNS: Pharmacological therapies
CL: Knowledge

91 One year ago, a client was in a plane crash and several people were killed. The client is now experiencing nightmares, insomnia, headaches, loss of appetite, and fatigue. The nurse considers that the client may be experiencing:
- [ ] 1. panic disorder.
- [ ] 2. posttraumatic stress disorder.
- [ ] 3. bipolar disorder.
- [ ] 4. conversion disorder.

CORRECT ANSWER: 2
The client is reliving the crash because it's close to the first anniversary of the accident. Option 1: Panic disorder isn't correct because the client is still able to function. Option 3: Bipolar disorder isn't appropriate because the client isn't exhibiting mania and depression. Option 4: Conversion disorder isn't correct because the client isn't exhibiting any physical symptoms, such as paralysis, that aren't supported by a medical diagnosis.
NP: Collecting data
CN: Psychosocial integrity
CNS: Coping and adaptation
CL: Application

92 The nurse is working in a psychiatric facility and is beginning shift activities. Which client should the nurse see first?
☐ 1. A 45-year-old male who is to be transferred from the locked unit to the open unit
☐ 2. A 33-year-old male who is having visual hallucinations of spiders on the walls
☐ 3. A 27-year-old male admitted after attempting suicide who has been taking amitriptyline (Elavil) for 2 weeks and now seems very calm
☐ 4. A 36-year-old male who is pacing the floor and talking to himself

CORRECT ANSWER: 3
The client who has been taking amitriptyline for 2 weeks and now seems very calm poses an increased risk for a suicide attempt as he begins to feel better and gains the energy to attempt suicide again. Option 1: The 45-year-old client obviously is improving due to being transferred to an unlocked unit but will need to be assessed early in the shift. Options 2 and 4: The client having visual hallucinations and the client who is pacing the floor and talking to himself pose no threat to the other clients or themselves at this time.
NP: Planning care
CN: Psychosocial integrity
CNS: Psychosocial adaptation
CL: Application

---

93 The nurse is reviewing a client's medication administration record and notes that the client received a monoamine oxidase (MAO) inhibitor for 3 weeks before beginning a selective serotonin reuptake inhibitor (SSRI) regimen 1 week ago. This information alerts the nurse to watch for signs of:
☐ 1. serotonin syndrome.
☐ 2. hyporeflexia.
☐ 3. bradycardia.
☐ 4. urinary frequency.

CORRECT ANSWER: 1
Administering an SSRI too close to an MAO inhibitor causes serotonin syndrome, which is a life-threatening emergency. Symptoms include confusion, disorientation, mania, myoclonus, hyperreflexia, diaphoresis, shivering, tremors, nausea, diarrhea, and headache. Option 2: This client would exhibit hyperreflexia, not hyporeflexia. Option 3: Tachycardia is more likely than bradycardia. Option 4: Extrapyramidal adverse effects aren't associated with these drugs.
NP: Planning care
CN: Psychosocial integrity
CNS: Psychosocial adaptation
CL: Knowledge

---

94 A 40-year-old male client is recovering from an exacerbation of severe depression and a suicide attempt. The nurse is aware that the client's risk for a suicide attempt at this time is:
☐ 1. increased.
☐ 2. decreased.
☐ 3. unchanged.
☐ 4. absent.

CORRECT ANSWER: 1
The client's risk for a suicide attempt is increased because he's attempted suicide before. As the client begins to improve, increased energy and concentration levels may allow the client to devise and act on a suicide plan. Options 2, 3, and 4: The client's risk for a suicide attempt at this time isn't unchanged or absent and may not be reduced until several weeks after medications are begun.
NP: Planning care
CN: Psychosocial integrity
CNS: Psychosocial adaptation
CL: Application

95 The nurse is caring for a client who is pacing the halls, continuously wringing her hands, and telling herself how worthless she is. Which of the following nursing actions is appropriate?
- ☐ 1. Ignore the behavior.
- ☐ 2. Reassure her that things will get better soon.
- ☐ 3. Walk and talk with her as she paces.
- ☐ 4. Greet her with a friendly and cheerful smile.

CORRECT ANSWER: 3
Walking and talking with the client shows concern for her and fosters a therapeutic nurse-client relationship. Option 1: Behavior should never be ignored. Option 2: Reassuring the client that things will get better soon would provide the client with false reassurance. It could take some time for her to feel things are better. Option 4: Greeting the client with a friendly, cheerful smile could make the client feel intimidated and more worthless.
NP: Implementing care
CN: Psychosocial integrity
CNS: Psychosocial adaptation
CL: Application

96 A 61-year-old female client who was widowed 7 months ago is admitted to the psychiatric unit. Her family reports that she seemed to be coping well until 1 week ago, when she spoke of attempting suicide due to loneliness. Her son remarks that she's had enough time to grieve and needs to move on with her life. The nurse's appropriate response is:
- ☐ 1. "Seven months is long enough to grieve for anybody."
- ☐ 2. "How can you help her?"
- ☐ 3. "I think you need to give her support."
- ☐ 4. "Perhaps she needs more time; grieving can take 1 year or more."

CORRECT ANSWER: 4
The client needs to grieve in her own way, at her own pace. Option 1: Seven months might be enough time for some to work through the grieving process but isn't appropriate for all clients. Options 2 and 3: By asking family members how they can help the client or instructing them to give the client support the nurse incorrectly presumes that the client has had enough time to grieve and needs help to move on.
NP: Evaluating care
CN: Psychosocial integrity
CNS: Coping and adaptation
CL: Application

97 A 71-year-old male client is admitted to the psychiatric unit with a diagnosis of dementia. The client tells the nurse, "I have a date tonight. It's New Year's Eve you know." What is the nurse's most appropriate response?
- ☐ 1. "Oh, really. Who is your date?"
- ☐ 2. "It isn't New Year's Eve. You're silly."
- ☐ 3. "Today is Friday, April 7, 2000. We'll have lunch soon."
- ☐ 4. "Let me bring you some more medicine."

CORRECT ANSWER: 3
The nurse needs to reorient the client with reality. Option 1: Continuing the false conversation doesn't provide reality orientation. Option 2: Telling the client that he's silly pokes fun at the client. Option 4: By dismissing or ignoring the client's statement, the nurse isn't addressing the need to communicate with the client.
NP: Implementing care
CN: Psychosocial integrity
CNS: Psychosocial adaptation
CL: Application

98 The nurse is working in a psychiatric facility and is reviewing the clients' histories. The client with the highest suicide risk is:
- ☐ 1. middle-aged, married, unemployed, and plans to take an overdose.
- ☐ 2. adolescent, single, employed, and has no definite plan.
- ☐ 3. elderly, widowed, retired, and plans to shoot herself in the head.
- ☐ 4. middle-aged, divorced, chronically ill, and says she might kill herself.

CORRECT ANSWER: 3
The elderly client who plans to shoot herself in the head has the most definite and deadly plan. Option 1: An overdose isn't always deadly, making this client's plan less definite and deadly. Options 2 and 4: The clients described in these options have no definite plan for suicide.
NP: Collecting data
CN: Psychosocial integrity
CNS: Psychosocial adaptation
CL: Comprehension

99 The nurse finds a suicidal client trying to hang himself in his room. In order to preserve self-esteem and safety, the nurse should:
☐ 1. place the client in seclusion with checks every 15 minutes.
☐ 2. assign a nursing staff member to remain with the client at all times.
☐ 3. make the client stay with the group at all times.
☐ 4. refuse to let the client in his room.

CORRECT ANSWER: 2
Implementing a one-to-one staff-to-client ratio is the nurse's highest priority. This allows the client to maintain his self-esteem and keeps him safe. Option 1: Seclusion would damage the client's self-esteem. Options 3 and 4: Forcing the client to stay with the group and refusing to let him in his room doesn't guarantee his safety.
NP: Implementing care
CN: Psychosocial integrity
CNS: Psychosocial adaptation
CL: Application

100 A newly admitted client is diagnosed with schizophrenia. The client tells the nurse that the police are looking for him and will kill him if they find him. The nurse recognizes this as a delusion of which type?
☐ 1. Paranoid
☐ 2. Religious
☐ 3. Grandiose
☐ 4. Somatic

CORRECT ANSWER: 1
This client is exhibiting paranoid delusions, which are excessive or irrational suspicions or distrust of others. Option 2: A religious delusion is the belief that one is favored by a higher being or is an instrument of a higher being. Option 3: A grandiose delusion is the belief that one possesses greatness or special powers. Option 4: A somatic delusion is the belief that one's body or parts of one's body are distorted or diseased.
NP: Collecting data
CN: Psychosocial integrity
CNS: Psychosocial adaptation
CL: Knowledge

101 The nurse is assessing a 53-year-old male client and notes that he's having severe muscle contractions of the face and neck. Which nursing action is appropriate?
☐ 1. Obtain an order for physiotherapy.
☐ 2. Place the client in seclusion.
☐ 3. Place the client in Trendelenburg's position.
☐ 4. Administer an ordered anticholinergic.

CORRECT ANSWER: 4
The client needs immediate medication to treat the muscle rigidity, which is a part of acute dystonia. Options 1, 2, and 3: Obtaining an order for physiotherapy, placing the client in seclusion, and placing the client in Trendelenburg's position aren't appropriate actions and wouldn't be used to treat this client.
NP: Planning care
CN: Psychosocial integrity
CNS: Psychosocial adaptation
CL: Application

102 A client on the psychiatric unit is receiving lithium therapy and has a lithium level of 1 mEq/L. The nurse notes that the client has fine tremors of the hands. What should the nurse do?
☐ 1. Hold the client's next lithium dose.
☐ 2. Notify the physician immediately.
☐ 3. Have the lithium level repeated.
☐ 4. Realize that a fine tremor is expected.

CORRECT ANSWER: 4
Fine tremors of the hands are considered normal with lithium therapy. Options 1, 2, and 3: The lithium level is within normal limits so there is no need to hold a dose, notify the physician, or repeat the blood work.
NP: Implementing care
CN: Psychosocial integrity
CNS: Psychosocial adaptation
CL: Application

103 The nurse is caring for an 80-year-old male client who was admitted with a diagnosis of delirium secondary to drug toxicity. Which of the following is true about this client's diagnosis?
☐ 1. Metabolism in older clients is slower and allows medication to build up to toxic levels.
☐ 2. Older males experience delirium more frequently than older females.
☐ 3. The client is also probably diabetic.
☐ 4. The state of delirium is expected to last indefinitely.

CORRECT ANSWER: 1
Metabolism of drugs slows as the client gets older, allowing toxicity to build up. Older clients usually require lower doses of medications. Option 2: Males don't experience delirium more frequently than females. Option 3: It hasn't been established that the client is diabetic. Option 4: Delirium is classified as a reversible condition.
NP: Evaluating care
CN: Psychosocial integrity
CNS: Psychosocial adaptation
CL: Knowledge

104 A 31-year-old female client with a diagnosis of schizophrenia walks with the nurse to the dayroom but refuses to speak. What is the most therapeutic nursing intervention?
☐ 1. Ignore the refusal to speak and talk about something such as the weather.
☐ 2. Tell the client that the refusal to speak is making others uncomfortable.
☐ 3. Plan to spend time with the client, even in silence.
☐ 4. Make the client attend therapy with others so the other clients can encourage talking.

CORRECT ANSWER: 3
Spending time with the client lets her know that the nurse cares. Although sitting in silence can be awkward, it's therapeutic. Option 1: Ignoring the behavior and using small talk encourages the silence. Option 2: Telling the client about making others uncomfortable usually has no effect on the behavior. Option 4: Coercing the client to attend therapy with others would increase the silence.
NP: Implementing care
CN: Psychosocial integrity
CNS: Coping and adaptation
CL: Application

105 The nurse is having an interaction with a 38-year-old male delusional client. Which is the best nursing action?
☐ 1. Tell the client the delusions aren't real.
☐ 2. Explain the delusion to the client.
☐ 3. Encourage the client to remain delusional.
☐ 4. Begin to develop a trusting relationship with the client.

CORRECT ANSWER: 4
Developing a trusting relationship gives the nurse more therapeutic time with the client. Option 1: Never argue with or try to talk the client out of a delusion. The delusions are very real to them. Option 2: Explaining the delusions helps the nurse, not the client. Option 3: Encouraging the client to remain delusional isn't therapeutic.
NP: Implementing care
CN: Psychosocial integrity
CNS: Psychosocial adaptation
CL: Application

106 The nurse is caring for a 45-year-old female client who is having alcohol withdrawal delirium. Which nursing action has the highest priority?
☐ 1. Orientation to reality
☐ 2. Application of restraints
☐ 3. Replacement of fluids and electrolytes
☐ 4. Identification of support system

CORRECT ANSWER: 3
Alcohol withdrawal delirium is a medical emergency of paranoia, disorientation, delusions, hallucinations, elevated vital signs, vomiting, diarrhea, and diaphoresis. Fluid and electrolyte replacement is the nurse's top priority. Option 1: Orientation to reality is important but not the highest priority. Option 2: Restraints aren't always needed or appropriate for a client with alcohol withdrawal delirium. Option 4: Identifying the client's support system can be done later.
NP: Planning care
CN: Psychosocial integrity
CNS: Psychosocial adaptation
CL: Application

107 The nurse is instructing a client who is to receive disulfiram (Antabuse). Which substance would be safe for the client?
- ☐ 1. Aftershave lotion
- ☐ 2. Mouthwash
- ☐ 3. Back rub preparations
- ☐ 4. Antacids

CORRECT ANSWER: 4
Antacids don't interact with disulfiram. Options 1, 2, and 3: The client should avoid anything containing alcohol, including aftershave lotion, cough medicine, back rub preparations, and some mouthwashes.
NP: Planning care
CN: Psychosocial integrity
CNS: Psychosocial adaptation
CL: Comprehension

---

108 A 14-year-old female client is admitted to the psychiatric unit with a diagnosis of anorexia nervosa. She's emaciated and refuses to eat. Which nursing diagnosis has top priority?
- ☐ 1. *Imbalanced nutrition: Less than body requirements*
- ☐ 2. *Impaired urinary elimination*
- ☐ 3. *Anxiety*
- ☐ 4. *Interrupted family processes*

CORRECT ANSWER: 1
The nursing diagnosis with the highest priority refers to the client's nutritional status because it involves an issue that affects maintenance of life. Options 2, 3, and 4: The client might have many other problems related to the diagnosis of anorexia nervosa, such as impaired urinary elimination, anxiety, and interrupted family processes, but these don't take top priority.
NP: Planning care
CN: Psychosocial integrity
CNS: Psychosocial adaptation
CL: Comprehension

---

109 A 20-year-old female client is in the emergency department after being sexually assaulted by a stranger. Which nursing intervention has the highest priority?
- ☐ 1. Assist her in identifying which of her behaviors placed her at risk for the attack.
- ☐ 2. Make an appointment for her in 6 weeks at a local sexual assault crisis center.
- ☐ 3. Encourage discussion of her early childhood experiences.
- ☐ 4. Assist her in identifying family or friends who could provide immediate support for her.

CORRECT ANSWER: 4
The client needs a lot of support to help her through this ordeal. Option 1: Identifying behaviors that placed her at risk for the attack places the blame on the client. Option 2: The local crisis center needs to be called immediately. Option 3: Some psychiatric disorders are related to early childhood experiences but rape isn't.
NP: Implementing care
CN: Psychosocial integrity
CNS: Coping and adaptation
CL: Comprehension

---

110 The nurse is conducting a discharge planning session for a client diagnosed with mania. The client asks the nurse if he has to take his pills forever. Which is the nurse's most appropriate response?
- ☐ 1. "Yes, most likely you'll always have to take the medication."
- ☐ 2. "Yes, but only until you're symptom free."
- ☐ 3. "No, only until you're discharged."
- ☐ 4. "No, usually clients don't need medication after a year."

CORRECT ANSWER: 1
Clients with manic episodes usually must remain on medication for their entire lives to control the episodes. When a client is hospitalized, it's usually because the client has stopped taking his medicine. Options 2, 3, and 4: If the client stops taking the medication, his manic episodes will never be under control.
NP: Implementing care
CN: Psychosocial integrity
CNS: Psychosocial adaptation
CL: Comprehension

111 A 31-year-old male client with borderline personality disorder is instructed to stay in the game room. He asks the nurse to "bend the rules a little, just this one time." Which response is most appropriate?
☐ 1. "No."
☐ 2. "OK, but just this once."
☐ 3. Ignore the client.
☐ 4. "Let me explain the rules to you."

CORRECT ANSWER: 4
This allows the nurse to be firm but not confrontational with the client. Option 1: A simple "No" is too harsh by itself. The nurse's response needs more of an explanation. Option 2: By agreeing to bend the rules, the nurse would allow the client to manipulate the caregiver. Option 3: Ignoring the client would do nothing but frustrate him.
NP: Implementing care
CN: Psychosocial integrity
CNS: Psychosocial adaptation
CL: Application

112 The nurse is caring for a 33-year-old male client diagnosed with borderline personality disorder. The nurse tells the client that they'll be meeting for 1 hour every week on Monday at 1 p.m. The rationale for setting limits for a client with a personality disorder is to:
☐ 1. help the client clarify limits.
☐ 2. encourage the client to be manipulative.
☐ 3. provide the nurse with leverage against unacceptable behavior.
☐ 4. provide an opportunity for the client to assess the situation.

CORRECT ANSWER: 1
Clarifying limits and making clear what may be unclear to the client helps the client establish boundaries himself. This fosters a therapeutic, trusting relationship between the nurse and client. Option 2: The nurse should never encourage manipulation. Option 3: The nurse should never attempt to gather leverage against the client; that would be unprofessional. Option 4: The client needs to understand his behavior patterns before he can start assessing the situation.
NP: Implementing care
CN: Psychosocial integrity
CNS: Psychosocial adaptation
CL: Application

113 The nurse is caring for a client on the psychiatric unit who exhibits extrapyramidal adverse effects of antipsychotic medications. Which medication may be used to treat such extrapyramidal adverse effects?
☐ 1. chlorpromazine (Thorazine)
☐ 2. prochlorperazine (Compazine)
☐ 3. benztropine (Cogentin)
☐ 4. haloperidol (Haldol)

CORRECT ANSWER: 3
Cogentin is used to treat clients who exhibit such extrapyramidal adverse effects as motor abnormalities, including parkinsonism, pseudoparkinsonism, acute dystonia, and akathisia. Option 1: Thorazine is a phenothiazine antipsychotic medication. Option 2: Compazine is a phenothiazine and antiemetic. Option 4: Haldol is a butyrophenone antipsychotic medication.
NP: Planning care
CN: Psychosocial integrity
CNS: Psychosocial adaptation
CL: Knowledge

114 A 33-year-old female client diagnosed with bipolar 1 disorder is confrontational and rude to the other clients and staff. A positive nursing intervention for this behavior is to:
☐ 1. suggest that the nurse and the client go for a walk on the patio.
☐ 2. promise the client a trip to the movies if behavior improves.
☐ 3. explain why this behavior is inappropriate.
☐ 4. engage the client in a game of checkers.

CORRECT ANSWER: 1
The nurse should redirect negative behaviors in a calm, firm, and nondefensive manner. Accompany the client on walks and provide other gross motor activities in an open, secure area to expend and refocus energy and prevent escalation of the behavior. Option 2: The nurse should make only realistic promises that can be kept because a broken promise would elicit mistrust. Options 3 and 4: A client with bipolar 1 disorder commonly isn't able to understand long explanations and can't tolerate competitive games.
NP: Implementing care
CN: Psychosocial integrity
CNS: Psychosocial adaptation
CL: Application

115 The nurse is caring for a 39-year-old female client admitted to the chemical dependency unit for detoxification. The family reports that the client usually starts drinking early in the morning and continues at intervals all day. When would the first signs of alcohol withdrawal symptoms most likely occur?
- ☐ 1. 6 to 12 hours after the last drink
- ☐ 2. 48 to 72 hours after the last drink
- ☐ 3. 4 days after the last drink
- ☐ 4. 5 or more days after the last drink

CORRECT ANSWER: 1
When alcohol or any drug of abuse is terminated abruptly by a person who is physiologically dependent, a specific pattern of signs and symptoms begins within 6 to 12 hours after heavy alcohol use ceases. Options 2, 3, and 4: The symptoms of withdrawal begin much sooner than 2, 3, 4, 5, or more days after the last drink and may last 7 to 10 days.
NP: Collecting data
CN: Psychosocial integrity
CNS: Psychosocial adaptation
CL: Application

116 A 28-year-old male client with the diagnosis of schizophrenia tells the nurse that he constantly hears a voice that yells at him and tells him to do bad things. The nurse's best response is to:
- ☐ 1. say, "You know that can't be true."
- ☐ 2. say, "I realize the voices are real to you, but I don't hear anything."
- ☐ 3. send the client to his room for "time out."
- ☐ 4. immediately touch the client on the shoulder to show acceptance.

CORRECT ANSWER: 2
The nurse shouldn't reinforce the hallucination; saying "the voices" rather than "they" denies validation and lets the client know that you don't share the perception. Such early interventions may prevent an aggressive response to command hallucinations. Option 1: Saying "You know that can't be true" is demeaning to the client. Option 3: "Time out" may be perceived as punishment and isn't appropriate in this situation. Option 4: Avoid touching the client without warning. The client may perceive touch as threatening and respond aggressively.
NP: Implementing care
CN: Psychosocial integrity
CNS: Psychosocial adaptation.
CL: Application

117 The nurse is caring for a 51-year-old female client diagnosed with obsessive-compulsive disorder. She spends many hours each day counting everyone named Mary in the phone book. What is the most likely reason for this counting ritual?
- ☐ 1. It relieves the client's anxiety.
- ☐ 2. It gives the client some element of control over her life.
- ☐ 3. It gives the client a sense of pleasure.
- ☐ 4. It increases the client's self-esteem.

CORRECT ANSWER: 1
Compulsive acts tend to reduce a client's feeling of anxiety. The client recognizes that the behavior is excessive or unreasonable but because it promotes a feeling of relief from discomfort, she feels compelled to continue the act. Options 2, 3, and 4: Performing compulsive acts doesn't provide pleasure or gratification and doesn't give the client feelings of control over her life or increase her self-esteem. The client may instead feel controlled, weak, and ineffectual because she can't control the rituals.
NP: Collecting data
CN: Psychosocial integrity
CNS: Psychosocial adaptation
CL: Application

118 The nurse is caring for a 53-year-old male client with posttraumatic stress disorder who is experiencing a frightening flashback. The nurse can best offer reassurance of safety and security by:
- ☐ 1. encouraging the client to talk about the traumatic event.
- ☐ 2. assessing for maladaptive coping strategies.
- ☐ 3. staying with the client.
- ☐ 4. acknowledging feelings of guilt or self-blame.

CORRECT ANSWER: 3
The nurse should stay with the client during periods of flashbacks and nightmares. Offer reassurance of safety and security and assure the client that these symptoms aren't uncommon following a severe trauma. Options 1, 2, and 4: Although all of the options may be carried out in the future, the nurse's top priority during the flashback is to stay with the client.
NP: Implementing interventions
CN: Psychosocial integrity
CNS: Psychosocial adaptation
CL: Application

119 A 36-year-old male client diagnosed with bipolar 1 disorder is receiving lithium carbonate 900 mg daily in divided doses. During discharge teaching, the nurse instructs the client to:
☐ 1. limit his intake of dietary sodium.
☐ 2. increase his calorie intake.
☐ 3. discontinue the medication when his symptoms subside.
☐ 4. notify the physician if persistent nausea, vomiting, and diarrhea occur.

CORRECT ANSWER: 4
The physician should be notified of persistent nausea, vomiting, and diarrhea because these are signs of lithium toxicity. Options 1 and 2: Adequate sodium and other nutrients should be included in the diet while decreasing the number of calories. Option 3: The client should take the medication on a regular basis even when he feels well because discontinuation can cause the symptoms to return.
NP: Implementing care
CN: Physiological integrity
CNS: Pharmacological therapies
CL: Application

120 A few weeks after learning that she has a breast malignancy, a 42-year-old client lashes out at the nurse, saying, "I hate all of you. You aren't doing anything for me!" The nurse recognizes this as which stage of the grief process?
☐ 1. Stage I: Denial
☐ 2. Stage II: Anger
☐ 3. Stage III: Bargaining
☐ 4. Stage IV: Depression

CORRECT ANSWER: 2
The second stage of the grief process is when reality sets in. Self-blame or blaming others may lead to feelings of anger toward self and others. Option 1: Denial is the first stage of the grief process and the individual doesn't acknowledge that a loss has occurred. Option 3: Bargaining involves striking a bargain with God for a second chance. Option 4: In the depression stage of grief, the individual mourns for that which has or will be lost.
NP: Collecting data
CN: Psychosocial integrity
CNS: Coping and adaptation
CL: Application

121 A home health care nurse is caring for a client diagnosed with a conversion disorder manifested by paralysis in the left arm. An organic cause for the deficit has been ruled out. Which nursing intervention is most appropriate for this client?
☐ 1. Perform all physical tasks for the client to foster dependence.
☐ 2. Allot an hour each day to discuss the paralysis and its cause.
☐ 3. Identify primary or secondary gains that the physical symptom provides.
☐ 4. Allow the client to withdraw from all physical activities.

CORRECT ANSWER: 3
Primary or secondary gains should be identified because these are etiological factors that can be used in problem resolution. Option 1: The nurse should encourage the client to be as independent as possible and intervene only when the client requires assistance. Option 2: The nurse shouldn't focus on the disability. Option 4: The nurse should encourage the client to perform physical activities to the greatest extent possible.
NP: Implementing care
CN: Psychosocial integrity
CNS: Psychosocial adaptation
CL: Application

122 A 48-year-old male client is being maintained on clozapine (Clozaril) in the treatment of schizophrenia. Which of the following instructions in the client's discharge teaching plan takes top priority?
☐ 1. Report weekly to have blood levels drawn and obtain a weekly supply of the drug.
☐ 2. Rise slowly from a sitting or lying position to prevent a sudden decrease in blood pressure.
☐ 3. Don't consume over-the-counter medications without the physician's approval.
☐ 4. Take frequent sips of water, chew sugarless gum, or suck on hard candy if dry mouth is a problem.

CORRECT ANSWER: 1
Stressing the importance of weekly blood tests takes top priority in this client's discharge teaching plan because agranulocytosis (potentially lethal reduction of granulocytes) occurs in 1 to 2 percent of all clients taking clozapine. Options 2, 3, and 4: Although all of the listed instructions should be a part of the discharge teaching plan, the need for weekly blood tests has top priority.
NP: Implementing care
CN: Physiological integrity
CNS: Pharmacological therapies
CL: Application

123 A client who is taking haloperidol (Haldol) in the treatment of Tourette syndrome seems confused and complains of severe muscle rigidity. The nurse observes that the client is diaphoretic. The client's temperature is 105.8° F (41° C) and his pulse rate is 120 beats/minute. Which disorder should the nurse suspect?
☐ 1. Tardive dyskinesia
☐ 2. Neuroleptic malignant syndrome
☐ 3. Pseudoparkinsonism
☐ 4. Oculogyric crisis

CORRECT ANSWER: 2
The nurse should immediately suspect neuroleptic malignant syndrome. The symptoms of this disorder include parkinsonian muscle rigidity, diaphoresis, hyperpyrexia up to 107° F (41.7° C), and tachypnea; death may occur. Option 1: The symptoms of tardive dyskinesia include bizarre facial and tongue movements, stiff neck, and difficulty swallowing. Option 3: Pseudoparkinsonism is a reversible extrapyramidal adverse effect. Option 4: Oculogyric crisis is uncontrolled rolling back of the eyes.
NP: Collecting data
CN: Physiological integrity
CNS: Pharmacological therapies
CL: Application

---

124 The nurse is caring for a client who is to receive electroconvulsive therapy. Which statement by the client shows the need for further teaching by the nurse?
☐ 1. "I realize that this treatment will be painful but I know that it's necessary."
☐ 2. "I know that I'll have to sign a consent form."
☐ 3. "I can't eat or drink anything for several hours before the treatment."
☐ 4. "I'll have to remove my contact lenses before the treatment."

CORRECT ANSWER: 1
The client will be given a short-acting anesthetic by the anesthesiologist and won't feel any pain during the treatment. Options 2, 3, and 4 show that the client understands the preparation needed for the treatment.
NP: Collecting data
CN: Psychosocial integrity
CNS: Psychosocial adaptation
CL: Application

---

125 The nurse is caring for a 75-year-old man who is in the psychiatric unit with the diagnosis of depression. His wife was killed in an automobile accident that occurred while he was driving. The client states, "I have nothing to live for now." The nurse's best response is to say:
☐ 1. "You need to cheer up and get involved in unit activities."
☐ 2. "Everyone feels that way sometimes."
☐ 3. "Are you thinking about harming yourself?"
☐ 4. to say nothing and report the comment during a team conference.

CORRECT ANSWER: 3
The client's statement may be a verbal clue to suicidal intent. Asking a depressed person about suicide doesn't plant the idea in his mind and not asking the client may increase the risk. Options 1 and 2: Don't try to talk the client out of his sadness by being overly optimistic and inappropriately cheerful or by offering false reassurance. Option 4: If the nurse distances from or overtly rejects the client and his feelings, the client's belief that it isn't safe to express his feelings is reinforced.
NP: Implementing care
CN: Psychosocial integrity
CNS: Psychosocial adaptation
CL: Application

---

126 The nurse notices that a 33-year-old male client with borderline personality disorder is very manipulative and plays one staff member against another. The best way to deal with this behavior is to:
☐ 1. consistently enforce limits when the client attempts to manipulate.
☐ 2. seek the client's approval for any change in routine on the unit.
☐ 3. allow the client to bend the unit rules rather than entering into power struggles.
☐ 4. assign the client to the same staff member to maintain consistency.

CORRECT ANSWER: 1
The staff must be consistent in setting limits on all negative behaviors. Situations can escalate to crisis level when limit-setting is inconsistent. Option 2: The nurse should inform the client about changes in unit routines but shouldn't seek his approval. Option 3: Allowing the client to bend the unit rules is a form of manipulation and shouldn't be allowed. Option 4: Staff members should be rotated so that the client can learn to relate to more than one person.
NP: Implementing care
CN: Psychosocial integrity
CNS: Psychosocial adaptation
CL: Application

127 A client who is diagnosed with paranoid schizophrenia tells the nurse that a computer chip placed in his brain has informed him that his wife is cheating. What is the nurse's best response?
- ☐ 1. Attempt to disprove the delusion.
- ☐ 2. Ignore the client's statement and engage him in a game of pool.
- ☐ 3. Allow the client to write a letter to his wife expressing his thoughts.
- ☐ 4. Convey acceptance of the client's need for false belief but that you don't share the belief.

CORRECT ANSWER: 4
By conveying acceptance of the client's need for false belief, the nurse promotes trust with the client. The client must understand that the nurse doesn't view the idea as real. Option 1: Attempting to disprove the delusion may provoke agitation and doesn't foster trust or enhance the client's sense of safety and reality. Option 2: Provide noncompetitive activities and avoid aggressive games requiring close physical contact. Option 3: Allowing the client to write a letter to his wife expressing irrational thoughts would lead the client to think that the nurse shares the false belief and wouldn't be therapeutic.
NP: Implementing care
CN: Psychosocial integrity
CNS: Psychosocial adaptation
CL: Application

128 A 21-year-old female client undergoing treatment for schizophrenia becomes hostile and begins shouting obscenities while in the dayroom with other clients. What should the nurse do first?
- ☐ 1. Maintain a low level of stimulus in the client's environment.
- ☐ 2. Maintain and convey a calm attitude to the client.
- ☐ 3. Administer tranquilizing medications as ordered by the physician.
- ☐ 4. Discuss with the client alternate ways of handling frustration.

CORRECT ANSWER: 2
The nurse should first maintain and convey a calm attitude to the client because anxiety can be transferred from staff members to a client. Options 1, 3, and 4: Maintaining a low level of stimulus, administering ordered medications, and discussing ways to handle frustration are parts of the nursing plan of care but maintaining and conveying a calm attitude is the nurse's first priority.
NP: Implementing care
CN: Psychosocial integrity
CNS: Psychosocial adaptation
CL: Application

129 The nurse is instructing a 53-year-old female client about using the antianxiety medication lorazepam (Ativan). Which of the following statements by the client indicates a need for further teaching?
- ☐ 1. "I should get up slowly from a sitting or lying position."
- ☐ 2. "I shouldn't stop taking this medicine abruptly."
- ☐ 3. "I usually drink a beer every night to help me sleep."
- ☐ 4. "If I have a sore throat, I should report it to my physician."

CORRECT ANSWER: 3
The client shouldn't consume alcohol or any other central nervous system depressant while taking this drug. Options 1, 2, and 4: All of these statements indicate that the client understands the nurse's instructions.
NP: Collecting data
CN: Physiological integrity
CNS: Pharmacological therapies
CL: Application

130 A nurse on the psychiatric unit is caring for a 27-year-old male client who is experiencing a panic attack. The best initial nursing intervention in this case is to:
☐ 1. move the client to a less stimulating environment.
☐ 2. focus the client's energy on a repetitive or physically tiring task.
☐ 3. describe in detail what is happening to the client.
☐ 4. stay with the client.

CORRECT ANSWER: 4
It's important for the nurse to remain with the client during a panic attack because being left alone may further increase the anxiety. Option 1: Later, the client can be moved to a less stimulating environment to prevent further disruption of the perceptual field by sensory stimuli. Option 2: Repetitive tasks or physical exercise can help to drain off excess energy and may be used later. Option 3: The client is having difficulty focusing, so the nurse should use short, simple sentences.
NP: Implementing care
CN: Psychosocial integrity
CNS: Psychosocial adaptation
CL: Application

131 The nurse is caring for a 22-year-old female client with bulimia. The best way to assess the client for self-induced vomiting is to:
☐ 1. keep an accurate record of intake and output.
☐ 2. observe the client closely for 1 to 2 hours after meals.
☐ 3. weigh the client immediately after her first voiding.
☐ 4. observe the client for nausea after meals.

CORRECT ANSWER: 2
The client should be observed for at least 1 hour following meals; otherwise, this time may be used to discard food or engage in self-induced vomiting. The nurse may need to accompany the client to the bathroom if self-induced vomiting is suspected. Options 1 and 3: Strict documentation of intake and output is required to promote the client's safety and to plan nursing care but isn't the best way to assess for self-induced vomiting. Option 4: Self-induced vomiting isn't caused by nausea.
NP: Collecting data
CN: Psychosocial integrity
CNS: Psychosocial adaptation
CL: Application

132 A 34-year-old male client who is being maintained on the monoamine oxidase (MAO) inhibitor phenelzine (Nardil) is experiencing a hypertensive crisis. The physician writes all of the following orders for the client. Which one should the nurse carry out first?
☐ 1. Administer short acting antihypertensive medication.
☐ 2. Monitor vital signs.
☐ 3. Use external cooling measures to control hyperpyrexia.
☐ 4. Discontinue phenelzine.

CORRECT ANSWER: 4
The MAO inhibitor phenelzine should be discontinued immediately, as ordered, in the client experiencing a hypertensive crisis. Options 1, 2, and 3: The client's vital signs should be monitored, external cooling measures to control hyperpyrexia should be started, and short-acting antihypertensive medication should be administered according to a physician's order.
NP: Implementing care
CN: Physiological integrity
CNS: Pharmacological therapies
CL: Application

133 The nurse is caring for a client admitted to the psychiatric unit following an automobile accident in which his wife and child were killed. The client is unable to remember details of the accident. The nurse recognizes this as:
- ☐ 1. projection.
- ☐ 2. isolation.
- ☐ 3. repression.
- ☐ 4. regression.

CORRECT ANSWER: 3
Repression is the involuntary forcing of unacceptable ideas and impulses into the unconscious. Option 1: In projection, emotions, behaviors, and motives that are consciously intolerable are denied and then attributed to others. Option 2: Isolation is the separation of the emotional component from a thought. Option 4: Regression is the return to patterns of behavior and gratification that are more typical of a child.
NP: Collecting data
CN: Psychosocial integrity
CNS: Psychosocial adaptation
CL: Comprehension

134 A nurse on the psychiatric unit is caring for a client with an antisocial personality disorder. Which behavior is the nurse most likely to observe?
- ☐ 1. Manipulation, shallowness, and the need for immediate gratification
- ☐ 2. Tendency to profit from mistakes or learn from past experiences
- ☐ 3. Expression of guilt and anxiety regarding behavior
- ☐ 4. Acceptance of authority and discipline

CORRECT ANSWER: 1
Due to the client's lack of scruples and underlying powerlessness, the nurse expects to see manipulation, shallowness, impulsivity, and self-centered behavior. Options 2, 3, and 4: This client doesn't profit from mistakes and learn from past experiences, lacks anxiety and guilt, and is unable to accept authority and discipline.
NP: Collecting data
CN: Psychosocial integrity
CNS: Psychosocial adaptation
CL: Application

135 The nurse is caring for a 43-year-old female client who has been on antidepressant medication for 3 weeks in the treatment of prolonged depression after the death of her 17-year-old son. Which behavior alerts the nurse to the possibility of suicide?
- ☐ 1. The client attends a grief group.
- ☐ 2. The client is more energetic and appears calm and satisfied.
- ☐ 3. The client verbalizes decreased desire for self-harm.
- ☐ 4. The client participates in forming a no-suicide contract with the nurse.

CORRECT ANSWER: 2
During the 2nd or 3rd week of antidepressant drug therapy, clients have increased energy but their depression hasn't been resolved. The nurse must be alert for suicide because the client's energy level is high enough to carry out a plan. Options 1, 3, and 4: Attending a grief group, expressing a decreased desire for self-harm, and forming a no-suicide contract with the nurse wouldn't alert the nurse to immediate suicidal behavior.
NP: Collecting data
CN: Psychosocial integrity
CNS: Psychosocial adaptation
CL: Application

136 The nurse is planning care for a client who was admitted with dementia due to Alzheimer's disease. The family reports that the client has to be watched closely for wandering behavior at night. Which nursing diagnosis is the nurse's top priority for this client?
- ☐ 1. *Disturbed sleep pattern*
- ☐ 2. *Activity intolerance*
- ☐ 3. *Disturbed sensory perception*
- ☐ 4. *Risk for injury*

CORRECT ANSWER: 4
Providing a safe, effective care environment takes priority in this case. Options 1, 2, and 3: Disturbed sleep pattern, activity intolerance, and disturbed sensory perception fall under physical integrity and, although important, they aren't as important as providing a safe, effective care environment.
NP: Collecting data
CN: Psychosocial integrity
CNS: Psychosocial adaptation
CL: Application

137 The nurse is caring for a client diagnosed with histrionic personality disorder. The client is observed tearing pages out of the books in the unit library and putting them into the ventilation system. The best initial nursing intervention is to:
- ☐ 1. place the client in a safe, secluded environment.
- ☐ 2. help the client develop more acceptable methods of seeking attention.
- ☐ 3. withdraw attention from the client at this time.
- ☐ 4. identify inappropriate behaviors to the client in a matter-of-fact manner.

CORRECT ANSWER: 1
If the client begins destroying property or presenting potential harm to self or others, it may be necessary to immediately place the client in a safe, secluded environment. Option 2: When the client regains control and ceases the behavior, then attempt to talk to him to explore more acceptable ways of handling frustration and expressing feelings. Option 3: Lack of attention from the nurse wouldn't reduce the client's attention-seeking behaviors. Option 4: When the client regains control and ceases the behavior, the nurse must make it clear which behaviors are inappropriate.
NP: Implementing care
CN: Psychosocial integrity
CNS: Psychosocial adaptation
CL: Application

138 The nurse is caring for a 58-year-old male client diagnosed with paranoid schizophrenia. When the client says, "the earth and the roof of the house rule the political structure with particles of rain," the nurse recognizes this as:
- ☐ 1. tangentiality.
- ☐ 2. perseveration.
- ☐ 3. loose associations.
- ☐ 4. thought blocking.

CORRECT ANSWER: 3
Loose associations refers to changing ideas from one unrelated theme to another. Option 1: Tangentiality is the wandering from topic to topic. Option 2: Perseveration is involuntary repetition of the answer to a question in response to a new question. Option 4: Thought blocking is having difficulty articulating a response or stopping midsentence.
NP: Collecting data
CN: Psychosocial integrity
CNS: Psychosocial adaptation
CL: Application

139 A client with a diagnosis of Alzheimer's-type dementia approaches the nurse and states, "There is nothing wrong with my mind. My physician put me here to help me get my disability check. Will you tell the physician that there is nothing wrong with my mind so I can go home?" Which is the most appropriate response by the nurse?
- ☐ 1. "I think you should try to make the best of the situation."
- ☐ 2. "I don't believe that. Why else would you be here?"
- ☐ 3. "Are you saying that your mind seems okay to you?"
- ☐ 4. "No one here would lie to you."

CORRECT ANSWER: 3
The most therapeutic response in this case puts into words what the client has implied. Option 1: By telling the client to make the best of the situation the nurse is giving nontherapeutic advice. Option 2: By expressing disbelief and asking the client for another explanation, the nurse is refusing to consider the client's ideas. Option 4: By telling the client that no one would lie, the nurse is rejecting the client's ideas.
NP: Implementing care
CN: Psychosocial integrity
CNS: Psychosocial adaptation
CL: Application

140 A 24-year-old male client is undergoing treatment for hallucinations with an antipsychotic medication. Which of the following symptoms should alert the nurse to the possibility of early agranulocytosis?
- ☐ 1. Pigmentation of the skin and eyes
- ☐ 2. Phototoxicity
- ☐ 3. Sedation
- ☐ 4. Severe sore throat, fever, and malaise

CORRECT ANSWER: 4
Agranulocytosis is the severe reduction of granulocytes and is a potentially lethal adverse effect of antipsychotic medications. It's suspected if severe sore throat, fever, and malaise develop. Option 1: Pigmentation of the skin and eyes is a temporary reaction to the antipsychotic medication and isn't permanent. Option 2: Phototoxicity is extreme sensitivity of the skin to sunburn. Option 3: Sedation is an adverse effect that usually resolves without treatment in 1 to 2 weeks.
NP: Collecting data
CN: Physiological integrity
CNS: Pharmacological therapies
CL: Application

141 The nurse is caring for a client who is undergoing treatment for acute alcohol dependence. The client tells the nurse, "I don't have a problem. My wife made me come here." What defense mechanism is the client using?
- ☐ 1. Projection and suppression
- ☐ 2. Denial and rationalization
- ☐ 3. Rationalization and repression
- ☐ 4. Suppression and denial

CORRECT ANSWER: 2
The client is using denial and rationalization. Denial is the unconscious disclaimer of unacceptable thoughts, feelings, needs, or certain external factors. Rationalization is the unconscious effort to justify intolerable feelings, behaviors, and motives. The client isn't using projection, suppression, or repression. Options 1 and 4: Emotions, behavior, and motives, which are consciously intolerable, are denied and then attributed to others in projection. Suppression is a conscious effort to control and conceal unacceptable ideas and impulses into the unconscious. Option 3: Repression is the unconscious placement of unacceptable feelings into the unconscious mind.
NP: Collecting data
CN: Physiological integrity
CNS: Physiological adaptation
CL: Application

142 The nurse finds a 78-year-old client with Alzheimer's-type dementia wandering in the hall at 3 a.m. The client has removed his clothing and says to the nurse, "I'm just taking a stroll through the park." What is the best approach to this behavior?
- ☐ 1. Immediately help the client back to his room and into some clothing.
- ☐ 2. Tell the client that such behavior won't be tolerated.
- ☐ 3. Tell the client it's too early in the morning to be taking a stroll.
- ☐ 4. Ask the client if he would like to go back to his room.

CORRECT ANSWER: 1
The nurse shouldn't allow the client to embarrass himself in front of others. Intervene as soon as the behavior is observed. Option 2: Scolding the client isn't helpful because it isn't something the client can understand. Option 3: Don't engage in social chatter. The interaction with this client should be concrete and specific. Option 4: Don't ask the client to choose unnecessarily. The client may not be able to make appropriate choices.
NP: Implementing care
CN: Psychosocial integrity
CNS: Psychosocial adaptation
CL: Application

143 The nurse is providing nursing care to a client with Alzheimer's-type dementia. Which nursing intervention takes priority?
- ☐ 1. Establish a routine that supports former habits.
- ☐ 2. Maintain physical surroundings that are cheerful and pleasant.
- ☐ 3. Maintain an exact routine from day to day.
- ☐ 4. Control the environment by providing structure, boundaries, and safety.

CORRECT ANSWER: 4
By controlling the environment and providing structure and boundaries, the nurse is helping to keep the client safe and secure, which is a top-priority nursing measure. Options 1, 2 and 3: Establishing a routine that supports former habits and maintaining cheerful and pleasant surroundings and an exact routine foster a supportive environment but keeping the client safe and secure takes priority.
NP: Implementing care
CN: Psychosocial integrity
CNS: Psychosocial adaptation
CL: Application

144 The nurse is caring for a client who is receiving fluoxetine (Prozac) in the treatment of depression. The client tells the nurse that the medication isn't doing him any good and he's going to stop taking it. Which response by the nurse would be the most therapeutic?
- ☐ 1. "Your physician has ordered the medicine and she knows what is best for you."
- ☐ 2. "Why do you think that? It has helped you before."
- ☐ 3. "We don't have time to discuss that; you're running late for group therapy."
- ☐ 4. "You don't think you should take your medicine because you feel it isn't doing you any good."

CORRECT ANSWER: 4
The nurse should repeat the main idea of what the client said. The client then knows whether the statement was understood and has a chance to continue or clarify if necessary. Option 1: Telling the client that his physician knows what is good for him is belittling and talking down to the client. Option 2: Asking why a client feels a certain way is intimidating and implies that he must defend his behavior or feelings. Option 3: Appearing too rushed to communicate with the client shows rejection and could cause the client to stop interacting with the nurse.
NP: Implementing care
CN: Psychosocial integrity
CNS: Psychosocial adaptation
CL: Application

145 The nurse is caring for a 25-year-old female who is exhibiting signs of very low self-esteem. Which client outcome is desirable?
- ☐ 1. The client will participate in new activities without voicing extreme fear of failure.
- ☐ 2. The client will sleep without interruption at night.
- ☐ 3. The client will be encouraged to confront fear of failure.
- ☐ 4. The nurse will spend time with the client.

CORRECT ANSWER: 1
A desired client outcome for a person with low self-esteem is participation in new activities without exhibiting extreme fear of failure. Options 2, 3, and 4: Allowing the client to sleep without interruption, encouraging the client to confront fear of failure, and spending time with the client are nursing interventions.
NP: Implementing care
CN: Psychosocial integrity
CNS: Psychosocial adaptation
CL: Application

146 The nurse is conducting a discharge evaluation on a 20-year-old female client with anorexia nervosa. Which outcome shows that the client's self-concept has improved?
- ☐ 1. The client has reached 80% of body weight for age and size.
- ☐ 2. The client doesn't describe herself as fat when looking in the mirror.
- ☐ 3. The client consumes adequate calories as determined by the dietitian.
- ☐ 4. The client understands how she has used maladaptive eating behaviors in an effort to control life events.

CORRECT ANSWER: 2
When the client's self-concept has improved, she would state that viewing her body as fat was a misperception. Options 1, 3, and 4: Reaching an appropriate body weight, consuming adequate calories, and understanding her use of maladaptive eating behaviors show that other goals of therapy have been met.
NP: Collecting data
CN: Psychosocial integrity
CNS: Psychosocial adaptation
CL: Application

147 The nurse is instructing a client who is being discharged on disulfiram (Antabuse). Which statement by the client indicates the need for further teaching by the nurse?
- [ ] 1. "I won't use liquid cough and cold preparations."
- [ ] 2. "This medicine will cure my alcoholism."
- [ ] 3. "I'll carry an identification card that says that I'm taking this drug."
- [ ] 4. "I'll continue to go to my Alcoholics Anonymous meetings."

CORRECT ANSWER: 2
Disulfiram therapy isn't a cure for alcoholism. It provides a measure of control for the individual who desires to avoid impulse drinking. Options 1, 3, and 4: These options show that the nurse's teaching was effective and that the client understands the purpose and appropriate use of the drug.
NP: Collecting data
CN: Physiological integrity
CNS: Pharmacological therapies
CL: Application

148 The nurse is caring for an 88-year-old female client in a nursing home. The client is confused and thinks she's in a train station. Which response to this behavior is the nurse's top priority?
- [ ] 1. Correct errors in the client's perception of reality in a matter-of-fact manner.
- [ ] 2. Have a conversation with the client when this behavior occurs.
- [ ] 3. Observe the client and know her whereabouts at all times.
- [ ] 4. Refer to the date, time, and place during interactions with client.

CORRECT ANSWER: 3
The nurse's top priority is to maintain safety and security for the client by observing her and knowing her whereabouts at all times, otherwise, the client may wander off and endanger herself. Options 1, 2, and 4: Correcting errors in the client's perception, conversing with her, and orienting her to date, time, and place are important but don't have the highest priority in this case.
NP: Implementing care
CN: Psychosocial integrity
CNS: Psychosocial adaptation
CL: Application

149 The nurse is caring for a 31-year-old male client who is receiving the tricyclic antidepressant amitriptyline (Elavil). Which anticholinergic adverse effects is this client most likely to develop?
- [ ] 1. Sedation and weight gain
- [ ] 2. Hypertension and anuria
- [ ] 3. Orthostatic hypotension and tachycardia
- [ ] 4. Dry mouth, constipation, and urinary hesitancy

CORRECT ANSWER: 4
Amitriptyline is one of the most potent anticholinergic agents. The client may develop such adverse effects as dry mouth, constipation, and urinary hesitancy. Options 1 and 3: Sedation, weight gain, orthostatic hypotension, and tachycardia are common adverse effects of this medication but aren't anticholinergic adverse effects. Option 2: Hypertension and anuria aren't commonly seen adverse effects of tricyclic antidepressants.
NP: Collecting data
CN: Psychosocial integrity
CNS: Pharmacological therapies
CL: Application

150 A client is exhibiting anxiety, which is evidenced by muscle tension, hypervigilance, distractibility, and increased vital signs. Which nursing intervention has top priority?
- [ ] 1. Remain with the client and use a soft voice and reassuring approach.
- [ ] 2. Assist the client to identify factors that contribute to anxiety.
- [ ] 3. Teach relaxation techniques such as deep breathing and muscle relaxation.
- [ ] 4. Administer antianxiety medications as appropriate.

CORRECT ANSWER: 1
The priority nursing intervention is to remain with the client and use a soft voice and reassuring approach. Remaining with the client provides for his safety and a soft voice is calming and reassuring, which will add to his feelings of safety and protection. Options 2, 3, and 4: Interventions such as identifying factors that contribute to anxiety, teaching relaxation techniques, and administering antianxiety medications are included in the client's plan of care but should be addressed later.
NP: Implementing care
CN: Psychosocial integrity
CNS: Psychosocial adaptation
CL: Application

151 The nurse on the psychiatric unit is caring for a 51-year-old male client who is suicidal. Which nursing intervention takes priority?
- [ ] 1. Discourage sleeping except at bedtime.
- [ ] 2. Make a verbal contract with the client to notify the staff of suicidal thoughts.
- [ ] 3. Limit time spent alone by encouraging the client to participate in group activities.
- [ ] 4. Create a safe physical and interpersonal environment.

CORRECT ANSWER: 4

Creating a safe environment is the nurse's highest priority intervention. This includes removing obvious hazards, recognizing nonobvious and emerging hazards, maintaining close observation, serving as a client advocate in interpersonal situations, and communicating concern to the client in both verbal and nonverbal ways. Options 1, 2, and 3: Other interventions, such as discouraging sleep except at bedtime, making a verbal contract, and encouraging participation in group activities, should be included in the client's plan of care but don't have top priority.

NP: Implementing care
CN: Psychosocial integrity
CNS: Psychosocial adaptation
CL: Application

---

152 A 34-year-old female in a homeless shelter tells the nurse, "I lost my job, my house, and my car. All my friends have turned their backs on me." What is the nurse's best response?
- [ ] 1. "Anyone can have a run of bad luck."
- [ ] 2. "It sounds as if you've really been hurt."
- [ ] 3. "Every cloud has a silver lining."
- [ ] 4. "You should learn a new trade; then you can find a job."

CORRECT ANSWER: 2

By saying, "It sounds as if you've really been hurt," the nurse is paraphrasing the content and feeling of the client's message. Paraphrasing helps to highlight important parts of the client's message that may otherwise be lost. Option 1: This is a stereotypical comment. Option 3: This statement gives false reassurance. Option 4: Giving job advice at this time is nontherapeutic.

NP: Implementing care
CN: Psychosocial integrity
CNS: Psychosocial adaptation
CL: Application

---

153 A 46-year-old male client undergoing treatment for paranoia refuses to take his fluphenazine (Prolixin) because he says he thinks it's poisoned. The nurse's response should be to:
- [ ] 1. omit the dose and notify the physician.
- [ ] 2. tell him that he'll receive an injection if he refuses the oral medication.
- [ ] 3. put the medication in his juice without informing him.
- [ ] 4. allow him to examine the medication to see that it isn't poisoned.

CORRECT ANSWER: 1

The nurse's best response is to omit the dose and notify the physician because insisting that the client take the medication will only increase his paranoia and agitation. Options 2 and 3: Forcing injections and tricking clients into taking medication is illegal. Don't put the medication in his juice without informing him. Option 4: A rational approach to irrational ideas seldom works.

NP: Implementing care
CN: Physiological integrity
CNS: Pharmacological therapies
CL: Application

---

154 A 51-year-old female client is being started on an antipsychotic medication. Which of the following should the nurse be aware of when administering antipsychotics?
- [ ] 1. Antipsychotic drugs have reduced absorption if taken with antacids.
- [ ] 2. Antipsychotic drugs don't generally cause sedation.
- [ ] 3. Antipsychotic drugs have few serious adverse effects.
- [ ] 4. Antipsychotic drugs raise the client's seizure threshold.

CORRECT ANSWER: 1

Antacids can decrease the absorption of antipsychotic drugs. Options 2, 3, and 4: Antipsychotic drugs can cause sedation and many other adverse effects. They should be given with caution to clients who have seizure problems because they lower the seizure threshold.

NP: Implementing care
CN: Physiological integrity
CNS: Pharmacological therapies
CL: Application

Psychiatric Nursing

155 A newly admitted client's medical diagnosis is obsessive-compulsive disorder. For several minutes, the nurse has observed the client pacing in the hallway. Repeatedly, the client takes three long steps, stops momentarily, and then takes three short steps. In planning an approach to the client, it's important for the nurse to recognize that the client's behavior:
☐ 1. shows a direct relationship to his awareness of the environment.
☐ 2. results from overwhelming feelings of depression.
☐ 3. can be an early sign of psychosis.
☐ 4. represents an attempt to reduce anxiety.

CORRECT ANSWER: 4
Ritualistic behaviors are used to increase the feelings of individual control and decrease anxiety. Even though the client may recognize that the activity is illogical, he feels compelled to carry out the behavior. Option 1: The stimulus for the behavior comes from within the individual, not the environment. Option 2: The client is responding to overwhelming effects but no symptoms of depression are suggested. Option 3: Obsessive-compulsive behavior is classified as an anxiety-related disorder. Unlike a psychotic client, this client retains reality orientation.
NP: Implementing care
CN: Psychosocial integrity
CNS: Psychosocial adaptation
CL: Application

156 Following an act of self-mutilation with a knife, a client diagnosed with borderline personality disorder has been an in-client for 1 week. The nurse understands that an important predischarge outcome to be achieved is that the client will:
☐ 1. voice plans to stop the intake of alcohol when feeling distressed.
☐ 2. identify three ways to reduce self-destructive ideation.
☐ 3. verbalize an understanding of his feelings preceding acts of self-mutilation.
☐ 4. state comprehension of possible causes of borderline personality disorder.

CORRECT ANSWER: 3
In clients with borderline personality disorders, self-mutilation is a response to increased feelings of anxiety and represents the inability to cope in a constructive or healthy manner. When the person can recognize a feeling as it's building in intensity and connect it to impulses toward self-mutilation or other acting out, this enables the person to seek assistance in identifying more constructive coping responses. Option 1: There is no indication that alcohol use is a problem for this client. Option 2: The client isn't manifesting self-destructive impulses, although accidental or impulsive suicide could occur. Option 4: While understanding the theories or causation may have some benefit for this client, the emphasis of interventions should be on helping the client change behaviors and cope more constructively and less dangerously.
NP: Evaluating care
CN: Psychosocial integrity
CNS: Psychosocial adaptation
CL: Application

157 A 31-year-old female client in the psychiatric unit is suicidal. The nurse asks the client to enter into a no-suicide contract and the client refuses. The next thing the nurse should do is:
☐ 1. restrict the client to her room.
☐ 2. promptly administer ordered antidepressant medications.
☐ 3. encourage the client to tell staff when she feels suicidal urges.
☐ 4. question the client about reasons for not signing the no-suicide contract.

CORRECT ANSWER: 3
The nurse's priority at this time is to protect the client from acting on her self-destructive impulses. Unwillingness to enter into a contract increases the suicide risk level and may indicate the absence of ambivalence about the suicide. Option 1: Confining the client to her room wouldn't provide protection and could increase her opportunity for acting on suicidal impulses unless close observation and supervision are included. Option 2: Antidepressant medications don't act immediately and may not be indicated because there is no information indicating that the client is depressed. Option 4: The client may feel overwhelmed or threatened by questions that challenge her decision. Questioning the client wouldn't provide protection, which is the nurse's first priority.
NP: Implementing care
CN: Psychosocial integrity
CNS: Psychosocial adaptation
CL: Application

158 The nurse sees a client who is taking phenelzine (Nardil) eating from another client's meal tray. Thirty minutes after the meal, the client complains of headache and nausea; 45 minutes after the meal, the client vomits. Before calling the physician, it's most important for the nurse to:
☐ 1. determine the client's blood pressure readings.
☐ 2. perform a capillary blood glucose test.
☐ 3. assess the client's breathing rate and rhythm.
☐ 4. auscultate for the client's bowel sounds.

CORRECT ANSWER: 1
Nardil is a monoamine oxidase inhibitor that, when combined with tyramine-containing foods, can cause hypertensive crisis, a potentially life-threatening condition. Headache, nausea, and vomiting are signs of this condition. Options 2, 3, and 4: Performing a capillary blood glucose test, assessing the client's breathing rate and rhythm, and auscultating the client's bowel sounds wouldn't help in determining the cause of hypertensive crisis.
NP: Implementing care
CN: Physiological integrity
CNS: Pharmacological therapies
CL: Application

---

159 A new client in the psychiatric unit has a medical diagnosis of bipolar affective disorder. The client and several others are in the common day-room, where several groups of clients and staff are playing card games. When the client begins laughing and talking loudly and interferes with other clients' activities, the appropriate initial nursing response is to:
☐ 1. tell the client to slow down and be quiet.
☐ 2. administer ordered sedatives promptly.
☐ 3. place the client in a quiet seclusion room.
☐ 4. accompany the client to a less stimulating area.

CORRECT ANSWER: 4
The client is showing behaviors associated with a state of elevated affect. In such circumstances, the individual is distracted by and responds to stimuli in the environment. Attempting to reduce the stimuli by environmental manipulation is an appropriate nursing intervention. Option 1: The client in a state of elevated affect is irritable and tends to respond to demands with hostility and increased affect. Option 2: While medications may be indicated for a more exaggerated state of elevated affect, this situation doesn't suggest the need for a chemical response. If medication is ordered, it's most likely an antianxiety agent or an antipsychotic agent. Nothing in the situation describes urgent circumstances. Option 3: The nurse can initiate therapeutic seclusion only if the facility's policy or physician orders allow for this type of intervention.
NP: Implementing care
CN: Physiological integrity
CNS: Reduction of risk potential
CL: Application

---

160 The nurse is instructing a client who is receiving bupropion (Wellbutrin) to help him quit cigarette smoking. Which statement should be included when the nurse teaches the client about this medication?
☐ 1. "The drug should be taken at bedtime."
☐ 2. "Diarrhea is a frequent adverse effect."
☐ 3. "Drinking alcohol should be avoided."
☐ 4. "Slowing of the heart rate is likely".

CORRECT ANSWER: 3
Bupropion is a selective serotonin reuptake inhibitor, which can also be given for its antidepressant effect. An addictive effect can also occur if this drug is taken with alcohol, other central nervous system depressants, and tricyclic antidepressants. Option 1: This drug should be taken during the morning to decrease the likelihood of insomnia. Option 2: Constipation is a more frequent adverse effect than diarrhea. Option 4: Tachycardia, not bradycardia, is a common cardiovascular adverse effect of bupropion.
NP: Implementing care
CN: Physiological integrity
CNS: Pharmacological therapies
CL: Application

Posttests

POSTTEST I

To assess your readiness for NCLEX-PN, take the following posttest, which contains 85 questions on the four subject areas covered on the actual examination. Then check your responses against the correct answers and rationales provided on pages 239 to 249.

QUESTIONS

1 A paranoid schizophrenic male client thinks that someone is trying to kill him by poisoning his food. The physician has just prescribed an antipsychotic medication to be administered immediately in liquid form. What is the best approach to take?
☐ 1. Mix the medication in his food.
☐ 2. Explain the action of the medication before giving it.
☐ 3. Allow a trusted staff member to administer the medication.
☐ 4. Delay giving the medication until a rapport with the client is established.

2 A boy with a patent ductus arteriosus was delivered 6 hours ago and is being held by his mother. As the nurse enters the room to assess the neonate's vital signs, the mother says, "The physician says that my baby has a heart murmur. Does that mean he has a bad heart?" Which response by the nurse would be most appropriate?
☐ 1. "He'll need more tests to determine his heart condition."
☐ 2. "He'll require oxygen therapy at home, for a while."
☐ 3. "He'll be fine. Don't worry about him".
☐ 4. "The murmur is caused by a natural opening that can take a day or so to close. It's a normal part of your baby's transition."

3 A client verbalizes that she's suffering from post-traumatic stress disorder as a result of a rape that occurred 6 months ago. She describes flashbacks that cause extreme distress and immobility. Which nursing action is best in this situation?
☐ 1. Avoid any discussion of the event.
☐ 2. Give the client an opportunity to discuss the rape.
☐ 3. Recommend a support group where she can talk about the rape.
☐ 4. Refer the client to a rape crisis specialist.

4 Hypertensive crisis is a possible adverse effect for a client receiving which type of antidepressant?
☐ 1. Tricyclic antidepressant
☐ 2. Monoamine oxidase inhibitor (MAO)
☐ 3. Atypical antidepressant
☐ 4. Typical antidepressant

5 A client underwent a transurethral prostatic resection for benign prostatic hypertrophy 24 hours ago and is receiving irrigations through a three-way catheter. He has received 500 ml of oral fluids, 800 ml of I.V. fluids, and 900 ml of irrigation fluid. His total output in the indwelling urinary catheter collection bag is 2,000 ml. What is the client's urine output?
☐ 1. 600 ml
☐ 2. 1,100 ml
☐ 3. 1,200 ml
☐ 4. 2,000 ml

6 The physician orders a sling for a client with a wrist fracture. The nurse knows that the sling has been applied correctly by observing that the elbow is flexed:
☐ 1. slightly greater than 90 degrees and the fingers are covered.
☐ 2. at a 90-degree angle and the fingers are covered.
☐ 3. slightly less than 90 degrees and the fingers are exposed.
☐ 4. at a 90-degree angle and the fingers are exposed.

7 Which precaution should the nurse take when caring for a client with myocardial infarction who has received a thrombolytic agent?
☐ 1. Avoid puncture wounds.
☐ 2. Monitor the potassium level.
☐ 3. Maintain a supine position.
☐ 4. Force fluids.

8 The nurse is scheduled to collect a 24-hour urine specimen from a client beginning at 8 a.m. The client voids at 8 a.m., and the nurse discards the urine. The nurse saves all the subsequently voided urine in an iced container. At 8 a.m. the next day, the client voids and the nurse adds the voided urine to the specimen container and sends it to the laboratory. Which statement regarding the procedure is correct?
☐ 1. The procedure was performed correctly.
☐ 2. The first voiding should have been saved.
☐ 3. The urine didn't have to be kept on ice.
☐ 4. The last voiding should have been discarded.

9 A client with a peptic ulcer is receiving Maalox and oral cimetidine (Tagamet). The nurse administers the drugs correctly by giving:
☐ 1. cimetidine with meals and Maalox 1 hour after meals.
☐ 2. Maalox and cimetidine together with meals.
☐ 3. Maalox and cimetidine together between meals.
☐ 4. Maalox and cimetidine together with other scheduled medications.

10 While transporting a client to the radiology department for an X-ray, the nurse notices that the client's chest tube has become disconnected from the drainage unit. Which action by the nurse is most appropriate?
☐ 1. Clamp the chest tube immediately with two clamps.
☐ 2. Place the end of the tube in a container of sterile saline solution.
☐ 3. Apply an occlusive dressing; then notify the physician.
☐ 4. Leave the tube disconnected until the client arrives at the radiology department.

11 A multipara client complains of severe afterpains whenever she breast-feeds her neonate. Which intervention should the nurse include in the client's plan of care?
☐ 1. Obtain a physician's order to administer an analgesic before breast-feeding.
☐ 2. Encourage the client to empty her bladder before breast-feeding.
☐ 3. Teach the client how to massage her fundus when afterpains occur.
☐ 4. Show the client how to hold the neonate to prevent any pressure on the uterus when afterpains occur.

12 Which form of exercise should be recommended to a client who was ruled out for a myocardial infarction and is scheduled for a complete cardiac workup in 2 weeks?
☐ 1. Exercising shouldn't be recommended.
☐ 2. Lifting weights at the local gym
☐ 3. Jumping rope to music
☐ 4. Doing sit-ups with bent knees

13 During the administration of an enema, a client begins to complain of cramping. What action should the nurse take next?
☐ 1. Discontinue the enema.
☐ 2. Increase the speed of the enema to finish more quickly.
☐ 3. Lower the bag to the level of the bed.
☐ 4. Slow the flow rate of the enema solution.

14 A male client is being discharged 8 days after a lumbar spinal fusion. He asks the nurse to explain any activity limitations he'll have. Which response by the nurse is appropriate?
☐ 1. When standing for long periods, keep your back and both legs straight.
☐ 2. When lifting, use the muscles of your back and stomach to support the weight of the object.
☐ 3. You may find it more comfortable to sleep in a recliner for the first few days when you return home.
☐ 4. Get out of bed by rolling to one side and pushing off the bed with your arms.

15 A 62-year-old female client has been admitted to the coronary care unit with a myocardial infarction. She appears anxious and states that she's afraid her life will never be the same. Which response by the nurse is best?
☐ 1. "We're taking good care of you now; you don't need to worry."
☐ 2. "Life is always changing; we'll help you adjust."
☐ 3. "You seem anxious; tell me more about how you're feeling."
☐ 4. "We'll teach you how to adjust to the necessary changes."

16 When caring for a client with increased intracranial pressure (ICP), which nursing procedure is correct?
☐ 1. Administer enemas to prevent constipation.
☐ 2. Turn on the television to stimulate the client.
☐ 3. Withhold baths until the increased ICP is reduced or stabilized.
☐ 4. Position the client flat in bed.

17 A 76-year-old male client with advanced parkinsonism and moderate physical disabilities is admitted to the rehabilitation unit. While assessing the client's abilities, the nurse would attribute which finding to Parkinson's disease?

☐ 1. Uncontrollable writing and twisting of the body
☐ 2. Pill-rolling tremors and muscle rigidity
☐ 3. Inability to understand speech
☐ 4. Recent weight gain

18 A 62-year-old male client is admitted to the hospital because of a 2-month history of cough and weight loss. The physician tentatively diagnoses tuberculosis. Which diagnostic test is most definitive for confirming active disease?
☐ 1. Tuberculin tine test
☐ 2. Mantoux skin test
☐ 3. Sputum culture for acid-fast bacilli
☐ 4. Chest X-ray

19 The nurse understands that the primary reason for teaching female clients breast self-examination (BSE) is that:
☐ 1. women are often reluctant to seek medical help.
☐ 2. most tumors are discovered during an annual breast examination.
☐ 3. women are embarrassed when physicians examine their breasts.
☐ 4. most tumors are discovered by clients while performing BSE.

20 Which skin care method should the nurse teach to a client whose leg cast was just removed?
☐ 1. Wash the skin in cool or tepid water and mild soap.
☐ 2. Avoid immersing the leg in water.
☐ 3. Rub the skin vigorously when drying.
☐ 4. Avoid lotions until the skin is healed.

21 What is the purpose of giving a vitamin K injection to a neonate immediately after delivery?
☐ 1. To prevent malnutrition
☐ 2. To prevent hypoglycemia
☐ 3. To boost the body's oxygen use
☐ 4. To prevent bleeding

22 The nurse chooses normal saline solution to irrigate a Levin tube because this solution will:
☐ 1. cause less distention.
☐ 2. prevent nausea.
☐ 3. prevent the loss of electrolytes.
☐ 4. remove hydrochloric acid.

23 Which nursing action best evaluates the effectiveness of incentive spirometry?
☐ 1. Assessing vital signs
☐ 2. Visually checking the volume displaced
☐ 3. Auscultating the upper airway
☐ 4. Observing for sputum production

24 Which action should the nurse take when a client's chest tube is accidentally pulled out of the pleural space?
☐ 1. Reinsert the chest tube into the pleural space.
☐ 2. Take vital signs and call the physician.
☐ 3. Have the client take deep breaths.
☐ 4. Cover the wound with a sterile occlusive dressing.

25 Which nursing action has the highest priority during the immediate postoperative period?
☐ 1. Recording vital signs every 15 minutes
☐ 2. Observing for hemorrhage
☐ 3. Recording intake and output
☐ 4. Maintaining a patent airway

26 The nurse is caring for a child who has a well-established tracheostomy and requires a routine tracheostomy tube change. Which intervention is most important before changing the tube?
☐ 1. Taking vital signs
☐ 2. Starting an I.V. line for emergency drugs
☐ 3. Restricting food and fluids for several hours before the tube change
☐ 4. Having a larger-size tracheostomy tube available to dilate the stoma

27 The nurse is planning care for a child who was severely burned 2 hours ago and is being transferred from a local hospital to the burn unit. Which intervention is critical during the first several hours after admission to the burn unit?
☐ 1. Providing fluid replacement
☐ 2. Administering antibiotics
☐ 3. Providing nutritional supplements
☐ 4. Culturing all wounds

28 An 11-year-old girl is admitted to the hospital for newly diagnosed diabetes mellitus. Nursing goals include controlling her blood glucose levels, teaching her about the disease and how to manage it, and advising her how to adjust her activities of daily living to cope with the disease. Which statement provides the most accurate information about insulin administration?
☐ 1. "Always clean the skin area and insert the needle holding the syringe at a 45-degree angle."
☐ 2. "Insert only half the needle to be sure that you don't hit the muscle."
☐ 3. "Always have someone help you give your injection."
☐ 4. "Clean the skin area and insert the needle holding the syringe at a 90-degree angle."

29 A boy with pertussis is placed in respiratory isolation. The nurse must wear a mask, gown, and gloves when caring for him. What is the reason for these precautions?

☐ 1. To protect the nurse from contracting the disease
☐ 2. To prevent transmission of the disease by body fluids
☐ 3. To prevent transmission of the disease by droplets from coughing
☐ 4. To provide respiratory isolation

30 The nurse caring for an 8-year-old boy with newly diagnosed diabetes mellitus is responsible for teaching him and his family about diabetes. The client mentions to the nurse that he likes only jelly beans. In teaching the child about nutrition, the nurse should:
☐ 1. tell him that he can't have jelly beans ever again.
☐ 2. take notes on his likes and dislikes in all food groups.
☐ 3. tell him that he'll need to take shots if he eats jelly beans.
☐ 4. avoid mentioning the jelly beans now because he has a lot to learn.

31 A 5-day-old jaundiced neonate is undergoing phototherapy. The physician prescribes a supplemental formula to be given after breast-feeding. The mother tells the nurse that she's worried her milk is no good and that maybe she should stop breast-feeding. Which response by the nurse is most appropriate?
☐ 1. It may be better if the baby were to formula-feed for a while.
☐ 2. The formula will add more liquids to replace those lost while your baby is under the phototherapy lights.
☐ 3. Breast-feeding can increase bilirubin production and should be stopped until the bilirubin levels are normal.
☐ 4. You may not have enough milk yet to satisfy the baby's needs.

32 Five pounds of traction was added to the left leg of a female client in bilateral skeletal traction 2 days ago. Two hours ago, the client started to complain of leg pain, and the physician prescribed Tylenol with codeine #2. The client continues to complain of pain to the nurse making rounds. Which action should the nurse take next?
☐ 1. Administer hydroxyzine hydrochloride (Vistaril) as prescribed.
☐ 2. Reposition the client's legs.
☐ 3. Tell the client that she can't receive any more medication.
☐ 4. Notify the physician of the client's continued complaints of pain.

33 A 6-year-old boy's indwelling urinary catheter was removed at 6 a.m. At noon, the child still hasn't voided. He appears uncomfortable, and the nurse palpates slight bladder distention. Which action should the nurse take first?

☐ 1. Insert a straight catheter, as ordered, for urine retention.
☐ 2. Consult the physician about replacing the indwelling urinary catheter.
☐ 3. Wait awhile longer to see if the client can void on his own.
☐ 4. Turn on the water faucet and provide privacy.

34 A 16-year-old boy underwent surgery 3 days ago to repair a fractured mandible. Because his mouth is wired shut, he has been placed on a liquid diet and must drink through a straw. He tells the nurse that he's very hungry. Which response by the nurse is best?
☐ 1. "I'm sorry. I'll bet you're just starving. I wish you were able to eat solid foods."
☐ 2. "You need to drink more fluids more frequently to keep your stomach full. That way, you won't feel so hungry."
☐ 3. "You need higher-calorie liquids to satisfy your hunger".
☐ 4. "I'll ask the dietitian to stop by and help you plan your meals."

35 The best long-term outcome for a female client with bulimia is that the client will:
☐ 1. be free from symptoms.
☐ 2. follow the prescribed medical regimen.
☐ 3. value herself as a worthy individual.
☐ 4. not harm herself by purging.

36 A client is admitted to the emergency department with signs of delirium tremens. Which nursing intervention is the priority?
☐ 1. Ensure the client's safety.
☐ 2. Provide adequate nutrition.
☐ 3. Notify the client's physician.
☐ 4. Provide adequate fluid intake.

37 Which finding would the nurse expect in a client with a nursing diagnosis of *Risk for injury related to acute intoxication?*
☐ 1. Orientation to person, place, and time
☐ 2. Stable vital signs
☐ 3. Calm, deliberate movements
☐ 4. Slowed reflexes and lack of coordination

38 A neonate's 1-minute Apgar score is 8. Which nursing intervention is most appropriate given the Apgar results?
☐ 1. Administer oxygen.
☐ 2. Prepare to administer stimulant medications.
☐ 3. Place the neonate in a warmed environment.
☐ 4. Provide a high-glucose feeding.

39 The nurse notes that a primipara's membranes had ruptured 36 hours before delivery. In view of this finding, which assessment information should the nurse determine first?

☐ 1. Does the client have a burning sensation when she urinates?
☐ 2. Does the client have an elevated temperature?
☐ 3. Is the client complaining of calf pain?
☐ 4. Is the client's perineal area edematous?

40 The admissions nurse is interviewing a male client with a history of chronic schizophrenia. The client reports that he has been taking fluphenazine decanoate (Prolixin Decanoate) and received his last dose 1 week ago. Which nursing action is most appropriate based on this medication history?
☐ 1. No action is necessary.
☐ 2. Call the physician for an immediate drug order.
☐ 3. Withhold all medication until further notice.
☐ 4. Watch the client closely for withdrawal symptoms.

41 A client is taking 300 mg of lithium carbonate three times daily. Which finding would require the nurse's immediate action?
☐ 1. Lithium serum level of 1.2 mEq/L
☐ 2. Increased appetite
☐ 3. Irregular pulse
☐ 4. Weight loss

42 A client is admitted to the hospital with the following arterial blood gas levels: pH, 7.27; PaO_2, 53 mm Hg; HCO_3^-, 25 mEq/L; $PaCO_2$, 50 mm Hg; and FIO_2, 21%. These findings indicate:
☐ 1. respiratory acidosis.
☐ 2. respiratory alkalosis.
☐ 3. metabolic acidosis.
☐ 4. metabolic alkalosis.

43 The nurse is preparing discharge instructions for a 3-year-old child who was hospitalized for acetaminophen intoxication. Which information is most important to include?
☐ 1. Explaining to the child the hazards of ingesting nonfood substances
☐ 2. Encouraging the parents to have syrup of ipecac available
☐ 3. Educating the parents about safe storage of poisons and drugs
☐ 4. Teaching the parents to always induce vomiting for any ingestion

44 Which symptom would indicate that a client taking a prescribed antianxiety medication is experiencing withdrawal?
☐ 1. Hypotension
☐ 2. Slurred speech
☐ 3. Insomnia and muscle tremors
☐ 4. Dry mouth

45 The nurse is caring for a primigravida who is in labor. Which action should the nurse take first when the membranes suddenly rupture?

☐ 1. Check the fetal heart rate.
☐ 2. Place the client on her left side.
☐ 3. Time the client's contractions.
☐ 4. Record the client's vital signs.

46 You're instructing an elderly client who is being discharged and has been started on two new medications. When teaching the client about new medications, the nurse should plan to:
☐ 1. give verbal instructions to the client in a high-pitched voice.
☐ 2. teach the client about the medications shortly before discharge, so the client won't forget.
☐ 3. begin teaching while the client is eating and relaxed and thus better able to understand the information.
☐ 4. give the client a copy of written instructions about the medications.

47 The nurse is caring for a 52-year-old female client diagnosed with a right-sided cerebrovascular accident who has expressive aphasia and left-sided weakness. When planning care for this client, which intervention should you delegate to a nursing assistant?
☐ 1. Accompany the client to speech therapy.
☐ 2. Perform active range-of-motion exercises to the client's upper extremities.
☐ 3. Turn and position the client every 2 hours.
☐ 4. Begin teaching the client simple sign language phrases.

48 The nurse is delivering a change-of-shift report. What information is most important to include?
☐ 1. The client hasn't voided since the catheter was removed 2 hours ago.
☐ 2. Several visitors have been seen during this shift.
☐ 3. The client's physician hasn't been in today to see the client.
☐ 4. The client was medicated for a headache 1 hour ago.

49 The nurse is caring for a 61-year-old male client diagnosed with a cerebrovascular accident. To determine if the client is experiencing right side hemianopsia, the nurse should check if the client:
☐ 1. uses only the right arm when eating.
☐ 2. pockets food in the right side of the mouth.
☐ 3. eats only food on the right side of the tray.
☐ 4. drools from the right side of the mouth.

50 The nursing assistant reports to the nurse that a client became short of breath while being bathed but is breathing better now. Which approach should the nurse take initially?
☐ 1. Instruct the nursing assistant to observe the client for any further shortness of breath.
☐ 2. Check the client and gather subjective and objective data related to the shortness of breath.

☐ 3. Tell the physician about the client's episode of shortness of breath.

☐ 4. Instruct the nursing assistant to complete the bath after allowing the client to rest.

51 While discussing a client's care with a nursing assistant, the nurse detects an odor of alcohol on the assistant's breath. The nurse should plan to:

☐ 1. report her observations to the charge nurse.

☐ 2. monitor the assistant closely to determine if performance is impaired.

☐ 3. tell the assistant she'll have to leave the unit immediately.

☐ 4. warn the assistant that she could loose her certification.

52 The nurse is beginning a shift and planning interventions. Which client requires minimized sensory deprivation?

☐ 1. A 45-year female admitted with pancreatitis

☐ 2. An 84-year-old woman admitted to the emergency department

☐ 3. A 23-year-old in the intensive care unit placed on a ventilator

☐ 4. A 16-year-old male admitted with a spinal cord injury

53 The nurse is preparing to determine how well a client understands his dietary restrictions but finds the client in a lot of pain. What is the most appropriate action by the nurse at this time?

☐ 1. Leave written materials with the client and come back later to review them.

☐ 2. Administer pain medication and come back to talk later.

☐ 3. Quickly gather as much information as possible by asking questions that require short answers.

☐ 4. Ask only the most essential questions to obtain the information needed.

54 A 45-year-old client confides to the nurse she's worried that her teenage son is socializing with other teens whom she suspects are using illegal drugs. What is the nurse's best response?

☐ 1. "Most young people experiment with drugs. You have cause to be concerned."

☐ 2. "You should forbid your son from associating with those teens."

☐ 3. "You should learn about the early signs of drug use and discuss your concerns with your son."

☐ 4. "I suggest you get your son into a treatment program as soon as possible."

55 The nurse is caring for a severely depressed client on the psychiatric unit. After 2 weeks of therapy, the client expresses feelings of happiness and begins to socialize with the other clients and staff. At this time the client should be watched closely for:

☐ 1. psychotic behavior.

☐ 2. a sudden depressive mood.

☐ 3. outbursts of anger toward others.

☐ 4. suicidal behavior.

56 The nurse is caring for a psychotic client who believes he's Jesus Christ and requests that the staff refer to him as the Messiah. Which type of delusion is this client experiencing?

☐ 1. Grandiose

☐ 2. Nihilistic

☐ 3. Persecutory

☐ 4. Paranoid

57 The nurse is assisting in the plan of care for a child being treated for Lyme disease. This treatment will include:

☐ 1. a high-protein, high-fat diet.

☐ 2. activity restrictions for 6 weeks.

☐ 3. antibiotic therapy.

☐ 4. transfusion of plasma.

58 The nurse is caring for a client who is on complete bed rest following complete hip replacement. In an effort to reduce sensory deprivation, the nursing assistant should be instructed to:

☐ 1. provide mouth care before meals.

☐ 2. monitor the client's urine output every 2 hours.

☐ 3. check bilateral hand grasps every 4 hours.

☐ 4. orient the client to date and time frequently.

59 A 41-year-old male client reports that he's having trouble sleeping. The nurse reviews the client's diet history. What finding is most likely responsible for the client's lack of sleep?

☐ 1. Eating toast at bedtime

☐ 2. Having chili at lunchtime

☐ 3. Enjoying coffee with breakfast

☐ 4. Drinking a cola beverage at supper

60 The nurse is planning to teach a client of a different culture. To determine the client's beliefs related to health and illness, the nurse should:

☐ 1. learn about the client's culture through reading and research.

☐ 2. ask the family if the client strongly identifies with any cultural group.

☐ 3. ask the client to describe what he believes influences and is important to health care.

☐ 4. check the client's medical record to determine the exact ethnic background of the client.

61 The nurse is caring for a client who is taking potassium-wasting diuretics in the treatment of hypertension and determines that the client doesn't know what foods are high in potassium. The nurse should plan nursing interventions for which nursing diagnosis?

☐ 1. *Ineffective cardiopulmonary tissue perfusion related to cardiac arrhythmias*
☐ 2. *Deficient knowledge related to inability to identify potassium-rich foods*
☐ 3. *Imbalanced nutrition: Less than body requirements related to low intake of potassium*
☐ 4. *Deficient knowledge related to lack of experience in taking diuretics*

62 The nurse is assisting a registered nurse with a teaching project. When selecting audiovisual and written materials, it's important for the nurse to:
☐ 1. provide the client with the materials before the planned learning experience.
☐ 2. ensure the materials are lengthy and provide in-depth coverage of the material.
☐ 3. review the materials for accuracy and appropriateness to the client's education level.
☐ 4. choose materials that are brief and to the point.

63 The nurse has just finished instructing a client with an open abdominal wound. The client participated in the dressing change. Which is the best example of documentation?
☐ 1. The client was instructed regarding proper care of wound and dressing change.
☐ 2. The client demonstrated correct technique of wound care, following instructions.
☐ 3. The client and family verbalize understanding of proper wound care.
☐ 4. Written instructions regarding wound care were given to the client.

64 The nurse is instructing the parents of a child who is allergic to dust mites and has frequent asthma attacks. Teaching about how to reduce exposure to allergens has been effective when the parents can state the importance of:
☐ 1. allowing the child to play only with soft stuffed animals.
☐ 2. maintaining a high humidity environment in the home.
☐ 3. dusting the child's room daily with a damp clean cloth.
☐ 4. vacuuming the bedroom carpet daily.

65 The nurse is assisting in a liver biopsy on a 50-year-old male client with suspected liver cancer. When the procedure is completed, the nurse's plan of care includes placing the client in which position?
☐ 1. High Fowler's
☐ 2. Left lateral
☐ 3. Right lateral
☐ 4. Supine with a pillow at the small of the back

66 The nurse is caring for a client after paracentesis for abdominal ascites due to cirrhosis. Which finding best indicates that the paracentesis was effective in relieving abdominal distention?

☐ 1. The client's respirations changed from 32 to 24 breaths/minute.
☐ 2. The client's blood pressure dropped from 160/90 mm Hg to 100/60 mm Hg.
☐ 3. The client reports relief from headache.
☐ 4. The client can ambulate without assistance.

67 A 31-year-old female client tells the nurse that she has a history of developing urinary tract infections. The nurse knows further teaching is needed when the client states:
☐ 1. "I always wipe myself from front to back after urinating."
☐ 2. "I try not to drink fluids after 6 p.m. so the urine won't be sitting in my bladder all night."
☐ 3. "I drink at least 1 to 2 glasses of cranberry juice every day."
☐ 4. "I empty my bladder whenever I feel the urge to urinate."

68 A male client with schizophrenia has been displaying sexual overtures toward a female physician. The client tells the nurse, "That doctor is in love with me; she's always flirting with me." Which defense mechanism is this client using?
☐ 1. Projection
☐ 2. Denial
☐ 3. Reaction formation
☐ 4. Displacement

69 The nurse has been working with an autistic child for several months. Which of the following outcomes would be most desirable?
☐ 1. Communication with the family is maintained.
☐ 2. The child becomes involved in extracurricular school activities.
☐ 3. The child eats a high-protein diet.
☐ 4. A trusting relationship is established.

70 The nurse is caring for a client with a fracture of the right femur due to a skiing accident. Which is an early sign of fat emboli?
☐ 1. Abdominal cramping
☐ 2. Fatty stools
☐ 3. Confusion
☐ 4. Numbness in the right foot

71 A 78-year-old male client is admitted with suspected upper GI bleeding. The nurse should monitor this client for:
☐ 1. hemoptysis.
☐ 2. hematuria.
☐ 3. passage of bright red blood in the stool.
☐ 4. black, tarry stools.

72 The nurse is caring for a 41-year-old male client with rheumatoid arthritis. The nurse plans to ambulate the client:

☐ 1. when the client first awakens in the morning.
☐ 2. after returning from physical therapy.
☐ 3. after the client has a bath.
☐ 4. just before the noontime meal.

73 A 27-year-old female client with hepatitis B is discussing her concerns about the outcome of the illness with the nurse. Which statement made by the client indicates a need for further teaching?
☐ 1. "I know this can lead to chronic hepatitis."
☐ 2. "At least I know I won't get liver cancer."
☐ 3. "I know I need to use some type of protection when having sex."
☐ 4. "I hope I don't become a carrier of hepatitis."

74 The nurse is caring for a 55-year-old male client with acute pancreatitis. When checking the client's nasogastric drainage, the nurse expects the drainage to be:
☐ 1. clear to white.
☐ 2. light pink with occasional small clots.
☐ 3. golden yellow to green.
☐ 4. clear with large amounts of mucus.

75 The nurse is instructing a client on how to do her own dressing change after abdominal surgery and the importance of proper hand washing before the dressing change. Which practice contributes most to asepsis?
☐ 1. Using warm water
☐ 2. Drying each hand with a separate paper towel
☐ 3. Using an antibacterial soap
☐ 4. Washing the nail beds and between the fingers

76 The nurse is caring for a client with a hiatal hernia. The nurse knows that teaching has been effective when the client says that he'll:
☐ 1. lie down for 30 minutes after eating.
☐ 2. avoid eating concentrated sweets.
☐ 3. sleep on his right side.
☐ 4. eat small, frequent meals.

77 A client has returned to the medical surgical unit after an esophagogastroduodenoscopy (EGD). The nurse knows the client shouldn't be allowed to consume anything by mouth until:
☐ 1. the results of the EGD are sent to the unit.
☐ 2. the client has a positive gag reflex.
☐ 3. the first dose of I.V. antibiotics is administered.
☐ 4. positive bowel sounds are heard.

78 A client with benign prostatic hypertrophy is scheduled for a transurethral resection of the prostate. The nurse expects the client to experience which of the following before the procedure?
☐ 1. Urinary hesitancy and urgency
☐ 2. Hematuria and painful urination
☐ 3. Bladder spasms
☐ 4. Flank pain

79 The nurse is caring for a client with deep vein thrombosis of the left leg who is receiving a continuous heparin infusion to prevent extension of the clot. Which finding can be attributed to the effects of the heparin infusion?
☐ 1. The client complains of a severe headache.
☐ 2. The abdomen is firm and distended.
☐ 3. The client has multiple ecchymotic areas on both arms.
☐ 4. The left calf is swollen and warm to the touch.

80 The nurse is evaluating the discharge teaching of a 55-year-old female client with peptic ulcer disease. One indication that the teaching was effective is that the client tells the nurse she'll avoid:
☐ 1. eating foods high in calcium.
☐ 2. drinking any fruit juices.
☐ 3. over-the-counter medications with aspirin.
☐ 4. foods that are ice cold or frozen.

81 The nurse is caring for a 9-month-old boy with Reye's syndrome. It's most important that the nurse plans to:
☐ 1. check the skin for signs of breakdown every shift.
☐ 2. perform range-of-motion exercises every 4 hours.
☐ 3. monitor the client's intake and output.
☐ 4. place the client in protective isolation.

82 The nurse is observing a mother who has been taught how to correctly administer eardrops to her 2-year-old child. The nurse determines that the mother is doing it correctly when she:
☐ 1. pulls the pinna of the ear down and back.
☐ 2. pulls the pinna of the ear up and back.
☐ 3. pulls the pinna of the ear directly toward the back of the head.
☐ 4. inserts the dropper as far as it will go into the ear canal.

83 The nurse is caring for a 45-year-old woman experiencing the manic phase of bipolar disorder. To help the client reduce her hyperactive behavior, the nurse should:
☐ 1. encourage her to engage in one-on-one games with another client.
☐ 2. encourage her to engage in group activities requiring a lot of physical activity.
☐ 3. allow her to set her own limits on her behavior.
☐ 4. provide a calm, quiet environment.

84 The nurse is instructing a client on the care of an arteriovenous fistula created in his left arm 1 week ago. The nurse knows that the client understands the teaching when he says:
☐ 1. "I'll keep this arm covered when I take a shower."
☐ 2. "I should avoid carrying heavy packages with my left arm."

3. "I'll keep my left arm in a sling until the fistula is ready for use in dialysis."
4. "I'll keep a dry, sterile dressing over the fistula at all times."

85 The nurse is caring for a 41-year-old male client on complete bed rest following a spinal cord injury. Which intervention should the nurse include in the plan of care to prevent thrombophlebitis?
1. Massage the client's legs while giving a bath.
2. Have the client tighten and relax the calf muscles several times daily.
3. Encourage the client to keep the knees bent as much as possible.
4. Dangle the client's legs over the side of the bed twice each shift.

ANSWERS AND RATIONALES

1 CORRECT ANSWER: 2
A paranoid client needs to be reassured that the nurse is trustworthy. The best way to begin establishing trust is to explain any treatment before initiating it. Option 1: Mixing the medication in the client's food and risking the chance that he'll discover it later is deceptive and would reinforce his paranoid ideation. Option 3: Allowing a trusted staff member to give the medication may help but this isn't the best approach. Option 4: Delaying administration of medication doesn't comply with the physician's order to give the medication immediately; also, the nurse can't be sure that a rapport will be established.
NP: Implementing care
CN: Psychosocial integrity
CNS: Psychosocial adaptation
CL: Application

2 CORRECT ANSWER: 4
Although the nurse may want to tell the mother not to worry, the most appropriate response would be to explain the neonate's present condition, to relieve the mother, and to acknowledge an awareness of the condition. A neonate's systemic vascular system changes with birth; certain factors help to reverse the flow of blood through the ductus and ultimately favor its closure. This closure typically begins within the first 24 hours after birth and ends within a few days after birth. Options 1, 2, and 3 don't address the mother's question.
NP: Implementing care
CN: Health promotion and maintenance
CNS: Growth and development through the life span
CL: Analysis

3 CORRECT ANSWER: 2
Part of the healing process associated with rape trauma is being able to confront the memories and replace the victim role with one of a healthy self-concept and lifestyle. Option 1: Avoiding the sub-

ject is nontherapeutic. Options 3 and 4 may be done after the client has a chance to discuss the experience.
NP: Implementing care
CN: Psychosocial integrity
CNS: Coping and adaptation
CL: Application

4 CORRECT ANSWER: 2
MAO inhibitors in combination with tyramine-containing foods will raise a client's blood pressure and can cause a hypertensive crisis. Options 1, 3, and 4 don't produce this adverse effect.
NP: Evaluating care
CN: Physiological integrity
CNS: Pharmacological therapies
CL: Comprehension

5 CORRECT ANSWER: 2
This client has a urine output of 1,100 ml. To get the urine output, the nurse would subtract the irrigation fluid (900 ml) from the total output (2,000 ml).
NP: Evaluating care
CN: Physiological integrity
CNS: Basic care and comfort
CL: Application

6 CORRECT ANSWER: 3
The elbow should be flexed at slightly less than 90 degrees so that the hand and fingers are higher than the elbow, helping to prevent dependent edema. The fingers should be exposed to assess circulation.
NP: Evaluating care
CN: Physiological integrity
CNS: Reduction of risk potential
CL: Application

7 CORRECT ANSWER: 1
Thrombolytic agents are declotting agents that place the client at risk for hemorrhage from puncture wounds. All unnecessary needle sticks and invasive procedures should be avoided. Option 2: The potassium level should be monitored in all cardiac clients, not just those receiving a thrombolytic agent. Option 3: Although no specific position is required, most cardiac clients seem more comfortable in semi-Fowler's position. Option 4: The client's fluid balance must be carefully monitored, so it may be inappropriate to force fluids at this time.
NP: Implementing care
CN: Physiological integrity
CNS: Reduction of risk potential
CL: Application

8 CORRECT ANSWER: 1
The nurse followed the correct procedure for collecting a 24-hour urine specimen. Option 2: The first voiding should be discarded because it was produced by the kidneys before the scheduled 8 a.m. collection time. Option 3: The urine should be kept

on ice to prevent deterioration of urine contents. Option 4: The last voiding should be saved because it was produced by the kidneys before 8 a.m. on the 2nd day.

NP: Implementing care
CN: Physiological integrity
CNS: Reduction of risk potential
CL: Application

9 CORRECT ANSWER: 1

Maalox should be given 1 hour after meals and at bedtime, whereas cimetidine should be given with meals and at bedtime. These drugs should be given at least 1 hour apart. Options 2, 3, and 4 are incorrect because Maalox and cimetidine shouldn't be administered simultaneously.

NP: Implementing care
CN: Physiological integrity
CNS: Pharmacological therapies
CL: Application

10 CORRECT ANSWER: 2

Current protocol calls for leaving the tube unclamped and inserting it quickly into a container of sterile water or normal saline solution. Option 1: Clamping the tube would place the client at risk for tension pneumothorax or cardiac tamponade. Option 3: This is appropriate if the chest tube is accidentally removed from the chest, not the drainage unit. Option 4: This would allow atmospheric air to enter the pleural space.

NP: Implementing care
CN: Physiological integrity
CNS: Reduction of risk potential
CL: Knowledge

11 CORRECT ANSWER: 1

Breast-feeding stimulates the uterus to contract. In a multipara client, these contractions are sometimes painful (afterpains); therefore, the nurse should obtain an order to administer a mild analgesic before breast-feeding to lessen the pain. Options 2 and 4 aren't helpful in this situation. Option 3 would increase discomfort because the uterus is already contracting.

NP: Planning care
CN: Physiological integrity
CNS: Pharmacological therapies
CL: Application

12 CORRECT ANSWER: 1

Until a complete cardiac workup is performed, exercise shouldn't be recommended. The workup provides information about the client's coronary circulation and ability to withstand exercise. Therefore, it isn't safe for the client to exercise until the results of the test are known. Option 2: Weight lifting is contraindicated for cardiac clients because performing Valsalva's maneuver decreases blood supply to the myocardium. Option 3: Although rope jumping generally provides a good cardiac workout, the client shouldn't attempt this activity until after the physician has performed a complete diagnostic workup. Option 4: Sit-ups may be too strenuous and can cause the client to perform Valsalva's maneuver; they shouldn't be attempted until after the complete diagnostic workup.

NP: Planning care
CN: Health promotion and maintenance
CNS: Prevention and early detection of disease
CL: Analysis

13 CORRECT ANSWER: 4

Whenever a client begins to feel cramps during the administration of an enema, the nurse should slow the flow rate or withhold the enema for a few minutes and then continue with administration. Option 1: Cramping doesn't warrant discontinuation of the enema. Option 2: Increasing the speed of administration will increase the cramping. Option 3: Lowering the bag to the level of the bed will result in siphoning of the enema solution.

NP: Implementing care
CN: Physiological integrity
CNS: Basic care and comfort
CL: Application

14 CORRECT ANSWER: 4

Keeping the lumbar area straight while avoiding pressure on the operative site is essential to this client's recovery. Therefore, the client should roll to the side of the bed and use his arms to rise. Option 1: During prolonged standing, the client should bend one knee to reduce the stress on his lower back. Option 2: When lifting, the client should bend the knees and use the leg muscles to lift. Option 3: The client should sleep fully reclined on a firm mattress.

NP: Implementing care
CN: Health promotion and maintenance
CNS: Prevention and early detection of disease
CL: Analysis

15 CORRECT ANSWER: 3

Emotional support is one of the key nursing interventions for a client with a myocardial infarction. The client and family should be encouraged to express their feelings and concerns and to ask questions. Options 1, 2, and 4: These statements block communication by making the client feel that she isn't understood and that the nurse isn't interested in hearing what she has to say.

NP: Implementing care
CN: Psychosocial integrity
CNS: Coping and adaptation
CL: Application

16 CORRECT ANSWER: 3

The nurse should help the client to avoid activities that raise ICP. All unnecessary activities, including baths, should be eliminated. Option 1: Enemas cause cramping and force the client to perform Valsalva's maneuver, which is contraindicated in clients with increased ICP. Option 2: Noxious stimuli cause an increase in ICP. Option 4: The head of the bed should be raised 30 degrees to promote venous drainage.

NP: Implementing care
CN: Physiological integrity
CNS: Physiological adaptation
CL: Application

17 CORRECT ANSWER: 2

One of the classic signs of Parkinson's disease is pill-rolling tremors, rhythmic motion of the thumb against the fingers that sometimes diminishes with movement. Another classic finding is widespread rigidity of the muscles throughout the body. Option 1: Choreiform movements are associated with Huntington's disease. Option 3: Aphasia isn't a problem typically associated with Parkinson's disease. Clients can understand verbal communications but have difficulty articulating words. Option 4: Clients with Parkinson's disease usually experience anorexia and difficulty swallowing; consequently, they tend to lose weight.

NP: Collecting data
CN: Physiological integrity
CNS: Physiological adaptation
CL: Comprehension

18 CORRECT ANSWER: 3

An acid-fast smear and a culture of *Mycobacterium tuberculosis* from the client's sputum or other body secretions are the only methods of confirming active disease. Option 1: The tuberculin tine test is a screening test for tuberculosis but it doesn't confirm active disease. Option 2: The Mantoux skin test is the most reliable skin test but this also doesn't confirm active disease. Option 4: A chest X-ray can detect old lesions or new ones when they're large enough to be seen but it can't detect active disease.

NP: Collecting data
CN: Physiological integrity
CNS: Reduction of risk potential
CL: Analysis

19 CORRECT ANSWER: 4

Most breast tumors are discovered during monthly self-examination. Option 1: Women generally aren't reluctant to seek medical help. However, many become anxious about the tumor's pathology, whether benign or malignant. Option 2: Fewer breast tumors are discovered during annual gynecologic examinations than during monthly self-examinations. Option 3: Although many women become embarrassed and uneasy during their yearly gynecologic examination, this isn't the primary reason for teaching breast self-examination. Nurses can advise female clients who are particularly embarrassed to switch to a female gynecologist.

NP: Collecting data
CN: Health promotion and maintenance
CNS: Prevention and early detection of disease
CL: Application

20 CORRECT ANSWER: 1

The amount of cellular debris and the condition of the skin under the cast depend on the overall skin integrity and the length of time in the cast. If the skin is intact, a cold-water enzyme wash is used to emulsify dead cells and fatty deposits on the skin. At home, the client should avoid hot water and harsh soaps. Water can be cool or slightly warm, and the soap should be mild. Option 2: Immersing the leg in a tub or basin helps to remove skin debris without causing irritation. Option 3: The skin should be patted dry, not vigorously rubbed. Option 4: Generous amounts of lotion may be applied gently to the skin. This helps to lubricate dry skin.

NP: Implementing care
CN: Physiological integrity
CNS: Basic care and comfort
CL: Application

21 CORRECT ANSWER: 4

Vitamin K is needed for adequate blood clotting. Because it's synthesized in the large intestine and the neonate has yet to take in oral nourishment, vitamin K is injected to ensure adequate building of blood clotting factors until the neonate begins to produce these factors internally. Options 1, 2, and 3: Vitamin K doesn't prevent malnutrition or hypoglycemia or boost the body's oxygen use.

NP: Implementing care
CN: Physiological integrity
CNS: Pharmacological therapies
CL: Application

22 CORRECT ANSWER: 3

Normal saline solution is isotonic and prevents the loss of electrolytes. Irrigating with sterile water would deplete electrolytes. Option 1: Distention is caused by fluid volume and wouldn't be affected by the choice of normal saline solution or sterile water. Option 2: Irrigation solution wouldn't cause nausea because it's removed or suctioned out. Nausea results when decompression doesn't occur. Option 4: Irrigation solution wouldn't remove hydrochloric acid.

NP: Implementing care
CN: Physiological integrity
CNS: Basic care and comfort
CL: Application

23 CORRECT ANSWER: 2

The goal of incentive spirometry is to increase inspiratory depth and volume. This can be measured directly by visualizing the volume displaced (with a volume-oriented incentive spirometer) or the number of plastic balls elevated (with a flow-oriented inspiratory spirometer). Option 1: This would be helpful for determining the client's oxygenation status, not for measuring the effectiveness of incentive spirometry. Option 3: If the goal is to increase inspiratory volume to maximum capacity, all lung lobes should be auscultated for inspiratory air exchange. Option 4: An increase in sputum production may be an indication for incentive spirometry; however, incentive spirometry doesn't affect the production of sputum and wouldn't be helpful in evaluating the effectiveness of this therapy.

NP: Evaluating care
CN: Physiological integrity
CNS: Basic care and comfort
CL: Application

24 CORRECT ANSWER: 4

Sealing the entry site is necessary so that air doesn't enter the pleural space and cause the lung to collapse. This should be done with a sterile, occlusive dressing. Option 1: This isn't within the nurse's scope of practice. Additionally, reinserting the same tube would put the client at risk for infection. Insertion of a chest tube is done only under sterile conditions. Option 2: The nurse would take vital signs and call the physician only after sealing the insertion site and assessing the client for respiratory difficulties. Option 3: This intervention would be done to establish maximum lung expansion and to promote relaxation if the client is anxious and is taking rapid, shallow breaths.

NP: Implementing care
CN: Physiological integrity
CNS: Physiological adaptation
CL: Application

25 CORRECT ANSWER: 4

Priorities are determined by the ABCs: airway, breathing, and circulation. Maintaining a patent airway is always the nurse's first priority. Option 1: Frequent assessment of vital signs is important but isn't the first priority. Option 2: Assessment and maintenance of circulation follow airway and breathing maintenance. Option 3: Assessing the client's kidney function and fluid balance is important but isn't the nurse's first priority.

NP: Implementing care
CN: Physiological integrity
CNS: Physiological adaptation
CL: Application

26 CORRECT ANSWER: 3

Even though a tracheostomy tube change is usually accomplished without incident in a client with a well-established tracheostomy, the possibility of aspiration still exists. Restricting the client's oral intake reduces this risk. Option 1: Taking vital signs isn't a priority in this case. Option 2 is unnecessary. Option 4: A smaller-size tube, not a larger one, should be available to make sure one will fit into the stoma.

NP: Planning care
CN: Physiological integrity
CNS: Physiological adaptation
CL: Application

27 CORRECT ANSWER: 1

Because clients suffer significant fluid loss within the first 24 hours after a burn, adequate fluid re-

placement is critical. Options 2, 3, and 4 are important aspects of care but aren't as critical as fluid replacement during the early recovery.

NP: Planning care
CN: Physiological integrity
CNS: Physiological adaptation
CL: Application

28 CORRECT ANSWER: 1

The correct procedure is to clean the area and then insert the syringe at a 45-degree angle because the injection is given subcutaneously. Option 2: As much as 5 units of insulin per drop can be lost to leakage. Inserting the needle all the way prevents leakage. Option 3: The client should learn to administer the insulin herself; however, she may need some assistance until she feels more comfortable giving the injections. Option 4: Recent studies have shown that 95% of insulin injections that are given at a 90-degree angle in the arms and legs are administered I.M., not subcutaneously; this is why teaching the 45-degree angle is important.

NP: Implementing care
CN: Physiological integrity
CNS: Pharmacological therapies
CL: Application

29 CORRECT ANSWER: 3

Pertussis is transmitted by droplets released during coughing episodes, not body fluids (option 2). Pertussis bacteria can be transferred to the nurse holding the child by means of drooling during and after coughing. Gowns are worn to prevent the nurse's clothing from transporting the disease to other clients. Wearing a mask can help prevent the inhalation of respiratory droplets; however, the chances of getting the disease (option 1) are slim as long as the nurse has already had the disease or immunizations are up-to-date. Option 4: These precautions don't conform with respiratory isolation protocols.

NP: Implementing care
CN: Safe, effective care environment
CNS: Safety and infection control
CL: Application

30 CORRECT ANSWER: 2

To discuss the treatment plan for diabetes, the client and family must be able to understand the importance of good nutrition and how foods are metabolized and used by the body. The nurse should obtain a list of all the client's likes and dislikes to help establish a good meal plan. Options 1 and 3: Threatening the client with increased shots or denying him his favorites for life heightens his anxiety and sets him up for noncompliance. Option 4: The client needs to understand what happens when he eats foods high in sugar and what substitutes he can use that will be just as satisfying.

NP: Implementing care
CN: Psychosocial integrity
CNS: Coping and adaptation
CL: Analysis

31 CORRECT ANSWER: 2

Supplemental formula is given during phototherapy to provide additional glucose and protein for albumin binding and the transport and conjugation of bilirubin. Option 4: Within 5 days after delivery, a breast-feeding mother should have enough milk to nurse effectively. Options 1 and 3 are factually inaccurate.

NP: Collecting data
CN: Physiological integrity
CNS: Physiological adaptation
CL: Analysis

32 CORRECT ANSWER: 1

The additional weight to the traction has exacerbated muscle spasms in the leg and increased the client's anxiety. Hydroxyzine hydrochloride helps to calm the client and potentiates the effect of Tylenol. Option 2: Although repositioning helps, the nurse must remember to reposition the torso as well to maintain correct body alignment. Option 3: Telling the client that she can't receive more medication would heighten anxiety and does nothing to ease the pain. Option 4: The nurse has options other than notifying the physician at this time.

NP: Implementing care
CN: Physiological integrity
CNS: Pharmacological therapies
CL: Application

33 CORRECT ANSWER: 4

Urine retention can result from many factors, including stress and use of opiates. Initially, the nurse should use independent nursing actions, such as providing the client with privacy, placing him in a sitting or standing position to enlist the aid of gravity and increase intra-abdominal pressure, and turning on the water faucet. Option 1: If these measures are unsuccessful and the physician has left standing orders for straight catheterization, the nurse can proceed with the catheterization. Option 2: Consulting the physician would involve the use of a dependent nursing action; independent actions should be attempted first. Option 3: Waiting longer will only increase the child's distention and pain.

NP: Implementing care
CN: Physiological integrity
CNS: Basic care and comfort
CL: Application

34 CORRECT ANSWER: 4

This response validates the client's feelings and reassures him that the nurse will attempt to seek help. Option 1: This acknowledges the client's feelings but provides no solution. Options 2 and 3: Although the client may need additional intake or higher-calorie liquids to satisfy his hunger, the dietitian must evaluate the situation before dietary changes are made.

NP: Planning care
CN: Physiological integrity
CNS: Basic care and comfort
CL: Analysis

35 CORRECT ANSWER: 3

Until the client begins to value herself, she'll continue to have an eating disorder. Options 1, 2, and 4: These don't reflect real changes in self-concept or self-value, which are the keys to recovery for someone with an eating disorder.

NP: Evaluating care
CN: Psychosocial integrity
CNS: Psychosocial adaptation
CL: Analysis

36 CORRECT ANSWER: 1

Delirium tremens, an acute condition that occurs with alcohol withdrawal, is characterized by gross memory disturbances, severe agitation, and hallucinations that are frightening and upsetting. Because clients experiencing delirium tremens may injure themselves or others, the priority is client safety. Options 2, 3, and 4: These are important but ensuring the client's safety is the priority in this case.

NP: Collecting data
CN: Safe, effective care environment
CNS: Safety and infection control
CL: Analysis

37 CORRECT ANSWER: 4

The nurse would expect to observe slowed reflexes and lack of coordination given this diagnosis. Other possible signs of acute intoxication include disorientation (option 1), vital sign fluctuations (option 2), involuntary movements (option 3), restlessness, slowed respirations, unintelligible speech, hyperthermia, dehydration, and aggressive or crying behavior when roused.

NP: Collecting data
CN: Safe, effective care environment
CNS: Safety and infection control
CL: Comprehension

38 CORRECT ANSWER: 3

A neonate with an Apgar score between 8 and 10 is considered vigorous and needs normal neonatal care, which includes providing warmth. Option 1: Administering oxygen would be inappropriate if the 5-minute Apgar score is 8. Option 2: Stimulant medications aren't called for with an Apgar rating of 8, which doesn't indicate that the neonate is depressed. Option 4: The Apgar rating doesn't determine the need for a high-glucose feeding.

NP: Planning care
CN: Health promotion and maintenance
CNS: Growth and development through the life span
CL: Application

39 CORRECT ANSWER: 2

When amniotic membranes have been ruptured longer than 24 hours, the risk of puerperal infection increases. The cardinal sign of puerperal infection is an elevated temperature. Options 1, 3, and 4 aren't related to an early rupture of membranes.

NP: Collecting data
CN: Physiological integrity
CNS: Physiological adaptation
CL: Comprehension

40 CORRECT ANSWER: 1

Fluphenazine decanoate, a long-acting antipsychotic medication, is administered I.M. once every 4 to 6 weeks. Because the client's last dose was 1 week ago, no action concerning his medication is necessary. Options 2, 3, and 4 would be inappropriate.
NP: Collecting data
CN: Physiological integrity
CNS: Pharmacological therapies
CL: Application

41 CORRECT ANSWER: 3

An irregular pulse is a sign of lithium toxicity, a life-threatening condition that occurs with serum levels above 3.5 mEq/L. Other symptoms of toxicity include altered level of consciousness, seizures, and coma. Option 1: A serum level of 1.2 mEq/L is considered within the therapeutic range for this drug. Options 2 and 4: Increased appetite and weight gain aren't signs of toxicity.
NP: Evaluating care
CN: Physiological integrity
CNS: Pharmacological therapies
CL: Application

42 CORRECT ANSWER: 1

Because the pH is low (less than 7.35) and the $PaCO_2$ is elevated (above 45 mm Hg), the client probably has respiratory acidosis with hypoxemia. Option 2: In respiratory alkalosis, the pH is above 7.45 and the $PaCO_2$ level is below 35 mm Hg. Option 3: In metabolic acidosis, the pH is below 7.35 and the $PaCO_2$ level may be less than 35 mm Hg. Option 4: In metabolic alkalosis, the pH is greater than 7.45 and the $PaCO_2$ may be above 45 mm Hg.
NP: Collecting data
CN: Physiological integrity
CNS: Physiological adaptation
CL: Analysis

43 CORRECT ANSWER: 3

Educating parents about the safe storage of drugs and other poisonous substances is vital to reduce the risk of future poisoning episodes. Option 1: A 3-year-old child would be incapable of understanding such an explanation. Option 2: Although having syrup of ipecac is important, teaching preventive measures is the priority. Option 4: This information is incorrect because vomiting is contraindicated for ingestion of some substances. The nurse should provide the parents with the telephone number of the local poison control center instead.
NP: Planning care
CN: Health promotion and maintenance
CNS: Growth and development through the life span
CL: Analysis

44 CORRECT ANSWER: 3

Insomnia, weakness, muscle tremors, anxiety, irritability, sweating, anorexia, fever, nausea, vomiting, headache, incoordination, and restlessness are common symptoms of the early stages of withdrawal. Options 1, 2, and 4: Hypotension, slurred speech, and dry mouth aren't associated with early withdrawal.
NP: Collecting data
CN: Physiological integrity
CNS: Pharmacological therapies
CL: Application

45 CORRECT ANSWER: 1

The nurse should check the fetal heart rate immediately after the membranes rupture to assess for fetal distress caused by a prolapsed cord. Option 2: Changing the client's position is unnecessary if there is no sign of fetal distress. Option 3: The contractions should be timed; however, this isn't the priority. Option 4: Maternal vital signs shouldn't be affected.
NP: Implementing care
CN: Health promotion and maintenance
CNS: Growth and development through the life span
CL: Application

46 CORRECT ANSWER: 4

Provide a copy of written instructions so that the client has something to refer to after discharge. Option 1: High-pitched tones are harder for the elderly to hear. Option 2: The client may be anxious to leave and busy getting everything ready for discharge and wouldn't be as receptive to teaching at this time. Option 3: Although the client may be more relaxed, he may also be more distracted when eating and not hear all of the instructions.
NP: Planning care
CN: Safe, effective care environment
CNS: Safety and infection control
CL: Comprehension

47 CORRECT ANSWER: 3

Nursing assistants are taught proper positioning skills, although this activity still needs to be supervised. Option 1: It isn't necessary to accompany the client to speech therapy and would take the assistant off the unit, reducing available help. Option 2: Not all nursing assistants are taught to perform active range-of-motion exercises. Option 4: It wouldn't be necessary to teach the client sign language.
NP: Planning care
CN: Safe, effective care environment
CNS: Coordinated care
CL: Comprehension

48 CORRECT ANSWER: 1

It's important to report when a catheter was removed so that the client can be monitored for urine retention. Option 2: It isn't vital to pass on information such as number of visitors but the client may be tired from all the activity. Option 3: The physician's absence isn't vital information. Option 4: It's important to report that the client was medicated for a headache but this isn't as critical as information about the client's catheter removal and voiding pattern.

NP: Planning care
CN: Safe, effective care environment
CNS: Coordinated care
CL: Application

49 CORRECT ANSWER: 3

Hemianopsia involves loss of one-half of the visual field. The client would only see the food on the right half of the tray. Options 1, 2, and 4: Using one arm only, pocketing food in one side of the mouth, and drooling aren't related to the visual fields.

NP: Collecting data
CN: Safe, effective care environment
CNS: Safety and infection control
CL: Application

50 CORRECT ANSWER: 2

The nurse needs to assess the client herself to determine what might have precipitated the episode and obtain a pulse oximetry reading if indicated. Option 1: Instructing the nursing assistant to observe the client for any further shortness of breath would be appropriate after the nurse has checked the client. Option 3: It wouldn't be necessary to inform the physician about the client's episode of shortness of breath. Option 4: After checking the client, the nurse may ask the nursing assistant to complete the bath after allowing the client to rest.

NP: Implementing care
CN: Safe, effective care environment
CNS: Coordinated care
CL: Application

51 CORRECT ANSWER: 1

The nurse is obligated to report any suspected substance abuse. Option 2: Allowing the assistant to continue to work could jeopardize client care. Option 3: It isn't the practical nurse's role to decide that the assistant must leave the unit immediately. Option 4: Warning the assistant that she could lose her certification doesn't address the issue sufficiently.

NP: Planning care
CN: Safe, effective care environment
CNS: Coordinated care
CL: Comprehension

52 CORRECT ANSWER: 4

Conditions affecting the spinal cord may lead to a reduction in sensory input. Sensory deprivation should be minimized in this case. Confinement secondary to traction, immobility, and bed rest also increase sensory deprivation and steps should be taken to minimize sensory deprivation in such cases. Option 1: Pancreatitis doesn't result in sensory de-

privation. Option 2: There isn't enough information to determine if an injury occurred to reduce sensory stimuli in the 84-year-old woman admitted to the emergency department. Option 3: The client on a ventilator in the intensive care unit (ICU) may be exposed to sensory overload while in the ICU.

NP: Planning care
CN: Safe, effective care environment
CNS: Safety and infection control
CL: Comprehension

53 CORRECT ANSWER: 2

To obtain the most accurate information, the client should be alert, relaxed, and pain-free. Option 1: If the client is in pain, he won't want to read the material. It's best to leave written materials after interviewing the client. Options 3 and 4: It's best to wait until the client is relieved of the pain so the nurse doesn't have to hurry through the interview and can obtain as much information as needed.

NP: Collecting data
CN: Physiological integrity
CNS: Basic care and comfort
CL: Comprehension

54 CORRECT ANSWER: 3

The best advice empowers the client to learn more about illegal drugs so she'll know what to watch for in her son. It also encourages her to keep lines of communication open with her son. Option 1: Telling the mother that she has cause to be concerned doesn't address how she can deal with her concern; it only confirms her concerns. Option 2: Telling the mother to forbid her son from associating with other teens doesn't address the potential problem of drug use; it avoids the issue and may be unrealistic. Option 4: It isn't known that the son is using drugs, so suggesting a treatment program isn't an appropriate response.

NP: Implementing care
CN: Health promotion and maintenance
CNS: Prevention and early detection of disease
CL: Application

55 CORRECT ANSWER: 4

When a severely depressed client suddenly begins to feel better, it often indicates the client has decided to kill himself or has developed a plan to commit suicide. He also has the energy now to carry out his thoughts. Option 1: Depression isn't always associated with psychotic behavior. Option 2: Improvement in mood doesn't indicate an increased depressive state. Option 3: Depressed clients have a tendency toward self-violence, not toward others.

NP: Collecting data
CN: Psychosocial integrity
CNS: Coping and adaptation
CL: Application

56 CORRECT ANSWER: 1

The client is experiencing grandiose delusions, which involve feelings of self-importance and uniqueness. Option 2: Nihilistic delusions are related to denial of self-existence. Option 3: Persecutory delusions are related to feelings of being conspired against. Option 4: Clients who are paranoid are suspicious and distrustful of others.

NP: Collecting data
CN: Psychosocial integrity
CNS: Psychosocial adaptation
CL: Comprehension

57 CORRECT ANSWER: 3

A current, effective therapy for Lyme disease involves treatment with tetracycline, erythromycin, or cephalosporin antibiotics. Option 1: No special diet is required in the treatment of Lyme disease. Option 2: Activity restrictions aren't indicated in the treatment of Lyme disease, although the infected person may experience flulike symptoms. Option 4: Plasma transfusions aren't necessary in the treatment of Lyme disease.

NP: Planning care
CN: Health promotion and maintenance
CNS: Prevention and early detection of disease
CL: Comprehension

58 CORRECT ANSWER: 1

Cleaning the mouth before meals enhances sensual stimuli and taste bud function. Option 2: Checking urine output doesn't affect sensory input. Options 3 and 4: Checking hand grasps and orienting the client would help to assess and stimulate neurologic deficits.

NP: Implementing care
CN: Safe, effective care environment
CNS: Coordinated care
CL: Application

59 CORRECT ANSWER: 4

Cola contains caffeine and may still be in the system at bedtime, interfering with sleep. Option 1: Eating toast at bedtime wouldn't interfere with sleep. Option 2: The effects of eating chili at lunchtime should be gone by bedtime. Option 3: The effects of drinking caffeine-containing coffee at breakfast would be gone by bedtime.

NP: Evaluating care
CN: Physiological integrity
CNS: Basic care and comfort
CL: Comprehension

60 CORRECT ANSWER: 3

The best way to obtain information about a client's cultural background and beliefs is to ask the client directly. Option 1: Don't assume that all members of an ethnic or cultural group share the same beliefs and practices. Option 2: The family may not know the client's specific beliefs and practices. Option 4: The medical record may not provide cultural or ethnic information and, even if it does, it can't

be assumed that the client subscribes to all the practices of the group.

NP: Collecting data
CN: Safe, effective care environment
CNS: Coordinated care
CL: Comprehension

61 CORRECT ANSWER: 2

The nursing diagnosis should specify the exact knowledge deficit, which is the client's lack of knowledge about foods high in potassium. Option 1: Although the client may be at risk for arrhythmias if potassium intake is insufficient, this isn't the appropriate diagnosis for the problem. Option 3: The client doesn't have imbalanced nutrition with low potassium intake. Option 4: The client's knowledge deficit is about food sources that are high in potassium.

NP: Planning care
CN: Physiological integrity
CNS: Reduction of risk potential
CL: Application

62 CORRECT ANSWER: 3

Educational materials that are of value to the client must be accurate. Learning is enhanced if the materials are also appropriate to the client's reading and education levels. Option 1: Providing the materials before the planned learning experience may be helpful but it doesn't ensure that the client will read or view them before teaching occurs. Option 2: Materials don't need to be lengthy. The client could be discouraged if it's overwhelming. Option 4: Materials shouldn't be too brief but should be accurate and cover all pertinent material.

NP: Collecting data
CN: Safe, effective care environment
CNS: Coordinated care
CL: Comprehension

63 CORRECT ANSWER: 2

The appropriate documentation indicates that client was instructed in and then demonstrated the correct technique of wound care. This signifies that the client understood and can apply the learning. Option 1: Only documenting that the client was instructed in proper wound care and dressing is too vague and doesn't specify what was learned. Option 3: Noting that the client and family verbalize understanding of proper wound care is a good way to evaluate learning but doesn't reflect that the client was able to do the wound care correctly. Option 4: Documenting that written instructions were given to the client is incorrect and doesn't reflect teaching or learning.

NP: Evaluating care
CN: Safe, effective care environment
CNS: Safety and infection control
CL: Comprehension

64 CORRECT ANSWER: 3

Dusting with a damp cloth picks up more dust and should be done daily to reduce dust mites. Option 1: Stuffed animals can harbor dust mites. Option 2: An environment high in humidity encourages growth of allergens and molds. Option 4: Carpeting should be removed when allergies are a problem.

NP: Evaluating care
CN: Health promotion and maintenance
CNS: Prevention and early detection of disease
CL: Application

65 CORRECT ANSWER: 3

Placing the client on the right side puts pressure on the liver to aid in preventing bleeding, because the liver is highly vascular. A pillow or blanket is placed along the costal margin. Options 1, 2, and 4: Other positions wouldn't put enough weight and pressure against the liver.

NP: Planning care
CN: Physiological integrity
CNS: Reduction of risk potential
CL: Application

66 CORRECT ANSWER: 1

Abdominal distention from ascites pushes upward on the diaphragm and can cause shortness of breath and labored breathing. A decrease in the respiratory rate indicates that this upward pressure has been relieved. Option 2: Such a decrease in blood pressure could indicate that the client is going into shock. The fluid removed from the abdomen is sometimes replaced by fluid in the vascular space, leading to hypovolemic shock. Option 3: Paracentesis wouldn't relieve a headache. Option 4: Reducing the abdominal fluid can make ambulating easier but this isn't the best indicator that the procedure was effective.

NP: Evaluating care
CN: Physiological integrity
CNS: Physiological adaptation
CL: Application

67 CORRECT ANSWER: 2

Restricting fluid intake contributes to urinary stasis, which in turn contributes to bacterial growth. Option 1: Wiping from front to back prevents spreading bacteria toward the urethra. Option 3: Drinking cranberry juice helps to maintain urine acidity, which retards bacterial growth. Option 4: Emptying the bladder frequently reduces the chance of urinary stasis and subsequent bacterial growth.

NP: Evaluating care
CN: Health promotion and maintenance
CNS: Prevention and early detection of disease
CL: Application

68 CORRECT ANSWER: 1

Projection involves attributing one's feelings or thoughts to another person. Option 2: Denial involves nonacceptance or lack of acknowledgement of reality. Option 3: Reaction formation involves substituting an unacceptable behavior or impulse into a socially acceptable one. Option 4: Displacement involves transferring feelings or behaviors to an acceptable object.

NP: Collecting data
CN: Psychosocial integrity
CNS: Coping and adaptation
CL: Comprehension

69 CORRECT ANSWER: 4

A priority when working with autistic children is establishing a trusting relationship. Option 1: Maintaining a relationship with the family is important but gaining the child's trust is the nurse's first priority. Option 2: It would be unrealistic to expect an autistic child to be involved in these types of school activities. Option 3: A high-protein diet isn't necessary.

NP: Evaluating care
CN: Psychosocial integrity
CNS: Coping and adaptation
CL: Application

70 CORRECT ANSWER: 3

Irritation and confusion are signs of hypoxia, which is caused by the fat emboli traveling to the lungs and producing an inflammatory response in lung tissue. Option 1: Abdominal cramping may be a sign of abdominal distention and constipation caused by immobility. Option 2: Fatty stools occur with pancreatitis. Option 4: Numbness may be secondary to neurovascular impairment.

NP: Collecting data
CN: Physiological integrity
CNS: Physiological adaptation
CL: Application

71 CORRECT ANSWER: 4

As blood from the upper GI tract passes through the intestines, bacterial action causes it to become black. Option 1: Hemoptysis involves coughing up blood from the lungs. Option 2: Hematuria is blood in the urine. Option 3: Bright red blood in the stools indicates bleeding from the lower GI tract.

NP: Collecting data
CN: Physiological integrity
CNS: Physiological adaptation
CL: Application

72 CORRECT ANSWER: 3

Warmth and the movement of the extremities during a bath eases the stiffness and pain of rheumatoid arthritis. Option 1: Ambulation when the client first awakens is the worst time because pain and stiffness are greatest after long periods of immobility. Option 2: The client may be too tired soon after returning from therapy. Option 4: There is no relationship between eating and ease of ambulation in rheumatoid arthritis.

NP: Planning care
CN: Physiological integrity
CNS: Basic care and comfort
CL: Comprehension

73 CORRECT ANSWER: 2
Hepatitis B can lead to cancer of the liver, especially if the person has chronic hepatitis. Options 1 and 4: Hepatitis B can become chronic or lead to a carrier state. Option 3: Hepatitis B is spread through blood and body fluids and persons should take precautions to prevent it from being spread through sexual activity.
NP: Evaluating care
CN: Physiological integrity
CNS: Physiological adaptation
CL: Application

74 CORRECT ANSWER: 3
A nasogastric tube is inserted to reduce stimulation of the pancreas. Drainage should be normal gastric and bile fluid, which is golden-yellow to green in color. Options 1 and 4: Clear to white or clear drainage with large amounts of mucus wouldn't indicate secretions from the stomach and small intestine. Option 2: Light-pink drainage with occasional small clots indicates abnormal bleeding.
NP: Collecting data
CN: Physiological integrity
CNS: Reduction of risk potential
CL: Comprehension

75 CORRECT ANSWER: 4
It's most important to clean the nail beds and between the fingers because they tend to harbor microorganisms and should be given special attention when hand washing. Option 1: It's desirable but not essential to use warm water. Friction is most responsible for removing microorganisms from the skin. Option 2: Drying each hand with a separate paper towel is desirable but not essential. Option 3: Antibacterial soap isn't required and may, over time, remove healthy normal flora on the skin.
NP: Collecting data
CN: Safe, effective care environment
CNS: Safety and infection control
CL: Comprehension

76 CORRECT ANSWER: 4
A small meal doesn't distend the stomach as much as a large meal, thereby preventing upward pressure of the stomach. Option 1: Lying down after eating would cause reflux of gastric contents into the esophagus. Option 2: Concentrated sweets should be avoided in diabetes mellitus and to prevent dumping syndrome after gastric resection. Option 3: Sleeping on the right side doesn't reduce symptoms of a hiatal hernia.
NP: Evaluating care
CN: Physiological integrity
CNS: Reduction of risk potential
CL: Comprehension

77 CORRECT ANSWER: 2
Because a local anesthetic is sprayed on the throat during an EGD, a positive gag reflex must be present before the client can have anything to eat or

drink. Option 1: It isn't necessary to wait for the report. Option 3: Antibiotics aren't routinely administered following an EGD. Option 4: An EGD shouldn't interrupt peristalsis.
NP: Collecting data
CN: Physiological integrity
CNS: Reduction of risk potential
CL: Application

78 CORRECT ANSWER: 1
As the prostate gland enlarges, it interferes with complete bladder emptying and the ability to initiate urination, which contributes to urgency and hesitancy. Option 2: Hematuria and painful urination might occur after the prostate resection because tissues have been cut and the urethra is tender and swollen from intubation. Option 3: Bladder spasms might occur after the procedure. Option 4: Flank pain is a sign of a kidney problem, not a prostate problem.
NP: Collecting data
CN: Physiological integrity
CNS: Physiological adaptation
CL: Application

79 CORRECT ANSWER: 3
Heparin is an anticoagulant and interferes with the conversion of fibrinogen to fibrin and prothrombin to thrombin, thus prolonging clotting time. As a result, the client bruises easily, as manifested by the ecchymotic areas. Option 1: Headaches wouldn't be related to heparin therapy. Option 2: A firm, distended abdomen could be a sign of constipation. Option 4: The deep vein thrombosis, not the heparin infusion, would cause fluid collection around the blood vessel and a local inflammatory response, resulting in swelling and warmth in the leg.
NP: Collecting data
CN: Physiological integrity
CNS: Pharmacological therapies
CL: Application

80 CORRECT ANSWER: 3
Aspirin is irritating to the stomach lining, possibly contributing to further ulceration and bleeding, and is contraindicated with peptic ulcer disease. Option 1: Foods high in calcium wouldn't be discouraged. Option 2: Fruit juices aren't contraindicated unless they're highly acidic and the client doesn't tolerate them. Option 4: Ice cold or frozen foods aren't contraindicated in clients with peptic ulcer disease.
NP: Evaluating care
CN: Physiological integrity
CNS: Reduction of risk potential
CL: Application

81 CORRECT ANSWER: 3
Monitoring intake and output alerts the nurse to the development of dehydration and cerebral edema, complications of Reye's syndrome. Option 1: Although checking the skin for signs of breakdown is important because the child may not be as active

as normal, it isn't as critical as monitoring the client's intake and output. Option 2: Active range-of-motion exercises may not be needed and aren't as important as monitoring the client's intake and output. Option 4: Placing the client in protective isolation isn't necessary.

NP: Planning care
CN: Physiological integrity
CNS: Reduction of risk potential
CL: Application

82 CORRECT ANSWER: 1

In children under age 3, the ear should be pulled down and back to straighten the ear canal and allow medication to flow easily to the eardrum. Option 2: Pulling the pinna of the ear up and back is appropriate for clients over age 3. Option 3: Pulling the pinna of the ear directly toward the back of the head is incorrect for inserting eardrops. Option 4: Inserting the dropper far into the ear canal could puncture the eardrum. The dropper should be inserted only as far as the edge of the ear canal.

NP: Evaluating care
CN: Physiological integrity
CNS: Basic care and comfort
CL: Application

83 CORRECT ANSWER: 4

Providing a calm, quiet environment reduces excessive stimuli and helps the client be less hyperactive. Option 1: During the manic phase, the client has difficulty concentrating, and playing games with another client might increase her agitation. Option 2: The manic client is easily overstimulated and group activities requiring a lot of physical activity would most likely be overstimulating. Option 3: Manic clients are unable to safely set their own limits.

NP: Planning care
CN: Psychosocial integrity
CNS: Psychosocial adaptation
CL: Application

84 CORRECT ANSWER: 2

Clients with arteriovenous fistulas should avoid having blood pressure readings, venipunctures, wearing anything restrictive on the arm, and carrying more than 5 to 10 lb of weight with the arm. The excess weight could cause constriction and occlude the fistula. Option 1: After 1 week, the suture line should be sufficiently healed and the site shouldn't be covered when showering. Option 3: It isn't necessary to keep the arm immobilized in a sling. Option 4: It isn't necessary to keep the site covered with a dressing.

NP: Evaluating care
CN: Physiological integrity
CNS: Reduction of risk potential
CL: Application

85 CORRECT ANSWER: 2

Tightening and relaxing the calf muscles increases circulation and promotes venous return, thereby preventing venous stasis, which contributes to thrombophlebitis. Option 1: Massaging the client's legs could dislodge a clot if present. Option 3: Keeping the knees bent encourages venous stasis by blocking venous return and arterial blood flow to the lower extremities. Option 4: Dangling the legs over the side of the bed leads to pooling of the blood in the lower legs, contributing to venous stasis and thrombus formation.

NP: Planning care
CN: Physiological integrity
CNS: Reduction of risk potential
CL: Application

POSTTEST 2

To assess your readiness for NCLEX-PN, take the following posttest, which contains 85 questions on the four subject areas covered on the actual examination. Then check your responses against the correct answers and rationales provided on pages 257 to 267.

QUESTIONS

1 Which nursing intervention would be most appropriate for a 2-week-old boy with a diagnosis of pyloric stenosis?
- ☐ 1. Provide clear liquids instead of formula.
- ☐ 2. Position the neonate on the left side after feeding.
- ☐ 3. Feed the neonate slowly.
- ☐ 4. Encourage the parents to hold and rock the neonate after feedings.

2 Which information is critical to include in the discharge plans for a client leaving the hospital in a leg cast?
- ☐ 1. Cast care procedures and devices to relieve itching
- ☐ 2. Skin care, mouth care, and cast removal procedures
- ☐ 3. Cast care, neurovascular checks, and hygiene measures
- ☐ 4. Cast removal procedures, neurovascular checks, and devices to relieve itching

3 The nurse is interviewing a client with a diagnosis of anorexia nervosa. Which type of family dynamics is the client likely to report?
- ☐ 1. Rigidity
- ☐ 2. Pattern of substance abuse
- ☐ 3. Pattern of overeating
- ☐ 4. Close-knit family life

4 A client with late-stage Alzheimer's disease who resides in an extended-care facility often misidentifies staff members as family or friends. How should the unit nurse instruct the ancillary nursing staff to prepare the client for his wife's visits?

☐ 1. Tell him that his wife is here to visit him.
☐ 2. Ask him if he remembers his wife each time she visits.
☐ 3. Ask him if he wants to visit with his wife when she arrives.
☐ 4. Refer to his wife by an endearing nickname in his presence.

5 The nurse is caring for a 4-month-old boy with a confirmed diagnosis of pertussis. The mother tells the nurse that the infant hasn't received his immunizations because her oldest child had a seizure after his first immunization and she feels that it's better to wait until infants are 6 months old to receive their first shot. She followed this same procedure with all five of her other children, and they never got sick. Which response by the nurse would be most appropriate?

☐ 1. "If you had listened to the pediatrician, your son wouldn't be here today."
☐ 2. "Even with the immunization, your son would have had a 50% chance of contracting pertussis."
☐ 3. "Now that your son has the disease, you won't have to worry about immunizations."
☐ 4. "Let's talk about how childhood diseases occur and how to protect your children from them."

6 A 3-week-old neonate has been receiving total parenteral nutrition (TPN) for the past week. The physician prescribed a blood transfusion to be given over the next several hours. The TPN is to be stopped during the blood transfusion. Which value is extremely important to monitor during the blood administration?

☐ 1. Hematocrit
☐ 2. Glucose
☐ 3. Specific gravity
☐ 4. Platelet count

7 Which response by a client best indicates an understanding of the adverse effects of phenytoin sodium (Dilantin)?

☐ 1. "I should take the medication with food to prevent nausea."
☐ 2. "I need to take this medication until my seizures stop."
☐ 3. "I need to see the dentist every 6 months."
☐ 4. "I need to report any drowsiness to the physician immediately."

8 A client with chronic obstructive pulmonary disease is receiving 2 L of oxygen/minute by way of a nasal cannula but continues to complain of shortness of breath despite having a respiratory rate of 35 breaths/minute. Which action should the nurse take?

☐ 1. Increase the oxygen to 6 L/minute.
☐ 2. Notify the physician immediately.
☐ 3. Instruct the client to breathe with pursed lips.
☐ 4. Administer morphine sulfate to slow the respiratory rate.

9 The nurse is instructing a client who is 7 months pregnant in ways to deal with her back pain. Which statement made by the client indicates that she understood the patient-teaching session?

☐ 1. "I'll do Kegel exercises when I have back pain".
☐ 2. "I'll do pelvic rocking exercises when I have back pain."
☐ 3. "I should wear support stockings now."
☐ 4. "I should wear nonconstrictive clothing."

10 Which postoperative position is best for a client who has had a supratentorial craniotomy?

☐ 1. High Fowler's
☐ 2. Semi-Fowler's
☐ 3. Lying flat with a small pillow
☐ 4. Side-lying

11 A client with a long history of bleeding esophageal varices has had a Sengstaken-Blakemore tube in place for 3 days. What should the nurse do first in preparing to remove the tube?

☐ 1. Deflate the esophageal balloon.
☐ 2. Deflate the gastric balloon.
☐ 3. Release the traction on the nose.
☐ 4. Deflate the gastric and esophageal balloons simultaneously.

12 The nurse is caring for a female client who has paraplegia as a result of a cerebrovascular accident. Nursing orders include turning the client at least every 2 hours during the day and no more than every 2 hours during the night. The nurse knows that turning this client too frequently during the night may:

☐ 1. interfere with rapid-eye-movement (REM) sleep and increase the client's confusion.
☐ 2. increase the nursing staff's nighttime workload.
☐ 3. increase the client's risk for injury due to shearing forces.
☐ 4. disturb other clients on the nursing unit.

13 A female client with a history of thrombophlebitis has started taking warfarin sodium (Coumadin) daily and asks the nurse why the medication is necessary. The nurse correctly explains that warfarin sodium:

☐ 1. thins the blood.
☐ 2. helps dissolve clots that are already present.
☐ 3. prolongs the time needed for the blood to clot.
☐ 4. will only be necessary while the client is on bed rest.

14 A full-length plaster cast was just applied to the left leg of a client with a fractured femur. The nurse realizes that the cast normally takes 10 to 48 hours to dry and hastens the drying process by:
☐ 1. suspending the cast by the foot to allow full air circulation.
☐ 2. using a hair dryer to speed the drying process.
☐ 3. wrapping the cast with towels to absorb the moisture.
☐ 4. resting the entire cast on pillows and turning the leg every 2 to 3 hours.

15 A neonate has a 5-minute Apgar score of 8. Which nursing measure is most appropriate?
☐ 1. Administer oxygen.
☐ 2. Prepare to administer stimulant medications.
☐ 3. Place the neonate in a warmed environment.
☐ 4. Provide a high-glucose feeding.

16 The membranes of a primigravida who is in labor suddenly rupture. Which action should the nurse take?
☐ 1. Check the fetal heart rate.
☐ 2. Place the client on her left side.
☐ 3. Time the client's contractions.
☐ 4. Determine the client's vital signs.

17 During the admission interview of a male client with a history of chronic schizophrenia, the client reports that he has been taking haloperidol decanoate (Haldol decanoate) and that he received his last dose 1 week ago. Which nursing intervention is most appropriate upon hearing this information?
☐ 1. Take no action.
☐ 2. Call the physician for an immediate drug order.
☐ 3. Withhold all medication until further notice.
☐ 4. Watch the client for withdrawal symptoms.

18 Which statement by a client is considered a presumptive sign of pregnancy?
☐ 1. "My breasts are so tender."
☐ 2. "I have a slight burning when I urinate."
☐ 3. "The brown spots on my face seem to be getting darker."
☐ 4. "I become nauseated and vomit when I eat French fries."

19 Which statement indicates that a client with rheumatoid arthritis understands how to control her disease?
☐ 1. "Pain medication will allow me to continue my activities as I always have."
☐ 2. "I should take my anti-inflammatory medication with food to prevent gastric irritation."
☐ 3. "If I exercise the affected joint a lot, it will be less painful."
☐ 4. "I should do all of my work in the morning so that I can rest in the afternoon."

20 A 14-year-old girl is in the 5th month of her pregnancy. Which factor places her at risk for the development of pregnancy-induced hypertension?
☐ 1. Her sexual partner's hypertension
☐ 2. Her mother's diabetes mellitus
☐ 3. Her hematocrit of 30%
☐ 4. Her age

21 A boy with diabetes has a blood glucose level of 58 mg/dl before breakfast. The nurse is to administer regular and NPH insulin as prescribed for his routine morning insulin dose. Which nursing action is appropriate?
☐ 1. Provide extra servings of food for breakfast.
☐ 2. Notify the physician and clarify the morning insulin order.
☐ 3. Wait about 15 minutes after the insulin injection before serving his breakfast.
☐ 4. Wait at least 45 minutes after the insulin injection before serving his breakfast.

22 Which finding in a 3-week-old full-term neonate is considered abnormal?
☐ 1. Mongolian spots
☐ 2. Milia
☐ 3. Generalized petechiae
☐ 4. Short, thick neck

23 Which statement by the nurse is most appropriate when dealing with a 7-year-old child in pain?
☐ 1. "I'm going to give you a needle to make the pain go away."
☐ 2. "You shouldn't need so much pain medicine."
☐ 3. "This medicine will take away anyone's pain."
☐ 4. "The needle will hurt a little but it'll make the pain better."

24 A client with active tuberculosis asks the nurse whether his wife and family are at risk for developing the disease if they visit him at the hospital. Which response by the nurse is best?
☐ 1. "No visitors will be permitted for the first few days to avoid transmission of the disease."
☐ 2. "You may have visitors, and they'll be instructed to wear masks while visiting."
☐ 3. "Tuberculosis is transmitted by touching clothing and other things in the room, so visitors are restricted."
☐ 4. "After you begin treatment, you'll no longer be infectious, so visitors will be permitted."

25 A client is being discharged with a prescription for a metered-dose inhaler of albuterol (Ventolin) with instructions to take two puffs every 6 hours. Which instruction should the nurse give the client?
☐ 1. Inhale quickly while depressing the inhaler.
☐ 2. Space each puff 1 to 2 minutes apart.
☐ 3. Take additional puffs with increased shortness of breath.
☐ 4. Try to hold each breath for 5 seconds after each inhaled puff.

26 A client has the following arterial blood gas levels: pH, 7.29; $PaCO_2$, 51 mm Hg; PaO_2, 60 mm Hg; and HCO_3^-, 25 mEq/L. These results are indicative of which acid-base imbalance?
☐ 1. Respiratory alkalosis
☐ 2. Respiratory acidosis
☐ 3. Metabolic alkalosis
☐ 4. Metabolic acidosis

27 A female client who was involved in a high-speed motor vehicle accident has an obvious deformed open fracture of the right femur that is bleeding significantly. She's alert and oriented and complains of severe pain. Which nursing intervention is the priority?
☐ 1. Align and splint the fracture.
☐ 2. Administer high-flow oxygen.
☐ 3. Apply direct pressure to the bleeding area.
☐ 4. Administer an analgesic as ordered.

28 Which changes in vital signs indicate that a client's intracranial pressure is increasing?
☐ 1. Increased pulse rate and decreased blood pressure
☐ 2. Increased pulse rate and increased blood pressure
☐ 3. Decreased pulse rate and decreased blood pressure
☐ 4. Decreased pulse rate and increased blood pressure

29 The physician orders forced fluids for a female client with lobar pneumonia who is producing thick, tenacious sputum. The nurse understands that encouraging the client to drink copious amounts of fluids helps to:
☐ 1. prevent a temperature elevation.
☐ 2. provide calories because the client's appetite is poor.
☐ 3. liquefy secretions.
☐ 4. maintain a patent airway.

30 A 70-year-old male client underwent a colostomy 5 days ago. The nurse teaches him how to irrigate the colostomy and explains that the primary purpose of the irrigation is to:
☐ 1. establish a regular elimination schedule.
☐ 2. eliminate bacteria in the bowel.
☐ 3. decrease flatus buildup in the bowel.
☐ 4. prevent constipation.

31 A nurse working in a local volunteer clinic is withdrawing blood from a client with suspected human immunodeficiency virus. While withdrawing the needle, blood splashes on the nurse's arm. What should the nurse do first?
☐ 1. Wash the area with bacteriostatic soap and water.
☐ 2. Scrub vigorously with povidone-iodine solution.
☐ 3. Rinse with water, then with isopropyl alcohol.
☐ 4. Wash the area with ammonia chloride.

32 A client with acute glomerulonephritis has received a lunch tray with spaghetti and meatless sauce, bread, fruit, and apple juice. The client complains to the nurse and asks why he can't have meat sauce. What should the nurse do?
☐ 1. Order a new tray with meat sauce for the client.
☐ 2. Offer to contact the dietitian immediately.
☐ 3. Explain that he needs to restrict his protein intake at this time.
☐ 4. Tell the client that he should consult his physician.

33 A 39-year-old client in her 14th week of pregnancy is scheduled for an amniocentesis. The purpose of this procedure at this time is to:
☐ 1. determine if the fetus has any chromosomal abnormalities.
☐ 2. calculate the expected date of delivery.
☐ 3. determine whether the placenta is secreting a sufficient amount of estriols.
☐ 4. estimate whether the composition of the amniotic fluid being produced is correct.

34 The nurse should advise a client taking monoamine oxidase (MAO) inhibitors to avoid eating:
☐ 1. cottage cheese.
☐ 2. avocados.
☐ 3. apples.
☐ 4. beans and rice.

35 When a client is experiencing a high level of anxiety, which nursing action is most appropriate?
☐ 1. Ask how the client handled anxiety in the past.
☐ 2. Determine the client's available social support.
☐ 3. Teach new coping skills.
☐ 4. Reduce the client's anxiety level.

36 A 13-year-old boy who suffered trauma to the liver and right lower lobe of the lung has a chest tube connected to a Pleur-evac system set at 20 cm of H_2O suction. At 10 a.m., the nurse notes that the Pleur-evac drainage level has increased by 400 ml since the 8 a.m. check. What should the nurse do next?
☐ 1. Notify the physician.
☐ 2. Check the client's vital signs and level of consciousness.
☐ 3. Reduce the amount of suction.
☐ 4. Do nothing because this is within normal limits.

37 During administration of a cleansing enema, a client complains of abdominal cramping. Which action by the nurse is most appropriate?
☐ 1. Tell the client that the enema must be given and continue the enema until completed.
☐ 2. Ask the client to try to relax and run the enema faster to complete it sooner.

3. Stop the enema flow, wait for the cramps to subside, and then resume the flow.
4. Stop the flow and discontinue the enema.

38 A client with acquired immunodeficiency syndrome needs help with repositioning in bed. Which infection-preventing barrier should be used by the nurse?
1. None necessary
2. Gloves
3. Gloves and a gown
4. Gloves, a gown, and a mask

39 The nurse is caring for a 30-year-old client who has full-thickness burns of the face and neck as a result of a flash burn. Which nursing diagnosis should be the nurse's highest priority when developing a plan of care?
1. *Impaired gas exchange*
2. *Ineffective airway clearance*
3. *Deficient fluid volume*
4. *Ineffective tissue perfusion*

40 A 25-year-old construction worker with a history of bipolar disorder is being considered for lithium therapy. Which risk factor would be a contraindication for this type of drug therapy?
1. Obesity
2. Diabetes mellitus
3. Acute cystitis
4. Under age 50

41 A child has been diagnosed with respiratory syncytial virus infection. Which findings would the nurse expect while checking this client?
1. Coughing, labored breathing, and stridor
2. Rhinorrhea, pharyngitis, cough, tachypnea, and low-grade fever
3. Runny nose, harsh cough, moderate fever, and irritability
4. Sore throat, high fever, and nasal congestion

42 A client with a fractured tibia and fibula is in a cast and complains of severe lower leg pain. What should the nurse do first?
1. Assess the client's neurovascular status.
2. Administer pain medication as ordered.
3. Elevate the leg above the level of the heart.
4. Prepare to assist with splitting the cast.

43 The nurse is discussing the signs of impending labor with a client who is in her third trimester of pregnancy. Which statement by the client indicates a need for further instruction?
1. "I may have an increase in Braxton Hicks contractions."
2. "I may feel a sudden desire to straighten my house."
3. "I won't feel the baby move for quite a while."
4. "I may have blood-tinged mucus in my vaginal discharge."

44 Which defense mechanism is most commonly used by clients with anorexia nervosa?
1. Reaction formation
2. Sublimation
3. Rationalization
4. Manipulation

45 A client arrives in the emergency department lethargic with paralysis of the left arm and leg. The nurse should focus primarily on assessing the client's:
1. alertness.
2. reflexes.
3. pupil accommodation.
4. motor function.

46 A mother brings her 10-year-old child to a family health clinic because she found several deer ticks on the child over the past 2 weeks. She's concerned that the child may have Lyme disease. The nurse checks the child for:
1. clear-fluid-filled blisters at the site of the tick bite.
2. a bull's-eye-shaped, red rash at the site of the tick bite.
3. pinpoint-size hemorrhagic areas around the tick bite.
4. a diffuse, flat, red rash in the area of the bite.

47 A client who was recently diagnosed with hepatitis B is being prepared for discharge in 1 to 2 days. Which statement by the client indicates a need for further teaching?
1. "It's OK if I have a glass of wine every other day."
2. "I should avoid using any over-the-counter medications for a headache."
3. "I know I need to increase my activity gradually."
4. "I'll be sure not to let anyone else use my razor."

48 The nurse is caring for a 2-year-old child with suspected cystic fibrosis. Which test is most likely ordered to confirm the diagnosis?
1. Sputum culture
2. Sweat test
3. Chest X-ray
4. Urine culture

49 The nurse is caring for a 26-year-old male client admitted to the mental health unit with a diagnosis of bipolar disorder. His wife reports he's been buying a lot of unnecessary things lately, has lost weight, and only sleeps 3 to 4 hours per day. You expect the client to exhibit which behavior?
1. Being quiet and reserved, keeping close to his room
2. Talking about himself at great length
3. Expressing feelings of hopelessness
4. Changing his bed linens several times per day

50 A client is experiencing alcohol withdrawal delirium tremens. The nurse plans to do which of the following?
☐ 1. Restrict fluid intake.
☐ 2. Maintain seizure precautions.
☐ 3. Keep the client occupied with things to do.
☐ 4. Keep the client restrained in bed.

51 The nurse is caring for a client with a cerebral vascular accident who has a diminished gag reflex. To minimize the risk of aspiration the nurse should plan to:
☐ 1. offer the client small sips of clear liquids frequently.
☐ 2. test the gag reflex every 4 hours.
☐ 3. massage the client's throat while feeding.
☐ 4. maintain the client in a side-lying position.

52 The Licensed Practical Nurse (LPN) has been assigned to a client who is scheduled to receive several medications and treatments. The nurse needs to request assistance from the RN in completing which of the following?
☐ 1. Checking blood glucose level with a finger stick
☐ 2. Administering furosemide (Lasix) 40 mg. I.V. push
☐ 3. Monitoring an I.V. infusion of lactated Ringer's solution
☐ 4. Changing a wet-to-dry dressing involving deep wound packing

53 A client who recently became incontinent due to pelvic surgery is being prepared for discharge. To help the client regain bladder continence, the nurse should teach the primary caregiver to:
☐ 1. limit the client's fluid intake.
☐ 2. change the client's diapers every 2 hours.
☐ 3. place the client on a bedpan on a routine schedule.
☐ 4. keep the call bell within easy reach of the client.

54 A 46-year-old female with a cerebrovascular accident has left-sided hemiparesis and facial drooping. She's tearful and tells the nurse that she's embarrassed by how she looks. Which nursing action can best help the client deal with her altered body image?
☐ 1. Encourage her to discuss her feelings.
☐ 2. Remind her she's right-handed and has that to her advantage.
☐ 3. Help her with her hairstyling and make-up.
☐ 4. Encourage her to focus on gaining reuse of her left side.

55 A client is returning to the floor after having a transurethral resection of the prostate under spinal anesthesia. The nurse instructs the nursing assistant to:
☐ 1. keep the client flat in bed for the rest of the shift.
☐ 2. give the client nothing by mouth until the next day.
☐ 3. encourage the client to urinate every 2 hours.
☐ 4. assist the client out of bed to ambulate.

56 A client is scheduled for a colon resection and tells you that he's having second thoughts about the operation. He realizes he has already signed the consent form but now he's unsure that he wants to have the operation. The nurse should:
☐ 1. explain to the client he's already on the operating room schedule.
☐ 2. reassure him that he's probably just nervous about the surgery.
☐ 3. tell him you'll notify the operating room and have his name removed from the schedule.
☐ 4. communicate this information to his physician.

57 While bathing a client, the nurse gathers information that should be documented in the client's chart. What information should be noted as subjective data?
☐ 1. The client's feet are cool and pale.
☐ 2. The client complains of a headache.
☐ 3. The client becomes short of breath while using the bedpan.
☐ 4. The indwelling catheter is draining dark orange-colored urine.

58 The nurse is caring for a 40-year-old client who was just told by the physician that his cancer has metastasized to his brain and liver. The nurse is aware that the client's behavior may reflect the initial stage of grief, which is:
☐ 1. awareness.
☐ 2. shock.
☐ 3. restitution.
☐ 4. acceptance.

59 The nurse is instructing a 53-year-old male client about a diet to prevent constipation. Which food choices indicate that the client understands the teaching?
☐ 1. Hamburger and mashed potatoes
☐ 2. Grilled cheese sandwich and applesauce
☐ 3. Chili and fresh fruit salad
☐ 4. Chicken breast sandwich and chocolate pudding

60 The nurse is caring for a 59-year-old male client recovering from an open cholecystectomy. Which comment by the client indicates successful preoperative and postoperative teaching?
☐ 1. "It hurts too much when I move, so it's better if I lie still on my back."
☐ 2. "I need to turn from side to side, even if it hurts my incision."
☐ 3. "I know the nurse will bring my pain medication every 3 hours."
☐ 4. " I'm afraid my incision will pop open if I move too much."

61 The nurse is caring for the following group of clients. Which of the clients is at the greatest risk of developing thrombophlebitis?
- ☐ 1. A 16-year-old girl admitted with exacerbation of asthma
- ☐ 2. A 27-year-old male being treated for a peptic ulcer
- ☐ 3. A 42-year-old female who underwent an abdominal hysterectomy
- ☐ 4. A 68-year-old man with lung cancer

62 A 35-year-old client is admitted with a diagnosis of Addison's disease. Which nursing intervention is most appropriate?
- ☐ 1. Provide frequent rest periods.
- ☐ 2. Administer diuretics.
- ☐ 3. Encourage a high-potassium diet.
- ☐ 4. Maintain fluid restrictions.

63 The nurse is instructing a client about prednisone, which she needs to take daily for immunosuppression following bilateral lung transplantation. The nurse knows the client understands how to take this medication correctly when she says:
- ☐ 1. "I should take this medicine on an empty stomach."
- ☐ 2. "I'll always take this medicine at bedtime."
- ☐ 3. "It's best if I take the pill with my evening meal."
- ☐ 4. "I should take this pill in the early morning."

64 The nurse is giving discharge instructions to a client who underwent eye surgery. Which safety precaution should be included?
- ☐ 1. Wear sunglasses at all times.
- ☐ 2. Sleep only on the operative side.
- ☐ 3. Wear a plastic eye shield when sleeping or napping.
- ☐ 4. Avoid watching television or using the computer.

65 The nurse is caring for a 21-year-old male client recovering from burn injuries received in a restaurant fire. The nurse watching for signs of Curling's ulcer, a common complication seen in clients with burns, should observe the client for:
- ☐ 1. purulent drainage from the burn sites.
- ☐ 2. black, tarry stools.
- ☐ 3. a decrease in blood pressure.
- ☐ 4. an irregular heart rate.

66 Which nursing diagnosis has the highest priority when caring for a client with an indwelling urinary catheter?
- ☐ 1. *Deficient knowledge related to first-time experience having an indwelling catheter*
- ☐ 2. *Anxiety related to concern that the catheter will become dislodged*
- ☐ 3. *Risk for infection related to the presence of the catheter*
- ☐ 4. *Acute pain related to irritation from the catheter*

67 The nurse is changing the dressing on a 17-year-old male client with an open abdominal wound received in a motorcycle accident 10 days ago. The nurse should check the wound for signs of granulation which include:
- ☐ 1. serosanguineous drainage.
- ☐ 2. pink, rounded wound edges.
- ☐ 3. pink to red tissue in the wound bed.
- ☐ 4. streaks of yellow tissue in the wound bed.

68 The nurse is instructing a nursing assistant on how to properly position a 45-year-old male client who underwent total hip replacement. The nurse explains that the client's hip needs to be:
- ☐ 1. straight with the knee flexed.
- ☐ 2. in an abducted position.
- ☐ 3. in an adducted position.
- ☐ 4. externally rotated.

69 The nurse in a family health clinic is caring for a 16-year-old female client with anemia. The nurse recognizes that the client:
- ☐ 1. needs to restrict activity as much as possible.
- ☐ 2. should be encouraged to eat foods high in calcium.
- ☐ 3. needs to have activities spaced to allow for rest periods.
- ☐ 4. should be supervised when ambulating.

70 A 54-year-old female client is scheduled for a cardiac catheterization. Before the procedure, the nurse should ask the client which of the following questions?
- ☐ 1. "Do you have any difficulty swallowing?"
- ☐ 2. "Do you have trouble being in a confined space?"
- ☐ 3. "Are you allergic to shellfish?"
- ☐ 4. "Can you tolerate lying on you left side for a long period of time?"

71 The nurse is caring for a client with hypovolemia. While monitoring for signs of impaired renal function, which observation should be reported to the primary nurse?
- ☐ 1. The client's urine output is 60 ml per hour.
- ☐ 2. The mucous membranes are dry and sticky.
- ☐ 3. The client gains 3 lb (1.4 kg) in 24 hours.
- ☐ 4. The client's skin turgor is inelastic.

72 A 60-year-old client tells the nurse she has a mammogram every year but they're always negative and no one in her family has ever had breast cancer. She states," I don't think I need to have them anymore." What is the nurse's best response?
- ☐ 1. "Mammograms can detect changes in your breast before you experience any symptoms."
- ☐ 2. "You really should talk to your physician about your thoughts."
- ☐ 3. "Do you do breast self-examinations every month?"
- ☐ 4. "Do you have any concerns that your insurance won't cover the test?"

73 The nurse is caring for a 61-year-old male client with heart failure. Which nursing action should the nurse's plan of care include?
☐ 1. Encourage the client to drink plenty of potassium rich juices.
☐ 2. Maintain the client on strict bed rest.
☐ 3. Accurately measure intake and output.
☐ 4. Keep the client in a recumbent position.

74 A 51-year-old female client who underwent a total gastrectomy is being prepared for discharge. The nurse recognizes the client needs further instruction regarding postoperative adjustments to surgery when she states:
☐ 1. "I know I should drink a lot of fluid with my meals."
☐ 2. "I'm going to increase my activity gradually when I get home."
☐ 3. "I wish I didn't have to take vitamin B_{12} injections for the rest of my life."
☐ 4. "I'm going to eat small, frequent meals from now on."

75 The nurse is caring for a 30-year-old female client after a bowel resection in the treatment of Crohn's disease. The client asks why she must have a nasogastric tube. The nurse explains that the purpose of the tube is to:
☐ 1. prevent abdominal peritonitis.
☐ 2. administer medications.
☐ 3. prevent distention of the abdomen.
☐ 4. facilitate measurements of gastric pH.

76 A 75-year-old client with Alzheimer's disease is admitted to an acute care setting. Which of the following should the nurse include in the client's plan of care?
☐ 1. Keep his room quiet and dark.
☐ 2. Encourage family members to bring a lot of visitors to see him.
☐ 3. Provide signs in the room to orient the client.
☐ 4. Place the client in a private room.

77 The nurse is caring for a 49-year-old male client diagnosed with diabetes insipidus. The nurse needs to closely monitor:
☐ 1. urine output.
☐ 2. blood glucose level.
☐ 3. heart rate.
☐ 4. bowel sounds.

78 The nurse is caring for a 40-year-old female client who is scheduled to undergo abdominal surgery to reattach the small intestine from a previous ileostomy. While the nurse is administering a cleansing enema, the client begins to complain of abdominal cramping. What should the nurse do next?
☐ 1. Stop the infusion and notify the charge nurse.
☐ 2. Encourage the client to relax and tell her the fluid is almost all inserted.

☐ 3. Instruct client to take slow, deep breaths and lower the infusion bag.
☐ 4. Raise the infusion bag a few inches and finish infusion quickly.

79 When returning from lunch break, the nurse is given a report on her clients from the primary nurse. Lunch trays have arrived on the floor and need to be given to the clients. Which client care need is the nurse's highest priority?
☐ 1. A diabetic client needs to have his blood glucose level checked by a finger stick.
☐ 2. An 88-year-old client needs assistance with feeding.
☐ 3. A client on an every-2-hour turning schedule is due to be turned.
☐ 4. A client who has been incontinent is requesting a bedpan.

80 A 77-year-old male client has been instructed to increase his dietary intake of foods high in zinc to aid in healing a leg ulcer. The client indicates that he understands the teaching by telling the nurse that he'll eat more:
☐ 1. dairy products.
☐ 2. eggs.
☐ 3. green vegetables.
☐ 4. fresh fruit.

81 The nurse is instructing a nursing assistant on the proper care of a client in Buck's extension traction following a fracture of his left fibula. Which observation indicates that the teaching was effective?
☐ 1. The weights are allowed to hang freely over the end of the bed.
☐ 2. The nursing assistant lifts the weights when assisting the client to move up in bed.
☐ 3. The leg in traction is kept externally rotated.
☐ 4. The nursing assistant instructs the client to do ankle rotation exercises.

82 A 20-year-old male client has just had a plaster cast applied to his right forearm following reduction of a closed radius fracture due to an in-line skating accident. It's most important for the nurse to check:
☐ 1. whether the cast is completely dry.
☐ 2. sensation and movement of the fingers.
☐ 3. whether the client is having any pain.
☐ 4. whether the cast needs pedaling.

83 The nurse is checking the laboratory values of a client with chronic renal failure who was just started on hemodialysis. The nurse should expect to find an improvement in:
☐ 1. complete blood count.
☐ 2. white blood cell count.
☐ 3. calcium level.
☐ 4. blood urea nitrogen level.

84 A 31-year-old female client undergoing treatment for alcoholism has received counseling and is ready for discharge. Which of the following best in-

dicates that the client has an adequate support system to help her to cope with recovery?
- ☐ 1. A neighbor of the client comes to visit every day and offers to do anything that will help the client.
- ☐ 2. The client's sister has made arrangements to attend Alcoholics Anonymous meetings with the client.
- ☐ 3. The client's spouse informed the staff that all alcohol has been removed from the house.
- ☐ 4. The client's pastor informs the staff that he'll remain in close contact with the client after discharge.

85 A 5-year-old client is admitted with arm fractures and multiple bruises and is reported to be a victim of abuse by family members. When observing the child's behavior, the nurse expects her to exhibit which of the following?
- ☐ 1. She has minimal interaction with peers.
- ☐ 2. She's able to complete developmental tasks above her age level.
- ☐ 3. She responds enthusiastically when asked to participate in floor activities.
- ☐ 4. She spends a lot of time with her parents and family.

ANSWERS AND RATIONALES

1 CORRECT ANSWER: 3
Although the definitive treatment for pyloric stenosis is surgery, nursing interventions are commonly aimed at helping the neonate retain food and maintain hydration before surgery. Slow feedings and frequent burping help to reduce the incidence of vomiting. Option 1: Feedings are typically thickened, not thinned. Option 2: Using the right side-lying position after feedings facilitates movement of food through the pylorus. Option 4: A neonate with pyloric stenosis should be placed on the right side in Fowler's position after feedings and handled as little as possible.
NP: Implementing care
CN: Physiological integrity
CNS: Basic care and comfort
CL: Application

2 CORRECT ANSWER: 3
Proper cast care procedures include observing the skin nearest the cast edges for signs of pressure ulcers, keeping the cast dry and intact, and avoiding the use of insertable devices (such as wire hangers or sticks) to relieve itching. Frequent neurovascular checks can reveal any evidence of pressure or impaired circulation to the leg under the cast. This includes checking the toes frequently for discoloration, swelling, or any lack of movement or sensation. Hygiene measures should focus on the client's normal elimination patterns and the importance of cleanliness after elimination as well as on the need

to maintain skin integrity by taking sponge baths and caring for dry skin. Options 1 and 4: Devices should never be inserted between the cast and the skin. Option 2: Although mouth care and cast removal are important issues, they aren't priority discharge instructions in this case.
NP: Implementing care
CN: Physiological integrity
CNS: Reduction of risk potential
CL: Application

3 CORRECT ANSWER: 1
Families of anorectic clients are typically composed of rigid, enmeshed people who have problems resolving conflicts. Options 2, 3, and 4: Substance abuse, overeating, and a close-knit family life aren't usually associated with this problem.
NP: Collecting data
CN: Psychosocial integrity
CNS: Psychosocial adaptation
CL: Comprehension

4 CORRECT ANSWER: 1
This simple response provides the best orientation regarding the client's wife. Option 2: This would further confuse the client and upset both him and his wife if he fails to remember. Option 3: This option is inappropriate because the client wouldn't be able to process this information intelligently and would be confused. Option 4: Using an unfamiliar name will only confuse and agitate the client.
NP: Planning care
CN: Safe, effective care environment
CNS: Coordinated care
CL: Application

5 CORRECT ANSWER: 4
Because pertussis vaccines are included in all childhood immunization programs in the United States, the number of children contracting this disease should be few. However, many children don't receive routine immunizations; consequently, outbreaks of pertussis and other childhood diseases are still a problem. The nurse should emphasize the importance of following the recommended schedule for pediatric immunizations, reinforcing the concept of preventing childhood disease. Option 1: Chastising the mother would do little to correct her misconception about the role of immunizations in preventing disease. Options 2 and 3 are factually incorrect and therefore inappropriate responses.
NP: Implementing care
CN: Health promotion and maintenance
CNS: Prevention and early detection of disease
CL: Application

6 CORRECT ANSWER: 2
A neonate has a limited glucose store. Stopping the total parenteral nutrition, a high-glucose I.V. fluid, to administer blood would cause the serum glucose to drop. Therefore, the nurse must monitor the glucose level closely. Options 1, 3, and 4: These levels

should also be monitored; however, they aren't as important as glucose in this situation.
NP: Collecting data
CN: Physiological integrity
CNS: Pharmacological therapies
CL: Application

7 CORRECT ANSWER: 3
Phenytoin sodium (Dilantin) can cause hypertrophy of the gums and gingivitis; therefore, regular dental checkups are essential. Option 1: Phenytoin doesn't need to be taken with food. Option 2: This drug should never be discontinued unless ordered by a physician. Option 4: Some drowsiness is expected initially; however, this usually decreases with continued use.
NP: Evaluating care
CN: Physiological integrity
CNS: Pharmacological therapies
CL: Analysis

8 CORRECT ANSWER: 3
This client can't exhale completely. Pursed-lip breathing prolongs exhalation and prevents air trapping. Option 1: Increasing the rate of oxygen administration in someone with a history of chronic respiratory disease may decrease the primary stimulus to breathe, which is a low PaO_2. Option 2: This client requires prompt treatment; waiting to notify the physician would take too long. Option 4: Morphine would decrease the respiratory rate and sedate the client, increasing the risk for hypoxia.
NP: Implementing care
CN: Physiological integrity
CNS: Physiological adaptation
CL: Application

9 CORRECT ANSWER: 2
Rocking the pelvis helps to relieve pressure and backache. Option 1: Kegel exercises strengthen the muscles of the pelvic floor and help prepare the pregnant client for delivery. Option 3: Support stockings are helpful for someone with varicose veins; however, they don't relieve backache. Option 4: Wearing nonconstrictive clothing can help ensure proper circulation but it doesn't relieve backache.
NP: Evaluating care
CN: Health promotion and maintenance
CNS: Growth and development through the life span
CL: Application

10 CORRECT ANSWER: 2
A client who has undergone a supratentorial craniotomy is placed in semi-Fowler's position to help maintain the airway and decrease cerebral edema. Option 1: High Fowler's position is contraindicated because the client may hyperflex the neck and block the airway. Option 3: Lying flat with a small pillow may increase cerebral edema in a client who has undergone a supratentorial craniotomy. Option 4: Side-lying is contraindicated for clients who un-

dergo supratentorial craniotomy because this position may increase intracranial pressure and doesn't help prevent cerebral edema.
NP: Implementing care
CN: Physiological integrity
CNS: Reduction of risk potential
CL: Application

11 CORRECT ANSWER: 3
When removing a Sengstaken-Blakemore tube, the traction on the nose that holds the balloon in place is removed first to prevent the tube from moving upward into the pharynx. Option 1: The esophageal balloon should be deflated first after the traction is removed to prevent airway obstruction. Option 2: Deflating the gastric balloon first may cause the tube to migrate upward and block the client's airway. Option 4: Only one balloon at a time is deflated, beginning with the esophageal balloon.
NP: Implementing care
CN: Physiological integrity
CNS: Physiological adaptation
CL: Application

12 CORRECT ANSWER: 1
Clients need at least 2 hours of uninterrupted sleep to achieve adequate REM sleep. Failure to get enough REM sleep may lead to increased confusion. Options 2 and 3: Although frequent turning would increase the staff's workload and the risk for injury from shearing forces, these aren't the reasons for the client's turning schedule. Option 4: Activity in the client's room may disturb other clients; however, this isn't the reason for limiting the client's turning during the night.
NP: Planning care
CN: Psychosocial integrity
CNS: Coping and adaptation
CL: Application

13 CORRECT ANSWER: 3
Warfarin sodium is given to those with thrombophlebitis because it prolongs the clotting time. Option 1: Warfarin sodium doesn't thin the blood. Option 2: Warfarin sodium doesn't dissolve clots that are already present. Option 4: Warfarin sodium will probably be continued after discontinuation of bed rest; and the client may require this drug for the rest of her life.
NP: Implementing care
CN: Physiological integrity
CNS: Pharmacological therapies
CL: Application

14 CORRECT ANSWER: 4
Supporting the cast fully with pillows and turning the leg every 2 to 3 hours allows the cast to dry while preventing impaired circulation to the skin and underlying tissue. Option 1: The cast will be pliable until dry and must be supported in a way that distributes the pressure evenly. Option 2: Using a hair dryer may dry the cast too quickly, caus-

ing it to crack. Option 3: The cast will dry faster when left open to the air.
NP: Implementing care
CN: Physiological integrity
CNS: Reduction of risk potential
CL: Application

15 CORRECT ANSWER: 3
A neonate with an Apgar score between 7 and 10 is considered vigorous and needs normal neonatal care, which includes providing warmth. Options 1, 2, and 4 are unnecessary.
NP: Planning care
CN: Health promotion and maintenance
CNS: Growth and development through the life span
CL: Application

16 CORRECT ANSWER: 1
The fetal heart rate should be checked immediately after the membranes rupture to identify any sign of fetal distress caused by prolapse of the cord. Option 2: There is no need to change the client's position unless fetal distress is evident. Option 3: The nurse would time the client's contractions as they occur. Option 4: The maternal vital signs shouldn't be affected with rupture of the membranes.
NP: Implementing care
CN: Health promotion and maintenance
CNS: Growth and development through the life span
CL: Application

17 CORRECT ANSWER: 1
Haloperidol decanoate, a long-acting antipsychotic medication that is given I.M., is usually administered every 4 weeks. Therefore, options 2, 3, and 4 would be unnecessary.
NP: Collecting data
CN: Physiological integrity
CNS: Pharmacological therapies
CL: Knowledge

18 CORRECT ANSWER: 1
The presumptive signs of pregnancy include tenderness, tingling, and swelling of the breasts. Option 2: Burning may be a sign of a urinary tract infection. Option 3: Chloasma is a bronze type of facial pigmentation that is unrelated to pregnancy. Option 4: The nausea and vomiting may be an aversion to greasy food.
NP: Collecting data
CN: Health promotion and maintenance
CNS: Growth and development through the life span
CL: Application

19 CORRECT ANSWER: 2
Aspirin and other nonsteroidal anti-inflammatory drugs should be taken with food to decrease gastric irritation. Option 1: The client with rheumatoid arthritis must learn to balance rest and activity. Option 3: Resting involved joints helps to reduce inflammation. Option 4: Rest periods should be planned between activities.

NP: Evaluating care
CN: Physiological integrity
CNS: Physiological adaptation
CL: Analysis

20 CORRECT ANSWER: 4
Pregnancy-induced hypertension is most common among teenagers and older primiparas. Options 1 and 2 have no bearing on pregnancy-induced hypertension. Option 3: A hematocrit of 30% may indicate that the client is anemic.
NP: Collecting data
CN: Health promotion and maintenance
CNS: Growth and development through the life span
CL: Comprehension

21 CORRECT ANSWER: 3
A diabetic client should normally wait about 30 minutes after insulin administration before eating. However, if the blood glucose level is less than 60 mg/dl, the client should eat within about 15 minutes after insulin injection. If the blood glucose level is greater than 240 mg/dl, the client should wait 45 to 60 minutes after insulin injection before eating. Regular insulin begins to act within 30 to 60 minutes after injection. Options 1 and 2: The blood glucose level isn't low enough to warrant extra food or notification of the physician. Option 4: The blood glucose level isn't higher than 240 mg/dl so waiting for breakfast wouldn't be appropriate.
NP: Planning care
CL: Physiological integrity
CNS: Pharmacological therapies
CN: Application

22 CORRECT ANSWER: 3
Petechiae are sometimes present over the head, neck, and back as a result of birth trauma; however, generalized petechiae may indicate a coagulopathy such as thrombocytopenia. Option 1: Mongolian spots are bluish pigmentations over the lower back buttocks, or extensor surfaces commonly found on dark-skinned neonates. Option 2: Milia are distended sebaceous glands that produce tiny whitish papules most commonly over the nose, chin, or cheeks; this finding is common among neonates. Option 4: Most infants have short, thick necks that are usually surrounded by skin folds.
NP: Evaluating care
CN: Health promotion and maintenance
CNS: Growth and development through the life span
CL: Application

23 CORRECT ANSWER: 4
Children are typically frightened of needles and often refuse pain medication because of their fear. Being truthful about the needle stick and focusing on the end result may help to lessen the child's apprehension. Options 1 and 3: These statements offer false reassurances and should be avoided. Option 2 is a negative statement and should also be avoided.

Posttests

259

NP: Implementing care
CN: Psychosocial integrity
CNS: Coping and adaptation
CL: Application

24 CORRECT ANSWER: 2

As long as the client is compliant with his treatment and disposes of his secretions properly, visitors wearing masks are allowed. Option 1: Tuberculosis is no longer treated by strict isolation; visitors are permitted if instructed properly in the transmission process. Option 3: Tuberculosis is transmitted by droplets through coughing and sneezing; it isn't carried on objects. Option 4: A variable period is needed before medications render the client noninfectious, so transmission precautions still need to be observed.
NP: Implementing care
CN: Safe, effective care environment
CNS: Safety and infection control
CL: Application

25 CORRECT ANSWER: 4

Holding the breath for 5 seconds allows the medication to keep the terminal bronchioles open for maximum drug distribution. Option 1: The client should inhale with a slow, sustained breath to attempt to achieve total lung capacity. Option 2: Each puff should be 3 to 5 minutes apart; this allows the first dose to dilate narrowed airways and the second puff to extend further through the airways. Option 3: Additional puffs can result in an overdose and should be done only with a physician's order.
NP: Implementing care
CN: Physiological integrity
CNS: Pharmacological therapies
CL: Application

26 CORRECT ANSWER: 2

The pH indicates an acidotic state, and the elevated $Paco_2$ levels indicate respiratory acidosis. Normal blood gas values include pH, 7.35 to 7.45; Pao_2, 80 to 100 mm Hg; $Paco_2$, 35 to 45 mm Hg; and HCO_3^-, 22 to 26 mEq/L. Option 1: In respiratory alkalosis, pH is above 7.45, $Paco_2$ is below 35 mm Hg, and HCO_3^- is less than 22 mEq/L. Option 3: In metabolic alkalosis, the pH is above 7.45, $Paco_2$ is above 45 mm Hg, and HCO_3^- is greater than 25 mEq/L. Option 4: In metabolic acidosis, the pH is below 7.45, $Paco_2$ is less than 35 mm Hg, and HCO_3^- is less than 22 mEq/L.
NP: Evaluating care
CN: Physiological integrity
CNS: Physiological adaptation
CL: Analysis

27 CORRECT ANSWER: 3

The first step in this situation is to control the obvious bleeding to prevent shock. Option 1: Realigning the fracture at this time may increase the bleeding and cause further tissue damage. Option 2: There is no indication that the client is in need of supple-

mental oxygen. Option 4: Although the client is in pain, the first priority is to control the bleeding.
NP: Implementing care
CN: Physiological integrity
CNS: Physiological adaptation
CL: Application

28 CORRECT ANSWER: 4

Signs indicative of increased intracranial pressure include bradycardia, increased systolic blood pressure, and a widening pulse pressure. Option 1: These vital signs are indicative of hypovolemic shock. Option 2: This change in vital signs is indicative of anxiety. Option 3: This change in vital signs indicates neurogenic shock.
NP: Collecting data
CN: Physiological integrity
CNS: Reduction of risk potential
CL: Comprehension

29 CORRECT ANSWER: 3

Adequate fluid intake maintains the client's hydration and helps to liquefy secretions. Option 1: Additional fluids may help reduce the body temperature but the primary reason for fluids in this case is to maintain hydration and liquefy secretions. Option 2: Fluids high in calories may help maintain nutrition but this isn't the primary reason for increasing fluids in this case. Option 4: Fluids alone won't maintain airway patency. However, increased fluids help to liquefy secretions, thereby preventing thick sputum from obstructing the airway.
NP: Implementing care
CN: Physiological integrity
CNS: Reduction of risk potential
CL: Application

30 CORRECT ANSWER: 1

The primary purpose of colostomy irrigation is to promote a regular elimination schedule. Options 2 and 3: Although irrigation may eliminate some bacteria as well as some flatus from the bowel, these aren't the primary reasons for a colostomy irrigation. Option 4: A colostomy irrigation may help relieve constipation and even prevent its occurrence if done frequently enough; however, the primary purpose of performing a colostomy irrigation at this time is to establish a regular elimination schedule.
NP: Implementing care
CN: Physiological integrity
CNS: Basic care and comfort
CL: Application

31 CORRECT ANSWER: 1

Washing the area with bacteriostatic soap and water is effective against human immunodeficiency virus (HIV). Option 2: Scrubbing vigorously may cause skin breakdown and should be avoided. Option 3: Alcohol isn't as effective as bacteriostatic soap and water. Option 4: Ammonia chloride won't kill HIV.
NP: Implementing care
CN: Safe, effective care environment

32 CORRECT ANSWER: 3
The nurse should explain that a low-protein diet is necessary to prevent any increase in the client's blood urea nitrogen level at this time. Option 1 would be inappropriate. Options 2 and 4 would be unnecessary because the nurse should possess adequate knowledge about the disease to deal with the situation.
NP: Implementing care
CN: Physiological integrity
CNS: Basic care and comfort
CL: Analysis

33 CORRECT ANSWER: 1
Amniocentesis performed early in pregnancy helps to detect any chromosomal abnormalities in the fetus. Options 2, 3, and 4 are all inaccurate statements about amniocentesis.
NP: Planning care
CN: Health promotion and maintenance
CNS: Growth and development through the life span
CL: Comprehension

34 CORRECT ANSWER: 2
Avocados, classified as both a fat and a fruit, are a tyramine-containing food. Eating avocados while taking MAO inhibitors may cause the client's blood pressure to rise inexorably, resulting in hypertensive crisis. Options 1, 3, and 4 are permitted with this type of drug.
NP: Collecting data
CN: Physiological integrity
CNS: Pharmacological therapies
CL: Comprehension

35 CORRECT ANSWER: 4
High levels of anxiety make the client vulnerable to accidental injury and self-inflicted harm and should be avoided at all cost. Reducing the level of anxiety will make the client more receptive to other forms of intervention. Option 1: A severely anxious client can't solve problems or respond to such a question. Option 2 would take too long and wouldn't be meaningful to the client in this high-anxiety state. Option 3: The client wouldn't be receptive to learning new coping skills until the anxiety is reduced or alleviated.
NP: Implementing care
CN: Psychosocial integrity
CNS: Coping and adaptation
CL: Application

36 CORRECT ANSWER: 2
This amount of drainage is excessive and the physician should be notified; however, the nurse should first assess the client's status to determine whether he's stable enough to be left alone or is in need of immediate help. Option 1: The physician should be called as soon as the vital signs are checked. Option

3: The rate of suction shouldn't be touched unless otherwise instructed by the physician. Option 4: Doing nothing would be negligent in this case.
NP: Collecting data
CN: Physiological integrity
CNS: Reduction of risk potential
CL: Analysis

37 CORRECT ANSWER: 3
When cramps occur, the nurse should stop the flow temporarily to allow the cramps to subside, and then continue with the enema. Options 1 and 2 would cause unnecessary discomfort for the client. Option 4 unnecessarily deprives the client of the treatment.
NP: Implementing care
CN: Physiological integrity
CNS: Basic care and comfort
CL: Application

38 CORRECT ANSWER: 1
When contacting the intact skin of an acquired immunodeficiency syndrome (AIDS) client, no protective barriers are necessary. Option 2: The nurse should wear gloves to protect the hands when contact with an AIDS client's blood or body fluids is possible. Option 3: A gown should be worn when the nurse's clothing may contact the blood or body fluids of an AIDS client. Option 4: A mask should be worn whenever the splashing of blood or body fluids is possible.
NP: Planning care
CN: Safe, effective care environment
CNS: Safety and infection control
CL: Application

39 CORRECT ANSWER: 2
The client with burns of the face and neck is at high risk for airway obstruction from respiratory tract edema. Options 1, 3, and 4 are important but not the priority.
NP: Planning care
CN: Physiological integrity
CNS: Physiological adaptation
CL: Application

40 CORRECT ANSWER: 2
The kidneys of a person with a diagnosis of diabetes mellitus are potentially compromised. Because lithium is excreted by the kidneys, use of the drug would further burden their function. Options 1, 3, and 4 aren't contraindications for lithium therapy.
NP: Collecting data
CN Physiological integrity
CNS: Pharmacological therapies
CL: Analysis

41 CORRECT ANSWER: 2
Manifestations of respiratory syncytial virus infection include pharyngitis, rhinorrhea, cough, tachypnea, low-grade fever, and dehydration. As the infec-

tion progresses, the nurse will be able to detect an audible wheezing with the child's breathing. Such wheezing can also be heard on auscultation. Options 1, 3, and 4: These aren't signs and symptoms of respiratory syncytial virus infection.

NP: Collecting data
CN: Physiological integrity
CNS: Physiological adaptation
CL: Comprehension

42 CORRECT ANSWER: 1

One potential complication of a lower leg or forearm fracture is the development of compartment syndrome as a result of swelling or bleeding into the tissues. Elevated compartment pressures can lead to vascular compromise and ischemia of the muscle tissue. Failure to detect this complication in a timely manner can lead to permanent injury or death of the tissue. Whenever a client has increasing pain or pain disproportionate to that expected for the injury, the nurse should always assess the neurovascular status and report the findings to the physician. Options 2, 3, and 4 may be appropriate interventions but they don't take priority over neurovascular assessment.

NP: Implementing care
CN: Physiological integrity
CNS: Physiological adaptation
CL: Application

43 CORRECT ANSWER: 3

A decrease in fetal activity may occur at any time during pregnancy. However, a prolonged decrease may indicate fetal distress. Options 1, 2, and 4 are signs of impending labor.

NP: Evaluating care
CN: Health promotion and maintenance
CNS: Growth and development through the life span
CL: Analysis

44 CORRECT ANSWER: 4

Manipulation is the most commonly used defense mechanism by clients with this disorder. Such clients typically are untruthful about their food intake and methods of losing weight and frequently attempt to manipulate staff and situations. Options 1, 2, and 3 may be used but they aren't as commonly used as manipulation.

NP: Collecting data
CN: Psychosocial integrity
CNS: Psychosocial adaptation
CL: Comprehension

45 CORRECT ANSWER: 1

This client may be experiencing a cerebrovascular accident. Checking the level of consciousness is imperative because this helps to determine the client's cerebral oxygenation status. Options 2, 3, and 4 should be performed secondarily in this situation.

NP: Collecting data
CN: Physiological integrity
CNS: Reduction of risk potential
CL: Analysis

46 CORRECT ANSWER: 2

A bull's-eye-shaped, red rash indicates infection from the spirochete that causes Lyme disease. The rash appears in 60% to 80% of cases in the first few weeks after the bite. Options 1, 3, and 4: The other lesions aren't specific to Lyme disease.

NP: Collecting data
CN: Health promotion and maintenance
CNS: Prevention and early detection of disease
CL: Comprehension

47 CORRECT ANSWER: 1

Clients recovering from hepatitis shouldn't consume alcohol because it's completely metabolized in the liver, which needs time to recover and regenerate from the hepatitis. Option 2: Most over-the-counter analgesics are metabolized in the liver. Option 3: Activity needs to be increased slowly to allow the liver to heal. Option 4: Hepatitis B is spread through blood and body fluids; blood could be spread on the razor.

NP: Evaluating care
CN: Physiological integrity
CNS: Reduction of risk potential
CL: Application

48 CORRECT ANSWER: 2

There are above-normal levels of sodium chloride in the sweat of children with cystic fibrosis. Option 1: Although the client has lung-related problems, a sputum culture isn't diagnostic for cystic fibrosis. Options 3 and 4: A chest X-ray and urine culture aren't diagnostic for cystic fibrosis.

NP: Collecting data
CN: Health promotion and maintenance
CNS: Prevention and early detection of disease
CL: Comprehension

49 CORRECT ANSWER: 2

Grandiosity and an exaggerated sense of self-worth are characteristics of the manic phase of bipolar disorders. Option 1: Being quiet and reserved and keeping close to his room would indicate withdrawal, which is seen more in depressed clients. Option 3: The client would express feelings of hopelessness in the depressive state of bipolar disorder. Option 4: Changing the bed linens several times per day is indicative of obsessive-compulsive disorders.

NP: Collecting data
CN: Psychosocial integrity
CNS: Coping and adaptation
CL: Comprehension

50 CORRECT ANSWER: 2

Clients experiencing delirium tremens are at high risk for developing seizures. Option 1: Fluid intake shouldn't be restricted because alcohol intake leads to dehydration. Option 3: Excessive environmental stimuli could trigger seizures and should be avoided. A quiet and calm environment is best. Option 4: Restraints could also trigger increased agitation,

contributing to seizures. The side rails should be padded.
NP: Implementing care
CN: Safe, effective care environment
CNS: Safety and infection control
CL: Application

51 CORRECT ANSWER: 4
A side-lying position is best to prevent aspiration if the client has difficulty swallowing his saliva. Option 1: If any liquids are allowed, they should be thickened. Clear liquids are harder to swallow and increase the risk of aspiration. Option 2: Testing the gag reflex wouldn't help to prevent aspiration and may be irritating. Option 3: The gag reflex is controlled by neuromuscular stimulation. A chin tuck is used when feeding to decrease the risk of aspiration.
NP: Planning care
CN: Physiological integrity
CNS: Reduction of risk potential
CL: Application

52 CORRECT ANSWER: 2
Administering I.V. push medications isn't within the scope of practice for the LPN. Options 1, 3, and 4: Checking the client's finger stick blood glucose level, monitoring an I.V. infusion of lactated Ringer's solution, and changing a wet-to-dry dressing are within the scope of the LPN's practice.
NP: Planning care
CN: Safe, effective care environment
CNS: Coordinated care
CL: Knowledge

53 CORRECT ANSWER: 3
Establishing a schedule is the first step to regaining bladder control. Option 1: Restricting fluids would decrease urine formation, which wouldn't help the client to establish a routine and would predispose the client to urinary tract infections. Option 2: The client should be checked every 2 hours and his skin should be kept clean and dry but this isn't the best aid to regaining bladder control. Option 4: Keeping the call bell in easy reach will help the client alert the caregiver but it isn't the best way to encourage a routine schedule.
NP: Collecting data
CN: Physiological integrity
CNS: Basic care and comfort
CL: Application

54 CORRECT ANSWER: 4
The nurse should focus on the client's abilities rather than disabilities. Encouraging the client to focus on gaining reuse of her left side focuses on something the client can do to help improve her condition and self-image. Option 1: The client has already expressed her feelings. Option 2: Reminding her that she's right-handed doesn't address the client's concern and wouldn't improve her self-

image. Option 3: Helping the client with hairstyling and make-up would aid her image but doesn't best address the issue of what the client can do to improve her condition and self-image.
NP: Implementing care
CN: Psychosocial integrity
CNS: Coping and adaptation
CL: Application

55 CORRECT ANSWER: 1
Because the client had spinal anesthesia, he needs to be kept flat for the next 8 to 12 hours. Option 2: The client won't need to stay away from consuming anything by mouth because he didn't have general anesthesia. Option 3: Immediately after a transurethral resection of the prostate, the client has an indwelling urinary catheter. Option 4: The client shouldn't be out of bed soon after spinal anesthesia.
NP: Implementing care
CN: Safe, effective care environment
CNS: Coordinated care
CL: Application

56 CORRECT ANSWER: 4
The client has the right to change his mind and may need to further discuss the operation with his physician. Option 1: Telling the client he's already on the operating room schedule would violate the client's right to refuse. Option 2: Reassuring him that he's probably just nervous about the surgery doesn't address the client's concern. It would be better to encourage the client to discuss his fears and concerns. Option 3: The decision to cancel the surgery hasn't been made. It's inappropriate to tell the client that you'll have his name removed from the operating room schedule.
NP: Collecting data
CN: Safe, effective care environment
CNS: Coordinated care
CL: Comprehension

57 CORRECT ANSWER: 2
Subjective data is data that is reported by the client. Options 1, 3, and 4 are examples of objective data that is observed or reported by the caregiver.
NP: Collecting data
CN: Safe, effective care environment
CNS: Coordinated care
CL: Comprehension

58 CORRECT ANSWER: 2
Shock and disbelief are the first steps in the grieving process. Option 1: Awareness is usually the second step. Options 3 and 4: Restitution and acceptance are the same and usually the final step in the grieving process.
NP: Evaluating care
CN: Psychosocial integrity
CNS: Psychosocial adaptation
CL: Knowledge

59 CORRECT ANSWER: 3
A meal of chili and fruit salad contains the highest amount of fiber, which should be included in the diet to prevent constipation. Options 1, 2, and 4: A hamburger and mashed potatoes, grilled cheese sandwich and applesauce, and chicken breast sandwich and chocolate pudding aren't as high in fiber as chili and fresh fruit salad.
NP: Evaluating care
CN: Physiological integrity
CNS: Basic care and comfort
CL: Comprehension

60 CORRECT ANSWER: 2
The client needs to change position and get out of bed postoperatively to prevent atelectasis and skin breakdown. Option 1: Saying that he'll lie still indicates that the client doesn't understand the importance of turning and changing positions. Option 3: The client will need pain medication to ease the pain and facilitate moving in bed but it won't be given automatically every 3 hours. Option 4: A fear such as this is a common concern with clients after surgery. Preoperative teaching should include information about splinting the incision and premedicating with pain medication before activities.
NP: Evaluating care
CN: Physiological integrity
CNS: Basic care and comfort
CL: Comprehension

61 CORRECT ANSWER: 3
The combination of decreased activity postoperatively and surgery to the pelvic region put this client at the greatest risk of developing thrombophlebitis. Options 1, 2, and 4: The other clients aren't limited in activity and aren't at as high a risk as the client who just underwent a hysterectomy.
NP: Collecting data
CN: Physiological integrity
CNS: Physiological adaptation
CL: Comprehension

62 CORRECT ANSWER: 1
A client with Addison's disease is dehydrated and hypotensive and very weak. Frequent rest periods are needed to prevent exhausting the client. Option 2: Diuretics wouldn't be given because the client is dehydrated. Option 3: Potassium levels are often elevated in Addison's disease because aldosterone secretion is decreased, resulting in decreased sodium and increased potassium. Option 4: The client is dehydrated; fluid intake would be encouraged, not restricted.
NP: Implementing care
CN: Physiological integrity
CNS: Physiological adaptation
CL: Analysis

63 CORRECT ANSWER: 4
It's best to take prednisone in the morning because it mimics the body's natural secretion of cortisol at that time. Option 1: Prednisone can be irritating to the stomach and should be taken with food. Option 2: Prednisone can disrupt sleep if taken at bedtime. Option 3: Taking prednisone with the evening meal isn't the best time to take the pill.
NP: Evaluating care
CN: Physiological integrity
CNS: Pharmacological therapies
CL: Comprehension

64 CORRECT ANSWER: 3
Wearing an eye shield while sleeping protects the eye from accidental injury. Option 1: Sunglasses should be worn when going outside but not at all times. Option 2: The client should sleep on the side that isn't affected by the operation. Option 4: Time spent watching TV or using a computer may need to be limited to prevent eyestrain but need not be totally restricted.
NP: Implementing care
CN: Safe, effective care environment
CNS: Safety and infection control
CL: Application

65 CORRECT ANSWER: 2
Black, tarry stools are a sign of a bleeding such as from a Curling's ulcer. Option 1: Purulent drainage would be a sign of wound infection at the burn sites. Option 3: A decrease in blood pressure could be a sign of fluid volume problems, complications from medications, or an electrolyte imbalance. Option 4: This would be indicative of shock and fluid volume loss.
NP: Collecting data
CN: Physiological integrity
CNS: Reduction of risk potential
CL: Application

66 CORRECT ANSWER: 3
Although nursing diagnoses involving risk usually don't take high priority, clients with indwelling catheters are at risk for developing urinary tract infections, one of the main causes of nosocomial infections. Options 1, 2, and 4: *Deficient knowledge, Anxiety,* and *Acute pain* are all appropriate diagnoses for a client with an indwelling catheter but aren't as high in priority.
NP: Planning care
CN: Safe, effective care environment
CNS: Safety and infection control
CL: Comprehension

67 CORRECT ANSWER: 2
Pink, rounded wound edges are evidence of new tissue growth and granulation. Option 1: Serosanguineous drainage is serum and blood draining from the wound and is associated with the exudative phase of wound healing. Option 3: The presence of pink to red tissue in the wound bed is a sign of healthy tissue. Option 4: Streaks of yellow tissue in the wound bed are fatty tissues.

NP: Evaluating care
CN: Physiological integrity
CNS: Physiological adaptation
CL: Comprehension

68 CORRECT ANSWER: 2
An abducted position keeps the new joint from becoming displaced out of the socket. Option 1: The client can keep his hip straight with the knee flexed as long as an abductor pillow is kept in place. Options 3 and 4: Keeping the hip adducted or externally rotated can dislocate the hip joint.
NP: Implementing care
CN: Physiological integrity
CNS: Basic care and comfort
CL: Application

69 CORRECT ANSWER: 3
Clients with anemia fatigue easily and need rest between activities to conserve energy. Option 1: Activities don't need to be severely restricted for clients with anemia. Option 2: The client needs to eat food that is high in iron, such as lean red meat and fortified breakfast cereal. Option 4: The client doesn't need close supervision when walking.
NP: Planning care
CN: Physiological integrity
CNS: Physiological adaptation
CL: Application

70 CORRECT ANSWER: 3
An iodine-based dye is injected during a cardiac catheterization. An allergy to shellfish indicates allergy to iodine and the client may need to be premedicated with an antihistamine. Option 1: The client doesn't have to swallow anything for the procedure. Option 2: Clients are confined during some imaging procedures but not cardiac catheterizations. Option 4: The client will be on her back for most of the procedure.
NP: Collecting data
CN: Safe, effective care environment
CNS: Safety and infection control
CL: Comprehension

71 CORRECT ANSWER: 3
A 3-lb weight gain in 24 hours indicates that the client is retaining fluid, which is a sign that the kidneys aren't excreting properly. Option 1: 60 ml/ hour is a satisfactory urine output; less than 30 ml/ hour is unsatisfactory. Options 2 and 4: Mucous membranes that are dry and sticky and inelastic skin turgor are signs of dehydration, probably secondary to the client's hypovolemia.
NP: Collecting data
CN: Physiological integrity
CNS: Physiological adaptation
CL: Analysis

72 CORRECT ANSWER: 1
The nurse needs to explain the importance of continuing with the yearly mammograms, as recom-
mended by the American Cancer Society. It's best to explain that a mammogram can be used to detect changes before the client experiences symptoms. Option 2: The nurse should address the client's concern while it's on the client's mind. Telling the client to discuss her thoughts with the physician doesn't address the issue but unnecessarily diverts it to the physician. Option 3: It's important for the client to do breast self-examinations but they aren't a substitute for mammograms and can't detect abnormalities as early as mammograms. Option 4: Asking about insurance concerns changes the subject. The client hasn't indicated that insurance is a concern.
NP: Implementing care
CN: Health promotion and maintenance
CNS: Prevention and early detection of disease
CL: Application

73 CORRECT ANSWER: 3
Accurate intake and output measurement is important in assessing whether the client is retaining fluid or responding to treatment. Option 1: The client most likely needs potassium supplements to replace potassium lost with diuretic therapy. Also, fluids are restricted in clients with heart failure. Option 2: The client's activities should be spaced to allow for frequent rest periods. Option 4: Keeping the client in a recumbent position would cause dyspnea; the semi-Fowler's position is better.
NP: Planning care
CN: Physiological integrity
CNS: Physiological adaptation
CL: Application

74 CORRECT ANSWER: 1
Clients who undergo total gastrectomy often experience the dumping syndrome when eating. This causes food and fluids to move into the jejunum too rapidly. To help reduce this effect, the client should drink fluids separately from meals. Option 2: The client needs to increase activity slowly while recovering from major surgery. Option 3: Vitamin B_{12} injections are required for life after total gastrectomy because the client no longer has the intrinsic factor needed to absorb vitamin B_{12} from foods. Option 4: Eating smaller, more frequent meals reduces the effects of the dumping syndrome.
NP: Evaluating care
CN: Physiological integrity
CNS: Physiological adaptation
CL: Analysis

75 CORRECT ANSWER: 3
The purpose of the nasogastric (NG) tube is to drain gastric and duodenal fluids until peristalsis resumes. Option 1: The tube doesn't prevent peritonitis. Option 2: The tube isn't used to administer medications. Option 4: Gastric pH can be measured by aspirating some of the NG drainage but this isn't the purpose of a postoperative NG tube.

NP: Implementing care
CN: Physiological integrity
CNS: Basic care and comfort
CL: Comprehension

76 CORRECT ANSWER: 3
Posting signs (such as the day of the week and month) helps to orient the Alzheimer's client and reduce problems due to forgetfulness. Option 1: The room should be well lit to help orient the client and prevent accidents. Option 2: Too many visitors could cause excessive stimulation and confusion. Option 4: The client doesn't need a private room.
NP: Planning care
CN: Psychosocial integrity
CNS: Psychosocial adaptation
CL: Application

77 CORRECT ANSWER: 1
Clients with diabetes insipidus have decreased or absent vasopressin secretion, resulting in polyuria. Option 2: Blood glucose levels are closely monitored in clients with diabetes mellitus. Option 3: Heart rate changes could be seen secondary to the fluid imbalances caused by diabetes insipidus but urine output has the highest priority. Option 4: Bowel sounds should also be monitored but not as closely as urine output.
NP: Collecting data
CN: Physiological integrity
CNS: Physiological adaptation
CL: Application

78 CORRECT ANSWER: 3
Lowering the bag slows the infusion and deep breathing helps the client to relax and better tolerate the procedure. Option 1: It may not be necessary to stop the infusion if cramping subsides with a slower infusion. Option 2: The client should be instructed on what to do to help her relax. Option 4: Raising the bag would speed up the infusion and increase abdominal cramping.
NP: Implementing care
CN: Physiological integrity
CNS: Basic care and comfort
CL: Application

79 CORRECT ANSWER: 1
Because lunch trays are due to be given to clients, the diabetic client needs to have the blood glucose level checked in case insulin administration is needed before eating. Options 2, 3, and 4: The other clients' needs don't have the highest priority and could be delegated to ancillary nursing staff.
NP: Planning care
CN: Safe, effective care environment
CNS: Coordinated care
CL: Comprehension

80 CORRECT ANSWER: 2
Foods rich in zinc include poultry, fish, whole grains, and eggs. Options 1, 3, and 4: The other foods listed aren't high in zinc.
NP: Evaluating care
CN: Physiological integrity
CNS: Basic care and comfort
CL: Knowledge

81 CORRECT ANSWER: 1
In Buck's extension traction, the weights should hang freely without touching the bed or floor. Option 2: Lifting the weights would break the traction. The client should be moved up in bed, allowing the weights to freely move along with the client. Option 3: The leg should be kept in straight alignment. Option 4: Doing ankle rotation exercises could cause the leg to go out of alignment.
NP: Evaluating care
CN: Physiological integrity
CNS: Reduction of risk potential
CL: Application

82 CORRECT ANSWER: 2
Neurovascular checks are most important because they're used to determine if any impairment exists after cast application and reduction of the fracture. Option 1: Checking to see if the cast is completely dry isn't the nurse's highest priority. Option 3: Checking to see if the client has pain is important but not the highest priority. Option 4: Pedaling to smooth the cast edge is done when the cast is completely dry.
NP: Collecting data
CN: Physiological integrity
CNS: Reduction of risk potential
CL: Application

83 CORRECT ANSWER: 4
The blood urea nitrogen (BUN) level reflects the amount of urea and nitrogenous waste products in the blood. Dialysis removes excess amounts of these elements from the blood, which is reflected in a lower BUN level. Options 1 and 2: Hemodialysis doesn't affect the white blood cell count. Option 3: Calcium levels are usually low in clients with chronic renal failure. They're corrected by giving calcium supplements, not through hemodialysis.
NP: Evaluating care
CN: Physiological integrity
CNS: Physiological adaptation
CL: Comprehension

84 CORRECT ANSWER: 2
The client's sister indicates a definite plan for the client to attend Alcoholics Anonymous meetings and become a part of a support group. Options 1, 3, and 4: The other options indicate support for the client but aren't as specific and don't include an actual plan to do something.

NP: Evaluating care
CN: Psychosocial integrity
CNS: Coping and adaptation
CL: Comprehension

85 CORRECT ANSWER: 1

An abused child is commonly withdrawn and avoids interaction with peers. Option 2: An abused child is commonly developmentally delayed. Option 3: An abused child commonly has a fear of socialization and demonstrates anxiety. Option 4: The abused child commonly is fearful of the abuser and tends to avoid contact with them.

NP: Collecting data
CN: Psychosocial integrity
CNS: Psychosocial adaptation
CL: Application

SELECTED REFERENCES

Abrams, A.C., and Goldsmith, T.L. *Clinical Drug Therapy: Rationales for Nursing Practice,* 6th ed. Philadelphia: Lippincott Williams & Wilkins, 2000.

Black, J. *Medical-Surgical Nursing: Clinical Management for Continuity of Care.* Philadelphia: W.B. Saunders, Co., 1999.

Bryant, R. *Acute and Chronic Wounds: Nursing Management,* 3rd ed. St. Louis: Mosby–Year Book, Inc., 2001.

Corrigan A., et al. *Intravenous Nurses Society Core Curriculum for Intravenous Nursing,* 2nd ed. Philadelphia: Lippincott Williams & Wilkins, 2000.

Craven, R.F., and Hirnle, C.J. *Fundamentals of Nursing: Human Health and Function,* 3rd ed. Philadelphia: Lippincott Williams & Wilkins, 2000.

DeLaune, S.C., and Ladner, P.K. *Fundamentals of Nursing Standards and Practice.* Albany, N.Y.: Delmar Pubs., 1999.

Diseases, 3rd ed. Springhouse, Pa.: Springhouse Corp., 2001.

Doenges, M.E., and Moorhouse, M.F. *Maternal/Newborn Plans of Care: Guidelines for Individualizing Care,* 3rd ed. Philadelphia: F.A. Davis Co., 1999.

Doenges, M.E., et al. *Nursing Care Plans: Guidelines for Individualizing Patient Care,* 5th ed. Philadelphia: F.A. Davis Co., 1999.

Elkin, M.K., et al. *Nursing Interventions and Clinical Skills,* 2nd ed. St. Louis: Mosby–Year Book, Inc., 2000.

Feigin, R.D., et al. *Textbook of Pediatric Infectious Diseases,* 4th ed. Philadelphia: W.B. Saunders Co., 1999.

Fischbach, F.T. *A Manual of Laboratory and Diagnostic Tests,* 6th ed. Philadelphia: Lippincott Williams & Wilkins, 2000.

Fortinash, K.M., and Holoday-Worret, P.A. *Psychiatric Mental Health Nursing,* 2nd ed. St. Louis: Mosby–Year Book, Inc., 2000.

Greenberg, M.D., and Rosen, C.L. "Evaluation of the Patient With Blunt Chest Trauma: An Evidence-Based Approach," *Emergency Medicine Clinics of North America* 17(1):41-62, viii, February 1999.

Handbook of Diagnostic Tests, 2nd ed. Springhouse, Pa.: Springhouse Corp., 1999.

Handbook of Geriatric Care. Springhouse, Pa.: Springhouse Corp., 1999.

Keltner, N.L., et al. *Psychiatric Nursing,* 3rd ed. St. Louis: Mosby–Year Book, Inc., 1999.

King, C., and Henretig, F.M. *Pocket Atlas of Pediatric Emergency Procedures,* Philadelphia: Lippincott Williams & Wilkins, 2000.

Kozier, B., et al. *Fundamentals of Nursing: Concepts, Process, and Practice,* 6th ed. Englewood Cliffs, N.J.: Prentice Hall, 2000.

Lowdermilk, D.L., et al. *Maternity Nursing,* 5th ed. St. Louis: Mosby–Year Book, Inc., 1999.

Maklebust, J., and Siegger, M. *Pressure Ulcers: Guidelines for Prevention and Nursing Management,* 3rd ed. Springhouse, Pa.: Springhouse Corp., 2001.

Mandeville, L.K., and Troiano, N.H. *AWHONN's High Risk and Critical Care Intrapartum Nursing,* 2nd ed. Philadelphia: Lippincott Williams & Wilkins, 1999.

Mastering Documentation, 2nd ed. Springhouse, Pa.: Springhouse Corp., 1999.

McKinney, E.S., et al. *Maternal-Child Nursing.* Philadelphia: W.B. Saunders Co., 2000.

National Council of State Boards of Nursing. Test Plan for the National Council Licensure Examination for Practical Nursing. Chicago: National Council of State Boards of Nursing, 1998.

Nursing Procedures, 3rd ed. Springhouse, Pa.: Springhouse Corp., 2000.

Nursing2001 Drug Handbook. Springhouse, Pa.: Springhouse Corp., 2000.

Phipps, W.J., et al. *Medical-Surgical Nursing: Concepts and Clinical Practice,* 6th ed. St. Louis: Mosby–Year Book, Inc., 1999.

Pillitteri, A. *Maternal & Child Health Nursing: Care of the Childbearing & Childrearing Family,* 3rd ed. Philadelphia: Lippincott Williams & Wilkins, 1999.

Smeltzer, A., and Bare, B. *Brunner and Suddarth's Textbook of Medical-Surgical Nursing.* Philadelphia: Lippincott Williams & Wilkins, 2000.

Springhouse Nurse's Drug Guide, 3rd ed. Springhouse, Pa.: Springhouse Corp., 2000.

Wong, D.L. *Whaley and Wong's Essentials of Pediatric Nursing,* 5th ed. St. Louis: Mosby–Year Book, Inc., 1999.

Yamada, T., et al., eds. *Textbook of Gastroenterology,* Volume 1 & 2, 3rd ed. Philadelphia: Lippincott Williams & Wilkins, 1999.

INDEX

A

Abandonment, borderline personality disorder and, 200
Abdomen, steps for assessing, 26
Abdominal binder, 27
Abdominal distention, 237, 247
Abdominal surgery, urine retention and, 20
Abduction, preventing hip dislocation with, 25
Abnormal involuntary movement scale, 194
Abortion, threatened, 132
Abruptio placentae, 125
Acetaminophen overdose, 151, 152, 160
Acquired immunodeficiency syndrome
  infants with, 177
  infection-preventing barrier and, 253, 261
  teaching client about transmission of, 104
Addison's disease, 255, 264
Adolescence, identity versus role confusion task of, 172
Adolescent mother, praising mothering skills of, 137
Aggressive behavior, setting limits on client with, 211
Aging client, genitourinary system of, 83
Agranulocytosis, 225
Airway
  postanesthetized client and, 80
  smoke inhalation and, 86
  suctioning infant's, 166
  unconscious client's, 85
Airway clearance, ineffective
  burn victim and, 253, 261
  chronic obstructive pulmonary disease and, 41
  laryngectomy and, 34
  mouth cancer and, 9
  suctioning and, 24
  tracheostomy and, 35
Albuterol (Ventolin), 163, 251, 260
Alcohol abuse and intake
  middle-stage addiction of, 202
  pregnancy and, 119

Alcohol treatment program
  collecting information from client in, 203
  family support for client in, 256, 266
Alcohol withdrawal
  fluid replacement for treating, 215
  onset of symptoms of, 218
Alertness, cerebral oxygenation and, 32
Allergy injections, 71
Alprazolam (Xanax), 201
Alzheimer's disease
  activities for client in middle stage of, 192
  ensuring safety of client with, 192
  mild, 192
  orienting client with, 256, 266
  therapeutic response to client with, 250, 257
Ambivalence, schizophrenic client and, 193
Ambulation, Miller-Abbott tube insertion and, 9
Ambulatory dialysis, 46
Amitriptyline (Elavil), 209, 212, 227
Ammonia levels, neurologic changes caused by high, 107
Amniocentesis, 252, 261
Amniotic membranes, ruptured, 128, 234, 243
Amphetamine use, symptoms of, 202
Amphotericin B, adverse effects of, 59
Analgesic administration, head injuries and, 145
Anemia
  aplastic, 181
  fatigue caused by, 255, 265
  in infants, 140
Anorexia nervosa. See Eating disorders.
Antacids
  antipsychotic medications and, 228
  constipation and, 7
Antianxiety drugs, 207, 235, 244
Antibiotic therapy, 175, 236, 246
Anticholinesterase, administration of, 102
Anticonvulsant medication, 16
Antidepressants, electroencephalogram and, 32

Antidiabetic drugs, 13
Antiembolism stockings, 17, 80
Antiemetics, intracranial pressure and, 99
Anti-inflammatory medication, 251, 259
Antirejection medication, 107
Antisocial personality disorder, 223
Antithyroid medication, 47
Anxiety
  client safety and, 210, 227
  compulsive acts by clients for reducing, 218, 229
  coping during hospitalization and, 150
  interventions for client exhibiting, 208
  moderate, 208
  reducing client's level of, 252, 261
Anxiety disorder, generalized, 197, 207
Anxiolytic overdose, 201
Apgar score, 130, 133
Aphasia, communicating with client with, 81
Apical pulse, 87
Arrhythmia, 37, 96, 191
Arterial insufficiency, 57
Arterial peripheral vascular disease, 57
Arteriovenous fistula, 107, 238, 249
Ascites, care for child with, 188
Aspiration
  reducing the risk of, 254, 263
  respiratory complications and, 130
Aspirin
  bleeding and, 18
  peptic ulcer disease and, 238, 248
Assessment of client, 26, 51, 168
Asthma, 58
Atelectasis, preventing postoperative, 140
Atropine sulfate
  cholinergic crisis and, 102
  for increasing cardiac transmission, 55
Auditory hallucination, 193, 204
Autistic client, desired outcome for, 237, 247
Autologous transplant, 109

Urinary catheter *(continued)*
    reducing the risk of infection
        from, 107
    risk for infection and, 255, 264
    safety precautions for inserting, 46
Urinary tract infection, 169, 237, 247
Urine output
    calculating, 231, 239
    fluid volume status and, 48
Urine retention
    abdominal surgery and, 20
    catheter removal and, 235, 244
    stress and, 234, 243
Urine specimen, 24-hour, collecting,
        48, 232, 239
UTI. *See* Urinary tract infection.

V

Vaccines for hepatitis A and B, 95
Vaginal delivery, 137
Vagotomy, purpose of, 106
Varicosities, definition of, 98
Venous insufficiency, 58
Venous stasis, 61
Ventricular fibrillation, 97
Vitamin K, purpose of adminis-
        tering, 119, 233, 241

WXY

Warfarin sodium (Coumadin),
        250, 258
Water-seal chamber, checking air
        leak in, 23
Water-seal drainage device, 142, 146
Weight gain, heart failure and, 76
Weight loss, hypertension and, 58
Wound
    care, 237, 246
    drainage system, 74
    management, 182
    preventing infection in, 73

Z

Zinc, food sources of, 256, 266
Z-track injection, 146